PRACTICAL DERMATOLOGY

SECOND EDITION

Practical Dermatology

BETH G. GOLDSTEIN, MD

Adjunct Clinical Assistant Professor
Department of Dermatology
University of North Carolina at Chapel Hill
Chapel Hill, North Carolina

ADAM O. GOLDSTEIN, MD

Clinical Assistant Professor
Department of Family Medicine
University of North Carolina at Chapel Hill
Chapel Hill, North Carolina

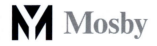

St. Louis Baltimore Boston Carlsbad Chicago Naples New York Philadelphia Portland
London Madrid Mexico City Singapore Sydney Tokyo Toronto Wiesbaden

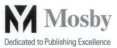

Dedicated to Publishing Excellence

⊤⊤ A Times Mirror
ᴗ Company

Vice President and Publisher: Anne S. Patterson
Editor: James F. Shanahan
Developmental Editor: Laura C. Berendson
Project Manager: Mark Spann
Production Editor: Beth Hayes
Book Design Manager: Judi Lang
Manufacturing Manager: Karen M. Boehme

SECOND EDITION
Copyright © 1997 by Mosby–Year Book, Inc.
Previous edition copyrighted 1992

Printed in the United States of America
Composition by TSI Graphics
Lithography/color film by TSI Graphics
Printing/binding by Von Hoffmann Press, Inc.

Mosby–Year Book, Inc.
11830 Westline Industrial Drive
St. Louis, Missouri 63146

Library of Congress Cataloging in Publication Data
Goldstein, Beth G.
    Practical dermatology / Beth G. Goldstein, Adam O. Goldstein.—2nd ed.
      p.   cm.—(Mosby–Year Book primary care series)
    Includes bibliographical references and index.
    ISBN 0-8151-3764-8 (pbk.)
    1. Skin—Diseases.   2. Dermatology.   I. Goldstein, Adam O.
  II. Title.   III. Series.
    [DNLM: 1. Skin Diseases—diagnosis.   2. Skin Diseases—therapy.
  WR 141 G624p   1997]
  RL71.G62   1997
  616.5—dc20
  DNLM/DLC   96-28852
  for Library of Congress   CIP

97 98 99 00 01/9 8 7 6 5 4 3 2 1

To Jared, Michael, Elianna, and Michael.

FOREWORD

There are few medical books that are sufficiently useful to the busy clinician that they end up with tattered edges and folded page corners to mark favorite information. The first edition of *Practical Dermatology* by Beth and Adam Goldstein is one of these rare gems. In the past 3 years I have relied on it once or twice every week to solve a dermatologic diagnostic dilemma, to jog my memory about treatment, or to copy pages to give to patients so they can better care for their chronic skin problems. The first edition was enthusiastically embraced by primary care clinicians because of its wonderful photographs, efficient style, and copyable patient handouts. With the second edition, the authors not only update the dermatologic science but also make the book even more useful than the first edition.

It is unusual for a book to be so "on target" for a primary care audience. This is no doubt the result of the unique collaboration between the two authors, Beth Goldstein, a dermatologist, and Adam Goldstein, a family physician. They bring together a unique collaboration between specialist and primary care physician that keeps the patient in focus at all times. I know of no other book that so nicely blends this unique knowledge and perception of the specialist and the generalist.

The emphasis in the second edition continues to be *practical* dermatology. The number of color photos has been greatly expanded. These will help you to "figure out a rash" and to explain to patients what they "have." There is nothing more reassuring than to have a patient look at a photograph and say "Oh yes, that does look exactly like what I have." The number of patient education handouts has been increased. The publisher encourages you to copy these for patient use. ICD-9 diagnoses are now included throughout the book. This will save your office staff time when trying to figure out how to code unusual diagnoses. A new chapter is included on tropical dermatology, which should appeal to a broader international audience and also help with the occasional patient who returns from vacation with an unusual rash.

Practical Dermatology is the perfect dermatology book to have close at hand when you are running between examination rooms on an especially hectic day and are stumped by a patient's rash. It is like having your favorite dermatology consultant on your bookshelf.

PAUL M. FISCHER, MD
University Family Medicine
Augusta, Georgia

PREFACE

Dermatology today remains both an art and a science. All clinicians, regardless of our levels of training, remain continuously challenged by the great number and variety of skin diseases. More importantly, our patients continue to come to our offices seeking relief from skin conditions that result in pain, itching, cosmetic deformity, emotional scars, frustration, and social isolation. There are few medical disciplines that can claim the high patient and clinician satisfaction seen when a dermatologic condition is successfully diagnosed and managed. Alternatively, when the diagnosis is unknown or when the treatment does not work, even the best of relationships may be strained. Such possibilities make the study and practice of dermatology very rewarding.

In our first edition of *Practical Dermatology,* we strove to provide a handbook that was particularly useful to the daily routine of busy clinical practice. We tried to design a text that would meet the unique needs of an expanding number of primary care clinicians (including family physicians, internists, pediatricians, OB–Gyns, physician assistants, and nurse practitioners), provide a quick reference for nondermatologic specialists who occasionally see and treat patients with skin disease, and to provide students at all levels of training with an inexpensive, yet comprehensive, dermatologic learning tool. We hope that our book does not sit on a reference shelf but rather that it finds a home in the clinical space we use on a daily basis. Like the first edition, this second edition strives to be the most practical dermatologic reference source by assisting clinicians in making the correct diagnosis when it is in doubt, developing a succinct differential diagnosis to expand clinical skills, choosing the optimal treatment regimen for satisfaction and cure, and empowering both patients and clinicians with patient education guidelines.

Changes in the medical marketplace, especially managed care, demand increased attention to outcomes at all levels of medical care. Such changes place new pressures on both dermatologists and nondermatologists in their approaches to treating and following all skin diseases. To assist in this challenge, we have continued to emphasize in our text the specific diagnostic and treatment details that are most needed by primary care clinicians, such as methods of application, sizes of medications, costs of therapies, treatment guidelines, algorithms, etc. The number of tables has been increased substantially to allow for quick review when needed. International Classification of Disease (ICD) codes are also now included throughout the text to allow the busy clinician to more efficiently code appropriate dermatologic diagnoses for billing purposes.

Other trends in medicine, including dermatology, reflect the growing importance of patient autonomy in medical decision making. To assist clinicians in this goal, the second edition of *Practical Dermatology* includes even more emphasis on patient education, including the addition of 12 more patient education handouts in the Appendix. Dermatologic support groups and World Wide Web sites are included where available. In particular, we encourage clinicians that have access to the Internet to visit the American Academy of Dermatology's World Wide Web site at http://www.aad.org/. This site maintains the most comprehensive electronic resource for dermatologic topics, new support groups, and policy issues.

The chapter on tropical diseases is new to this edition. Over the last few years, we were impressed by the paucity of practical information on tropical dermatology readily available to the nondermatologist. In addition, world travel continues to increase, as does an international audience for this text. Including these diseases provides a more comprehensive and global approach to practical dermatology. We sought out as guest authors of this section two renowned clinicians, Drs. Routh and Parrish, who have extensive experience and expertise on the topic.

Most importantly, we have updated, revised, and substantially expanded all sections of the book. The chapter on dermatologic therapeutics has been expanded by Dr. Ives, a pharmacologist with extensive dermatologic research, teaching, and clinical experience. Because of the many changes that have occurred since the first edition was published, we have attempted to incorporate all of the rapidly expanding advances in dermatologic therapeutics, without losing our basic focus on useful information for clinicians and their patients. Finally, we are fortunate to have the full support and wisdom of excellent publishers at Mosby, who recognize that the essential ingredient to any dermatologic text is the quality and quantity of its color images. To this end, we are excited that the text is entirely in color and that the number of color photographs has been substantially increased.

BETH G. GOLDSTEIN, MD
ADAM O. GOLDSTEIN, MD

ACKNOWLEDGMENTS

Our sincere thanks continue to go to our mentors, colleagues, and students for their supportive comments, criticism, and suggestions for improvement. We owe a large amount of gratitude to Paul Fischer, MD, for giving us the opportunity and encouragement to write the first edition of *Practical Dermatology*. We also sincerely appreciate the generous use of the slides that appear throughout the text and were made available by Robert A. Briggaman, MD, and his Department of Dermatology, University of North Carolina at Chapel Hill; Jack Lesher, MD, and his Division of Dermatology, Medical College of Georgia; Marshall Guill, MD; John Cook, MD; Steve Resnick, MD; Beverly Sanders, MD; Robert Clark, MD, PhD; and Elise Olsen, MD.

Equally important, we could not have finished this second edition without the continued support shown by our office staff, the love from our families, and, especially, the loyalty and encouragement of our patients.

CONTENTS

PART ONE

Art of Dermatology

A patient has a rash. What could be more straightforward? The clinician looks at the rash, sees that it looks familiar, and a few seconds later sends the patient home with a medication and instructions to return if the rash does not respond. For most clinicians, this ideal scenario rarely works out in practice the way it is imagined. *The art of dermatology involves understanding that dermatologic diagnosis and treatment are intuitively obvious but not intuitively simple.* What on the surface may look easy more often than not poses significant clinical or therapeutic dilemmas for many clinicians. For instance, a rash may not look familiar or may not respond to a chosen therapy, the therapy may be incorrect, the therapy may be correct but the medication strength or chosen vehicle may be wrong, the rash may be caused by two different but morphologically indistinguishable diseases, or there may be many different therapeutic options from which to choose. Such diagnostic and therapeutic dilemmas lie at the heart of dermatology and sometimes make a seemingly easy diagnosis complex and challenging for dermatologists and nondermatologists alike.

Dermatology is one of the least-studied disciplines in medicine, despite the fact that almost 10% of all outpatient visits to clinicians are for dermatologic problems. Eczematous dermatitis, acne, skin cancer, and warts alone account for 3%, or 22 million, outpatient visits each year. *The key to dermatologic diagnosis and treatment is practice.* Most clinicians can attain a high standard in dermatology by re-peated applications of the few principles outlined in Chapters 1 through 4.

Along with practice, clinicians must remember that excellence in dermatology involves far more than simple "diagnosis and treatment." Clinicians do not just treat skin diseases, they also care for patients. Although the science of dermatology involves experience with dermatologic diagnosis and techniques, the art of dermatology involves experience, practice, concern, and compassion for patients. What is the patient's main concern about a "rash?" Are there underlying fears of cancer, worries about contagion, or family stresses? A happy patient is more than someone who recovers from a bout of poison ivy after 2 weeks of partially relieved itching. Detailed patient education, concern about the cost of medication, reinforcing compliance with therapy, emphasizing prevention, and appropriate follow-up, including telephone calls, will complement all patient encounters.

In Part One, clinicians will find the tools and resources to learn, practice, and eventually master the basics of dermatologic practice. Terms, definitions, pitfalls in diagnosis and therapy, and broad differential diagnoses are discussed in Chapter 1. The art and science of dermatologic therapeutics are covered in Chapter 2. The most common and useful dermatologic procedures are outlined in a step-by-step format in Chapter 3. Finally, the increasingly important role of clinicians in preventing dermatologic disease is presented in Chapter 4.

Dermatologic Basics

TERMINOLOGY AND DEFINITIONS

All clinicians must learn and practice using the language of dermatology that is employed when describing dermatologic diseases. Using a standard language when describing lesions is important because it:

- Facilitates communications between physicians.
- Helps clinicians form a proper differential diagnosis.
- Allows for accurate documentation of potentially important changes that may occur during evolution of the disease.
- Helps students to learn and practitioners to teach dermatology in a comprehensive but succinct and organized way.

The dermatologic language includes lesions and their distribution and characteristics.

1. *Primary lesions* of the skin are either the first recognizable skin lesion or involve basic skin changes. Common primary skin lesions are shown in Box 1–1.

2. *Secondary lesions* of the skin evolve from primary skin lesions, either because of the natural history of a skin disorder (e.g., crusts in chicken pox) or because of scratching or infection. The common secondary lesions are shown in Box 1–2.

3. *Distribution* refers to where on the body lesions are found (e.g., hands, face, trunk). Some skin lesions have a characteristic distribution that involves several seemingly distinct but often related body areas, such as flexural body areas in adult atopic dermatitis, or fingerwebs, wrists, and waist in scabies.

4. *Distinguishing characteristics* are based on the epidemiology of the disease, the size of lesions, or associated systemic or laboratory findings.

MAKING THE RIGHT DIAGNOSIS

Clinicians often find that making a dermatologic diagnosis is either easy or impossible. Those who think dermatologic diagnosis is easy usually remember several common dermatologic conditions, such as acne, eczema, and contact dermatitis, but may fail to adequately consider the multitude of other diagnoses that may mimic or confuse simple pattern recognition. Such cases may lead to delayed diagnosis and treatment. On the other hand, those clinicians who avoid making a dermatologic diagnosis because of a feeling of hopelessness often miss many easily diagnosable

BOX 1–1.

Primary Skin Lesions

Macule: Small spot, different in color from surrounding skin, that is neither elevated nor depressed below the skin surface

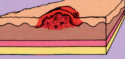

Papule: Small (≤5 mm diameter) circumscribed solid elevation on the skin

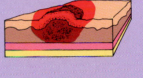

Plaque: Large (≥5 mm) superficial *flat* lesion, often formed by a confluence of papules

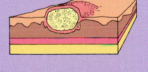

Nodule: Large (5–20 mm) circumscribed solid skin elevation

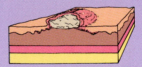

Pustule: Small circumscribed skin elevation containing purulent material

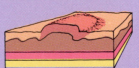

Vesicle: Small (<5 mm) circumscribed skin blister containing serum

Wheal: Irregular elevated edematous skin area, which often changes in size and shape

Bulla: Large (>5 mm) vesicle containing free fluid
Cyst: Enclosed cavity with a membraneous lining, which contains liquid or semisolid matter

Tumor: Large nodule, which may be neoplastic
Telangiectasia: Dilated superficial blood vessel

BOX 1–2.

Secondary Skin Lesions

Scale: Superficial epidermal cells that are dead and cast off from the skin

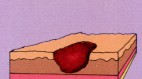

Erosion: Superficial, focal loss of part of the epidermis; lesions usually heal without scarring

Ulcer: Focal loss of the epidermis extending into the dermis; lesions may heal with scarring

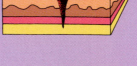

Fissure: Deep skin split extending into the dermis

Crust: Dried exudate, a "scab"

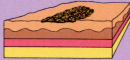

Erythema: Skin redness

Excoriation: Superficial, often linear, skin erosion caused by scratching

Atrophy: Decreased skin thickness due to skin thinning

Scar: Abnormal fibrous tissue that replaces normal tissue after skin injury

Edema: Swelling due to accumulation of water in tissue

Hyperpigmentation: Increased skin pigment

Hypopigmentation: Decreased skin pigment

Depigmentation: Total loss of skin pigment

Lichenification: Increased skin markings and thickening with induration secondary to chronic inflammation caused by scratching or other irritation

Hyperkeratosis: Abnormal skin thickening of the superficial layer of the epidermis

conditions. The truth lies somewhere between these two extremes. Dermatologic diagnosis requires both an appreciation for the variety of ways skin diseases present in different patients and an understanding of the types of skin diseases that should be included in the differential diagnosis of an unfamiliar skin disorder.

The first step in making the proper diagnosis involves taking a dermatologic history similar to the history that a clinician takes for diagnosing any medical disorder. The most important initial questions to ask patients with new rashes are given in Box 1–3,A. Remember to inquire about the patient's main concern and which treatments or medications may have been tried previously.

Subsequent questions that often are important in differentiating one disease from another are shown in Box 1–3,B.

The art of dermatologic diagnosis involves looking at and using all available information. For instance, many clinicians frequently fail to take a detailed drug history, including birth control pills, common over-the-counter (OTC) medications such as aspirin or ibuprofen, or "home-based" remedies. An outline for recording the combined dermatologic history and physical is shown in Table 1–1.

The second step in making the correct diagnosis is knowledge of which diseases help form a proper differential diagnosis for a new skin disorder. Most dermatologic diseases are distinguished by patient characteristics such as age or race, combined with morphologic characteristics and location of the disease. *Clinicians wishing to become more proficient in dermatologic diagnosis must practice making a differential diagnosis for every rash or lesion encountered, even when the diagnosis seems easy.*

BOX 1–3.
Dermatologic History

A. INITIAL QUESTIONS

1. When did the rash start?
2. What did it look like when it first started, and how has it changed?
3. Where did it start, and where is it located now?
4. What treatments, especially over-the-counter medications or self-remedies, has the patient tried? What was the effect of each of these treatments?
5. Are there symptoms (e.g., itching, pain)?
6. What is the patient's main concern about the rash (e.g., itching, pain, cancer)?
7. How is the rash affecting the patient's life?
8. Are other family members concerned or affected?
9. Has the patient ever had this rash before? If so, what treatment worked?
10. What does the patient think caused the rash?

B. FOLLOW-UP QUESTIONS

1. Does the patient have a history of chronic medical problems?
2. What is the patient's social history, including occupation (chemical exposures), hobbies, alcohol and tobacco use, and any underlying interpersonal or family stress?
3. What medications is the patient taking, acutely or chronically, including birth control pills and over-the-counter medications?
4. Does the patient have any underlying allergies?
5. Is there a family history of hereditary or similar skin diseases?
6. Will the patient's education or financial status influence treatment considerations?

TABLE 1–1.
Recording a Dermatologic History and Physical Examination

History	See Box 1–3.
Distribution	Where are the lesions located?
Primary features	What do the lesions look like?
Secondary features	Is there erythema, excoriation, crust, or pigmentary alterations?
Distinguishing features	What is the size of the lesion? Are there systemic findings? What are the laboratory findings? Are lesions altered by excoriation?
Diagnosis	Is the diagnosis certain or still undetermined?
Treatment	Are all treatments documented in the chart, including any sample medications given? When should the patient follow up?
Patient education	Are patient education handouts given to patients? Are potential side effects of treatments documented?

PITFALLS IN DIAGNOSIS

The skin has the ability to manifest lesions in varying locations and varieties, providing a constant challenge to clinicians in making a proper diagnosis. In addition, alterations from external sources such as excoriation, secondary infection, and self-medication may obscure even the most classic disease presentations. There are two basic diagnostic pitfalls:

- *Overdiagnosis* of certain disorders (e.g., bacterial pyoderma, superficial fungal infections, scabies, and herpes simplex infections)
- *Underdiagnosis* of others (e.g., contact dermatitis, nummular eczematous dermatitis, pityriasis rosea, psoriasis, perioral dermatitis, seborrheic dermatitis, stasis dermatitis, and pityriasis alba).

The failure to use basic, simple office procedures to confirm or rule out a diagnosis is the most common cause of both misdiagnosis and overdiagnosis. If simple, reliable methods are used whenever possible to confirm the diagnosis, most common pitfalls can be avoided. For example, treating an irritant dermatitis with an antifungal agent usually will not harm the patient, but the time, expense, and discomfort associated with delay in proper diagnosis and treatment could have been avoided by performing a simple laboratory procedure, the potassium hydroxide test (Fig. 1–1).

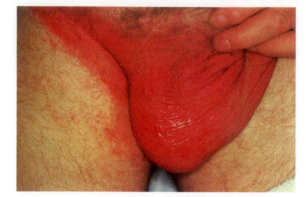

Fig. 1–1
Painful inflammatory eruption of the scrotum and groin in an adult with a primary irritant dermatitis. Tinea cruris does not involve the scrotum. Negative KOH test results will help rule out both candidiasis and tinea cruris. (Courtesy Marshall Guill, MD.)

Finally, every clinician needs to know when to seek consultation or referral on a particularly difficult case. Whether the consultant is a friend, colleague, or dermatologic specialist, a second opinion is almost always worthwhile if the diagnosis is in question. Referral is also indicated when the scope of disease exceeds the routine practice of the clinician. A major potential pitfall, malpractice because of failure to diagnose a cutaneous carcinoma, often can be avoided with appropriate, timely, and documented consultation and/or referral.

DIFFERENTIAL DIAGNOSES

Outlined on the inside front and back covers of this book are differential diagnoses for many kinds of dermatologic lesions. The outline is not all-inclusive but reviews the most likely diagnoses for a given eruption when the specific diagnosis is in doubt. These outlines are best used to form a differential diagnosis for an unknown skin condition or to help narrow the differential diagnosis to several conditions, which can then be further differentiated by specific physical or laboratory characteristics.

If, however, you already have one or two likely diagnoses in mind, then bypass this section and find the specific skin disease(s) in the table of contents or index. The appropriate section contains an abbreviated, disease-specific differential diagnosis.

The differential diagnoses listed on the inside front and back covers of this book are divided into three groups, which are *not* mutually exclusive:

1. *Lesions may be differentiated by their morphologic characteristics* (Fig. 1–2). Morphology is the key to communicating with other physicians. Although initially it may seem difficult to review and learn the lesions of papules, plaques, macules, and such, as discussed earlier in this chapter, such minimal terminology is indispensable.

2. *Lesions may be differentiated by their characteristic distribution.* Certain distributions are virtually diagnostic (Table 1–2). For example, excoriated, erythematous papules and plaques in the antecubital and posterior popliteal fossa of an infant almost always are atopic dermatitis.

3. *Lesions are often seen in particular age groups.* For example, tinea capitis is common in children but rare in adults, whereas tinea pedis is rare in children and common in adults.

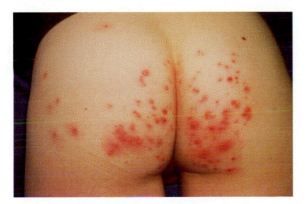

Fig. 1–2
Primary papules and pustules with secondary erythema in a patient with folliculitis. (Courtesy Beverly Sanders, MD.)

TABLE 1–2.
Classic Distribution of Common Skin Dermatoses

Acanthosis nigricans	Flexural areas
Atopic dermatitis	Extensor surfaces in infants; flexural areas in young children and adults
Bullous pemphigoid	Flexural areas
Hand and foot eczema	Palms, soles
Lichen planus	Wrists, ankles, mouth, sometimes genitalia
Psoriasis	Extensor surfaces, posterior scalp, sacral area
Scabies	Fingerwebs, wrists, axilla, waist, groin, feet
Seborrhea	Scalp, ears, central face, chest, groin
Xanthomas, eruptive	Extensor surfaces

SUGGESTED READING

Pariser RJ, Pariser DM: Primary care physicians' errors in handling cutaneous disorders, *J Am Acad Dermatol* 17:239–45, 1987.

Sober AJ, Fitzpatrick TB: *1995 Yearbook of dermatology*, St Louis, 1995, Mosby.

CHAPTER 2

Dermatologic Therapy

Successful dermatologic therapy requires an appreciation for the many potential interactions between the patient, the condition to be treated, and the potential pharmacotherapeutic choices. This chapter reviews factors that influence successful outcomes.

PATIENT-CENTERED THERAPEUTICS

When first selecting a therapy, consider issues that often influence compliance, patient satisfaction with the encounter, and, ultimately, the successful treatment of a skin disorder. Although the specifics of such guidelines will change from one patient to another, there are a few general rules to follow:

- Keep the treatment regimen as simple as possible.
- If the skin disease is chronic, choose a medication that is appropriate for long-term use and allow for refills.
- Determine whether a female patient is pregnant, trying to become pregnant, or currently breast-feeding a child.

TABLE 2–1.
Amount of Topical Medication to Dispense for Adult Use*

	bid/1 wk	tid/2 wk	bid/4 wk
Face and neck	15 g	45 g	60 g
Trunk	60 g	180 g	240 g
One arm	15 g	45 g	60 g
One leg	30 g	90 g	120 g
Hands and feet	15 g	45 g	60 g
Body	180 g	0.75–1 kg	1.25–2 kg

*For children, use one third to one half these amounts.

- Prescribe enough medication for the patient to cover all involved areas for the duration of the treatment (Table 2–1).
- Whenever possible, provide written instructions or make certain that they are available to the patient. Always be sure to determine literacy in every patient.
- When using topical medications, review with the patient how often to apply it, where

■Contributing author: Timothy J. Ives, Pharm D, MPH, Associate Professor of Pharmacy, School of Pharmacy, and Clinical Associate Professor of Family Medicine, University of North Carolina at Chapel Hill, Chapel Hill, North Carolina.

to apply it, how much to apply, and if any special application procedures (e.g., occlusion) are necessary.

• Have the patient repeat the instructions to ensure that they are fully understood, at both the time that they are initially prescribed and at follow-up office visits. This will help ensure adherence to the regimen.

• Patients should know what to do when an adverse reaction to a medication or cosmetic occurs (e.g., calling their physician or self-management). A patient education handout on general skin care can be found in Appendix H.

TOPICAL THERAPIES

Five components to the successful use of topical therapies are the (1) correct diagnosis, (2) type of lesion being treated, (3) medication, (4) vehicle (i.e., the base in which the active medication is delivered), and (5) the method used to apply the medication (Fig. 2–1). The characteristics of the ideal vehicle are shown in Box 2–1.

If the correct medication but the wrong vehicle is used, the response to therapy may be delayed, inadequate, or, in some cases, worsened. For example, use of a corticosteroid gel on hand

BOX 2–1.

Characteristics of the Ideal Vehicle

Easy to apply and to remove	Nondehydrating (overdrying leads to xerosis)
Nonallergenic	Nongreasy (overhydration leads to maceration)
Nontoxic	Pharmacologically inert and chemically stable
Nonirritating	Cosmetically appealing
Bacteriostatic	

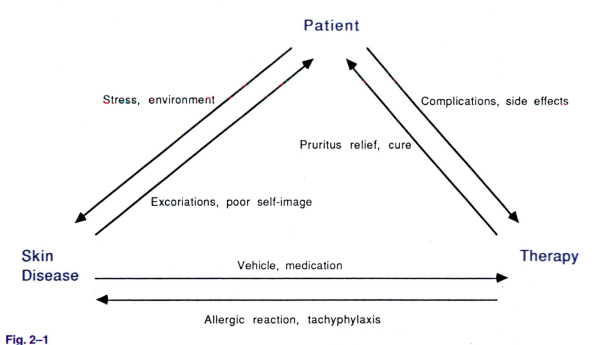

Fig. 2–1

Fig. 2–1
Relationships between dermatologic disease, therapy, and the individual patient may influence therapeutic success.

eczema with fissures will cause increased pain and stinging because of the alcohol base of the gel. Treating a moist lesion with an ointment may cause folliculitis secondary to the ointment's occlusive properties.

The type of lesion being treated is important, as exemplified by the time-honored adage: "If a lesion is wet, use agents to make it dry" (e.g., use a solution such as Burow's solution to allow a lesion to dry out) and "if a lesion is dry, make it wet" (e.g., use an ointment base such as yellow petrolatum [Vaseline] to increase hydration to the affected area). For example, in acute contact dermatitis from poison ivy, with moist weeping lesions, wet dressing changes or lotions will help "dry up" the dermatitis while providing cool, soothing relief. Therefore, for acute exudative dermatoses, bland treatments in liquid vehicles (e.g., solutions) are generally recommended. In contrast, when treating chronic psoriasis, therapeutic agents incorporated into creams or ointments may help to retain native moisture and provide relief to dry, pruritic skin.

In addition to the type of lesion being treated and the base of the treatment vehicle, topical drug penetration into the skin is determined by the method of topical application. For optimal absorption of most topical drugs, apply them to moist skin either immediately after bathing or after wet soaks. Occlusive dressings will also enhance drug absorption, often by a factor of 10. The site of an application is also important because variations in the epidermal layer will alter the extent of drug absorption.

Tachyphylaxis, a progressive decrease in clinical response as a result of repetitive application of a drug (e.g., topical corticosteroids), occurs when the body becomes tolerant to the pharmacotherapeutic effects of a particular medication. Even if the medication previously worked well, it may become ineffective, which influences the success or failure of many topical therapies. When prescribing medications for prolonged use, allow for drug-free intervals or switch at various intervals to alternative agents to help prevent this problem.

Vehicle Selection

Vehicles consist of three basic ingredients: powders, oils, and liquids (e.g., water). Powders aid in absorbing moisture, decrease friction, and help cover wide areas easily. Oils act as emollients and, because of their occlusive properties, often enhance drug penetration. Liquids in vehicles evaporate, providing a cooling, soothing sensation, while aiding exudative lesions to dry. Combinations of these three ingredients in varying proportions make up the most commonly used vehicles and are described below.

Ointments

Ointments are generally the most potent vehicles because of their increased occlusive effect. However, they are not useful in hairy areas, and the greasiness of the product may cause low patient acceptance. Ointments consist predominantly of water suspended in oil. This type of vehicle is an excellent lubricant, facilitates heat retention, decreases transepidermal water loss, provides enhanced medication absorption, and is semiocclusive. Ointments should be applied 2 to 3 times per day to dry, lichenified lesions, particularly after moistening the skin.

Creams

Creams are the most cosmetically appealing vehicle type for delivering topical medications. Although less potent than ointments, they are useful in most dermatoses. Creams are semisolid emulsions of oil in 20% to 50% water and can be washed off with water. For the same medication, cream formulations are usually stronger than lotions, but less potent than ointments.

Lotions

Lotions, aerosols, and solutions are the least potent vehicles, but are useful in hairy areas and in conditions in which large areas must be treated. Because lotions are powder-in-water preparations, to receive the desired therapeutic concentration with each application (and therefore the desired effect), patients must shake the container before each application. As the lotion evaporates, it provides a cooling and drying effect; lotions are therefore useful for treating moist dermatoses and pruritus.

Solutions

Solutions consist of water or water in combination with various medications or substances. *Solutions such as bath soaks and open wet dressings provide coolness and aid in drying exudative lesions by means of evaporation.* In addition, vasoconstriction results in decreased local blood flow and reduction in any local edema. Wet dressings allow for the cleansing of exudate while maintaining drainage in infected lesions (e.g., ulcers). Wet dressings should be changed every 6 hours for 2 to 3 days, before judging their effectiveness. Closed wet dressings consist of a wet dressing covered by an imper-

meable substance such as a polyurethane plastic (e.g., Saran Wrap, etc.), which allows heat to be retained, prevents evaporation, and causes maceration.

Gels

Gel formulations combine the best therapeutic advantages of ointments with the best cosmetic advantages of creams. Gels are transparent, colorless, semisolid emulsions that liquify on contact with the skin. They are oil-in-water emulsions with alcohol in the base, and they dry in a thin, greaseless, nonstaining film. Gels are an efficient method for delivering medications to hair-bearing areas and for treating acne.

A brief summary of topical pharmacotherapeutic preparations is shown in Table 2–2. The optimal vehicles for different body locations and lesions are shown in Table 2–3.

TABLE 2–2.

Topical Pharmacotherapeutic Preparations

Category	Examples	Special Considerations
Lotions	Calamine, Valisone, lindane	Cools and dries as it evaporates; useful for treating moist or pruritic skin
Creams	Nivea, Purpose, most topical corticosteroids, antifungal agents	Helps retain water; cosmetically appealing; useful in high-humidity environments; easily washed off
Gels	Benzoyl peroxide, Erygel, Topicort, Lidex	Becomes liquid on contact; cosmetically appealing; avoid on acutely inflamed skin because alcohol base may cause stinging
Ointments	Petrolatum, Aquaphor, Eucerin, most topical corticosteroids	Helps retain water, hydrating; avoid use in exudative, infected lesions; may be greasy; complications include folliculitis, maceration, and miliaria
Emulsions	Cetaphil, Unibase	Water-in-oil preparations that are less occlusive than ointments
Pastes	Zinc oxide paste	Less greasy than ointments, with some drying action; good as protective barrier
Wet dressings		
Open:	Apply 6-8 layers of gauze or a handkerchief, soaking wet, for 15 min 3 times daily	Antiinflammatory action and vasoconstriction aid in decreased edema and crust removal; evaporation and cooling offer relief of pruritus
Closed:	Same as for open, with plastic cover	Retains heat and causes maceration
Bath soaks	Aveeno, Alpha-Keri	Temperature should be lukewarm, not hot; limit to 20-30 min; oils may make tub slippery
Powder	Zeasorb, Micatin, Tinactin	Promotes drying; increases surface area; decreases maceration and moisture; avoid in open wounds
Fixed	Unna boot (zinc oxide gelatin boot)	Proper application will aid in decreasing edema; leave the dressing in place for 1 week, then remove by soaking in warm water

TABLE 2–3.

Optimal Vehicle Selection for Specific Body Sites

Vehicle	Smooth, nonhairy skin; thick, hyperkeratotic lesions	Hairy areas	Palms, soles	Infected areas	Between skin folds; moist, macerated lesions
Ointment	+++		+++		
Cream	++	+	++	+	++
Lotion		++		++	++
Solution		+++		+++	++
Gel		++		+	+

Tape: For use on small areas when occlusion is desired
Spray: Little clinical usefulness

+ = Infrequently used vehicle

++ = Acceptable vehicle

+++ = Preferred vehicle

CORTICOSTEROIDS

Corticosteroids are one of the most useful medications for treating a variety of skin diseases. The increase of available agents, strengths, and sizes has made the choice of a particular agent often complex or confusing. Along with the recent development of high-potency and ultra–high-potency topical corticosteroids, the potential for unpleasant adverse effects has increased, requiring clinicians to become familiar with many, often quite similar, medications. *Clinicians should become thoroughly familiar with the uses, costs, adverse effects, and contraindications of one or two preparations from each major corticosteroid class rather than trying to learn about 50 or more preparations.*

TABLE 2–4.

Classes of Topical Corticosteroids

Class	Potency	Examples	Indications
I	Ultra high	0.05% betamethasone dipropionate 0.05% clobetasol propionate	Severe inflammatory dermatoses unresponsive to standard treatment. Two-week use restriction; never use on the face or groin.
II	Very high	0.05-0.25% desoximetasone 0.2% flucinolone acetonide 0.5% triamcinolone acetonide	Severe inflammatory dermatoses (e.g., psoriasis, severe atopic dermatitis, or severe contact dermatitis)
III	High	0.025% betamethasone benzoate 0.025% fluocinolone acetonide 0.1% triamcinolone acetonide	Moderate cutaneous dermatoses
IV	Intermediate	0.025% triamcinolone acetonide 0.01% fluocinolone acetonide	Moderate cutaneous dermatoses
V	Low	2.5% hydrocortisone 0.2% betamethasone	Mild cutaneous dermatoses
VI	Very low	0.25 – 1.0% hydrocortisone (i.e., OTC strengths)	Very mild, self-limiting dermatoses

Topical Corticosteroids

The major effects of topical corticosteroids on skin are an antiinflammatory response, as a result of vasoconstriction, and decrease in collagen synthesis. These agents come in an array of strengths and vehicles (Tables 2–4 and 2–6), with short-term and long-term adverse effects (Table 2–5). Topical corticosteroids, particularly class I agents (the strongest), can cause significant hypothalamic–pituitary axis suppression with as little as 2 g/day when used for 2 or more weeks. The use of topical corticosteroids on nonintact skin increases the vehicle penetration. Increased vehicle penetration also occurs when these drugs are used under occlusion. The best time for application is when the skin is moist (e.g., after a bath or wet soak). The choice among topical corticosteroids for different body regions is based on the variability in skin thickness and the presence or absence of occlusion. Regional differences in percutaneous absorption (percentage of the total dose absorbed across the body) are as follows: sole of foot (0.14%), palm (0.83%), forearm (1.0%), scalp (3.5%), forehead (6.0%), jaw (13%), and genitalia (42%). Start with the lowest-potency agents needed, use for as short a time as possible, and try to avoid fluorinated products for extended use because of the risk of adverse effects such as perioral dermatitis, steroid acne, and atrophy (Figs. 2–2 and 2–3).

Factors that affect the response to therapy include differences in dermatologic disease states (e.g., acute vs. chronic lesions), potency, concentration, frequency of application, occlusive dressing, vehicle and patient acceptance. With especially dry or chronic lesions, the use of an occlusive dressing will help to maintain the skin's hydration.

Intralesional Corticosteroids

Intralesional corticosteroids, in a variety of concentrations, are used to treat keloids, acne cysts, stubborn psoriatic plaques, and alopecia areata. Intramuscular injections are indicated rarely (only with severe inflammatory disorders) and should be avoided in patients with psoriasis. Triamcinolone acetonide (2.5 to 60 mg/day), triamcinolone diacetate (5 to 40 mg/day), methylprednisolone sodium succinate (10 to 40 mg/day), and methylprednisolone acetate (40 to 120 mg/day) are used commonly. Adverse drug effects include local reactions and systemic absorption with problems similar to those of systemic corticosteroids. In addition, localized

TABLE 2–5.

Adverse Effects of Topical Corticosteroids

Short-term	Long-term
Local burning or irritation	Atrophy
Allergic reaction to vehicle	Telangiectasia
Allergic reaction to	Purpura
corticosteroid	Hypertrichosis
	Tinea incognito
	Acneiform eruption
	Perioral dermatitis
	(Fig. 2–2)
	Pigmentary alteration
	Striae (Fig. 2–3)
	Ocular hypertension
	Hypothalamic–pituitary
	axis suppression

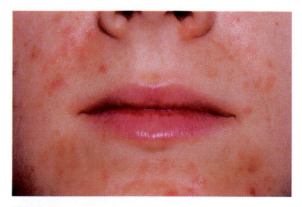

Fig. 2–2
Perioral dermatitis may occur as a result of prolonged use of topical corticosteroids on the face.

TABLE 2–6.

Topical Corticosteroid Potency, Strongest (Class I) to Weakest (Class VI)

Brand Name	Generic Name	Preparation	Size
Class I (ultra high)	*Unresponsive severe inflammatory dermatoses*		
Cordran tape 4 μ/sq cm^2	Flurandrenolide	Tape	2 × 3 in, 24 × 3 in, 80 × 3 in
Diprolene 0.05%	Betamethasone dipropionate*	Cream, ointment, gel	15, 45 g
		Lotion	30, 60 ml
Diprolene AF 0.05%	Betamethasone dipropionate	Cream	15, 45 g
Psorcon 0.05%	Diflorasone diacetate	Cream, ointment	15, 30, 45, 60 g
Temovate E 0.05%	Clobetasol propionate*	Cream, ointment	15, 30, 45 g
		Lotion	25, 50 ml
		Gel	15, 30, 60 g
		Emollient cream	15, 30, 60 g
Ultravate 0.05%	Halobetasol propionate	Cream, ointment	15, 50 g
Class II (very high)	*Severe inflammatory dermatoses*		
Aristocort 0.5%	Triamcinolone acetonide*	Cream, ointment	15, 240 g
Cyclocort 0.1%	Amcinonide	Cream, ointment	15, 30, 60 g
		Lotion	20, 60 ml
Diprosone 0.05%	Betamethasone dipropionate*	Cream, ointment	15, 45 g
		Aerosol	85 g
		Lotion	30, 60 ml
Florone 0.05%	Diflorasone diacetate	Cream, ointment	15, 30, 60 g
Halog 0.1%	Halcinonide	Cream, ointment	15, 30, 60, 240 g
		Solution	20, 60 ml
Lidex 0.05%	Fluocinonide*	Cream, ointment	15, 30, 60, 120 g
		Solution	20, 60 ml
		Gel	15, 30, 60, 120 g
		Solution	60 ml
Lidex E 0.05%	Fluocinonide	Cream	15, 30, 60, 120 g
Kenalog 0.05%	Triamcinolone acetonide*	Cream, ointment	20 g
Maxiflor 0.05%	Diflorasone diacetate	Cream	30, 60 g
		Ointment	15, 30, 60 g
Topicort 0.25%	Desoximetasone*	Cream	15, 60, 120 g
		Ointment	15, 60 g
		Gel 0.05%	15, 60 g
Class III (high)	*Moderate cutaneous dermatoses*		
Aristocort 0.1%	Triamcinolone acetonide*	Cream, ointment	15, 60, 240, 2520 g
Aristocort A 0.1%	Triamcinolone acetonide*	Cream	15, 60, 240 g
		Ointment	15, 60 g
Cutivate 0.05%	Fluticasone propionate	Cream	15, 30, 60 g
0.005%		Ointment	15, 30, 60 g
Dermatop 0.1%	Prednicarbate	Cream	15, 60 g
Elocon 0.1%	Mometasone furoate	Cream, ointment	15, 45 g
		Lotion	30, 60 ml

Continued.

TABLE 2–6 (cont.).

Brand Name	Generic Name	Preparation	Size
Kenalog 0.1%	Triamcinolone acetonide*	Cream	15, 60, 80, 240, 2520 g
		Ointment	15, 60, 80, 240 g
		Lotion	15, 60 ml
Synalar 0.025%	Fluocinolone acetonide*	Cream, ointment	15, 30, 60, 425 g
		Solution 0.01%	20, 60 ml
Synemol 0.025%	Fluocinolone acetonide*	Cream	15, 30, 60 g
Valisone 0.1%	Betamethasone valerate*	Cream	15, 45, 110, 430 g
		Ointment	15, 45 g
		Lotion	20, 60 ml
		Powder	5, 10 g
Class IV (intermediate)	*Moderate cutaneous dermatoses*		
Aristocort 0.025%	Triamcinolone acetonide*	Cream	15, 60, 2520 g
Kenalog 0.025%	Triamcinolone acetonide*	Cream	15, 80, 240, 2520 g
		Lotion	60 ml
		Ointment	15, 80, 240 g
Locoid 0.1%	Hydrocortisone butyrate	Cream, ointment	15, 45, g
		Solution	30, 60 ml
Valisone 0.01%	Betamethasone valerate*	Cream	15, 60 g
Westcort 0.2%	Hydrocortisone valerate	Cream	15, 45, 60, g
		Ointment	15, 45, 60 g
Class V (low)	*Mild cutaneous dermatoses*		
Aclovate 0.05%	Aclometasone dipropionate	Cream, ointment	15, 45, 60 g
Derma-Smoothe/FS 0.01%	Fluocinolone acetonide	Oil	120 ml
DesOwen 0.05%	Desonide*	Cream	15, 60, 90 g
		Ointment	15, 60 g
		Lotion	60, 120 ml
FS Shampoo 0.01%	Fluocinolone acetonide	Shampoo	180 ml
Synalar 0.01%	Fluocinolone acetonide*	Cream	15, 30, 60, 425 g
		Solution	20, 60 ml
Tridesilon 0.05%	Desonide*	Cream, ointment	15, 60 g
Class VI (very low)	*Very mild, self-limiting dermatoses*		
Hytone 1%	Hydrocortisone*	Cream, ointment	30, 120 g
		Liquid	45, 75, 120 ml
		Lotion	120 ml
		Roll-on stick	14 g
Hytone 2.5%	Hydrocortisone*	Cream	30, 60 g
		Ointment	30 g
		Lotion	60 ml
Pramosone 1%	Hydrocortisone with pramoxine HCl 1%	Cream	30, 60 g
		Ointment	30 g
		Lotion	60, 240 ml
Pramosone 2.5%	Hydrocortisone with pramoxine HCl 1%	Cream	30 g
		Ointment	30 g
		Lotion	60, 120 ml

*Available generically, but may not be so predictably effective. In most cases, however, is much less expensive.

atrophy, hypopigmentation, telangiectasia, and sterile abscesses may occur in relation to intralesional injections.

Systemic Corticosteroids

The systemic (i.e., oral) corticosteroid used most commonly to treat skin disorders is *prednisone*. The most frequent indications for its short-term use include allergic contact dermatitis and allergic drug eruption; indications for long-term use include bullous pemphigoid, pemphigus vulgaris, sarcoidosis, vasculitis, and systemic lupus erythematosus. *With chronic systemic corticosteroid use, the goal is to control the condition at the lowest effective dose.* If prolonged therapy (i.e., greater than 14 to 21 days) is indicated, the use of an alternate-day regimen will reduce the risk of adrenal suppression associated with chronic corticosteroid use. Oral corticosteroids (e.g., prednisone) should be taken as a single dose in the morning. Follow-up of patients receiving long-term corticosteroid therapy is demanding and requires careful monitoring. Patient flowcharts can be used to aid in patient follow-up (see Fig. 2–4). Some absolute and relative contraindications to the use of systemic corticosteroids are listed in Table 2–7, and the multiple skin and general complications in Table 2–8.

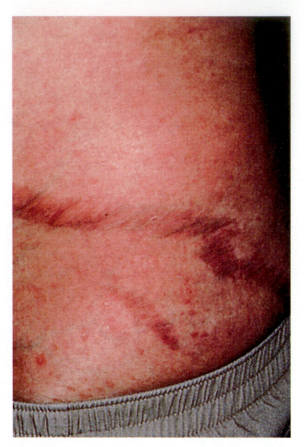

Fig. 2–3
Striae on the abdomen of a man as a result of prolonged use of triamcinolone acetonide 0.1% under occlusion to treat psoriasis.

TABLE 2–7.

Contraindications to Systemic Corticosteroid Use

Absolute	Relative
Psoriasis	Diabetes mellitus
Ocular herpes simplex infection	Hypertension
	Osteoporosis
Untreated tuberculosis	Renal insufficiency
	Congestive heart failure
	Psychotic tendencies
	Recent intestinal surgery
	Pregnancy or nursing
	Other infections (e.g., opportunistic)

TABLE 2–8.

Complications from Chronic Systemic Corticosteroids

Glucose intolerance	Aseptic necrosis of large joints
Myopathy	Increased susceptibility to infection
Personality disturbances	Posterior subcapsular cataracts
Electrolyte imbalances	Glaucoma
Striae	Cushingoid habitus
Weight gain	Excretion in breast milk
Growth retardation in children	Acne
Hypothalamic–pituitary axis suppression	Hypertension

Long-Term Corticosteroid Use Flow Sheet

Patient name:_____

Date:					
Preparation/dosage:					

Vital signs:

Weight					
Blood pressure					

Every 1–3 months

Glucose					
Na/K					
BUN/Cr					
Hgb/Hct					

Every 6 months

PPD					
Chest x-ray					
Eye examination					
Supplemental therapy:					
(e.g. potassium,					
estrogen, calcium)					

Fig. 2–4

Long-term corticosteroid use flow sheet. (Modified from Holland E, Taylor T: *J Fam Pract* 32:518, 1991.)

PITFALLS OF TREATMENT

Assuming that a proper diagnosis is made, the most common treatment errors are (1) *suboptimal medication use,* related to either too low or too high medication strength, improper vehicle, or insufficient dosage; (2) *lack of patient adherence* as a result of inadequate patient education or potential adverse drug events; (3) *clinically significant drug interactions;* and (4) *disregard of medication costs* to the patient.

Suboptimal Medication Use

The most frequent example of suboptimal medication use is the patient with extensive or facial contact dermatitis who is given a 5- to 7-day prednisolone dose pack (i.e., a tapering dose over 5 to 7 days) along with a 30-g tube of hydrocortisone 1% cream. The patient does well for 2 or 3 days at the highest dosage of prednisolone, but new lesions continue to develop. A better treatment regimen involves using prednisone as the oral corticosteroid, given in high enough dosage (e.g., 1 mg/kg of ideal body weight) for a long enough time to cover the 10-14 days of lesion outbreak (i.e., 50 mg; decrease by 5 mg/day over 10 days). In addition, in this example, the hydrocortisone 1% cream is not strong enough to treat cases of moderate inflammation, and the quantity prescribed is sufficient to cover the involved areas for only 3 days.

Other common examples include selecting the incorrect fungal agent for a documented fungal infection (e.g., using nystatin for a dermatophyte infection when the drug is active only against *Candida*) or using topical antifungal agents for tinea capitis when oral therapy is the correct route of administration. Another problem is using a medication for too short of a time to effectively treat the condition (e.g., using oral griseofulvin for tinea capitis for less than a month when it must be used for a minimum of 2 to 3 months).

When prescribing a medication, the *amount* to be dispensed needs to be considered carefully. An insufficient amount of medication used by the patient will lead most often to an inadequate therapeutic response. When considering the amount used per application, the number of applications to be given daily, and the duration of therapy, the prescription can be written so the patient will not run out of medication prematurely (Table 2–1). The Fingertip Unit (FTU) is a convenient method to estimate the amount of a topical preparation to be used per application. Each FTU is approximately equivalent to 0.5 and 0.4 g of ointment in men and women, respectively. An estimate of the number of FTUs required to cover various areas of the body is as follows: head and neck = 4.5, trunk (front or back) = 7, one arm = 3, one hand = 1, one leg = 6, and one foot = 2.

Patient Compliance

Proper patient adherence to the prescribed treatment includes receiving thorough patient education about the nature of the problem and proper use of the medication. For example, one of the most difficult conditions to successfully manage is urticaria. Patients are miserable, and the unpredictable nature of the outbreaks requires that the physician provide extra emotional support. Patients expect the urticaria to resolve while medications are taken "as necessary." If the patient understands that taking antihistamines (e.g., diphenhydramine, hydroxyzine, terfenadine, or cyproheptadine) "around the clock" is an essential aspect in management, both the physician and patient are more likely to be satisfied with the outcome.

Although not directly causal in nature, *several dermatologic conditions, including urticaria, psoriasis, acne vulgaris, alopecia areata, and rosacea, can be exacerbated by stress or other psychiatric disorders*. Selection of the most appropriate medications is important for a successful outcome; however, it is also important to consider therapies such as individual counseling, group therapy (e.g., support groups), stress management, cognitive–behavioral therapy, or psychopharmacotherapies (i.e., anxiolytics, antidepressants, or antipsychotic agents) as adjuncts in the management of psychodermatologic conditions.

Patients with chronic conditions such as acne or atopic dermatitis must be educated about the natural history of exacerbations and remissions and about the time needed to see any improvement *after* initiating the designated pharmacotherapy. Otherwise, patients may relate that the medication was working, but the desired effect did not persist after discontinuing its use. The parent of a teenager may call a clinician to report that the tetracycline prescribed 2 weeks before is making the child's acne worse. Tetracycline may not show any beneficial effects for 6 to 8 weeks; therefore it is helpful to explain to the parent the natural course of acne and arrive at mutual, realistic expectations.

If the skin condition is not responding, remember that the diagnosis and treatment may be correct, but the patient may not be following your recommendations. Ask your patients to bring all of their medications (both prescription and OTC) with them to every office visit. Are the tubes of cream still full? Are there as many pills used as expected? Are there reasons for not complying with medication use, such as cost or adverse drug effects?

Drug Interactions

The incidence of drug interactions ranges from 2% to 17% of all prescriptions, and interactions are experienced in 6% to 42% of older patients. The risk for a drug interaction increases with an increased number of drugs taken. The basic types of drug interactions are:

1. *Pharmacokinetic drug with drug* (e.g., decreased metabolism of theophylline as a result of the concurrent administration of ketoconazole, leading to elevated serum theophylline levels and potential toxicity)
2. *Pharmacodynamic drug with drug* (e.g., decreased thiazide or loop diuretic action because of antagonism from concurrent administration of NSAIDs)
3. *Drug with disease* (e.g., beta-blockers can worsen psoriasis, lithium can cause acne lesions)
4. *Drug with food* (e.g., a decrease in tetracycline absorption with concurrent oral calcium administration)

5. *Drug with alcohol* (e.g., increase in hepatic toxicity and decrease in therapeutic efficacy with alcohol and isoniazid or rifampin.)

Be aware that drug interactions are commonly experienced in primary care dermatologic practice (i.e., astemizole and erythromycin).

Medication Costs

Dermatologic agents vary tremendously in cost. Be aware of the average cost of medications prescribed and what patients can afford. As an ongoing exercise, contact several pharmacies to determine the average cost to the patient for the medications that you commonly prescribe. Although generic medications may differ in potency and vehicle component, the cost differential may negate any differences in therapeutic effectiveness. Generic topical medications are effective for treating the majority of skin disorders seen in primary care. Because the price difference between pharmacies may vary significantly, encourage patients to call several pharmacies for the cost of their prescription. Examples of medication costs to the patient for an entire course of various dermatologic pharmacotherapies are noted in Table 2–9.

TABLE 2–9.

Medication Costs to the Patient for Selected Dermatologic Medications

Drug	Dose	Duration	Cost
Fluconazole (Diflucan)	300 mg PO q wk	9 months	$689.79
Griseofulvin (Fulvicin P/G)	250 mg PO bid	3 months	186.79
Griseofulvin (generic ultramicrosize)	250 mg PO bid	3 months	134.49
Itraconazole (Sporanox)	200 mg PO bid 1 wk/mo	3 months	480.00
Azithromycin (Zithromax)	500 mg PO on day 1, then 250 mg PO on days 2-5	5 days	39.19
Erythromycin (E-Mycin)	500 mg PO bid	30 days	15.89
Tetracycline (generic)	500 mg PO bid	30 days	8.90
Doxycycline (generic)	100 mg PO qd	30 days	13.49
Minocycline (generic)	100 mg PO qd	30 days	55.69
Astemizole (Hismanal)	10 mg PO qd	1 month	63.16
Cetirizine (Zyrtec)	10 mg PO qd	1 month	56.91

Continued.

TABLE 2–9 (cont.).

Drug	Dose	Duration	Cost
Chlorpheniramine (generic, OTC)	4 mg PO q 4-6 hr prn	1 month (i.e., # 100)	3.99
Diphenhydramine (generic, OTC)	25 mg PO q 6 hr prn	1 month (i.e., # 100)	6.99
Loratadine (Claritin)	10 mg PO qd	1 month	63.56
Terfenadine (Seldane)	60 mg PO q 12 hr	1 month	61.85
Benzoyl peroxide (generic, OTC)	10% gel applied bid	1 year	7.88
Clindamycin (topical)	1% solution applied qd	1 year	62.37
Erythromycin (topical)	2% solution applied qd	1 year	35.37
Tretinoin (Retin-A)	0.05% cream applied qd	1 year	115.92
Isotretinoin (Accutane)	40 mg × 10/week	20 weeks	974.00

NOTE: Prices were determined at community pharmacies in Chapel Hill, N.C. on Nov. 2, 1996.

SUGGESTED READING

Crosby IA: My skin is only the top layer of the problem, *Arch Dermatol* 131:783–785, 1995.

Gupta AK, Sauder DN, Shear NH: Antifungal agents: an overview, *J Am Acad Dermatol* 30:677–98, 911–933, 1995.

Koo JYM, Pham CT: Psychodermatology. Practical guidelines on pharmacotherapy, *Arch Dermatol* 128:381–388, 1992.

Long CC, Findlay AY: The finger-tip unit: a new practical measure, *Clin Exper Dermatol* 16:444–447, 1991.

McKenzie AW: Percutaneous absorption of steroids, *Arch Dermatol* 86:611–614, 1992.

Olsen EA: A double-blind controlled comparison of generic and trade-name topical steroids using the vasoconstriction assay, *Arch Dermatol* 127:197–201, 1991.

Piacquadio DJ: Topical corticosteroids in clinical practice: focus on fluticasone propionate, *Cutis (Suppl 2S)* 57:4–9, 1996.

CHAPTER 3

Diagnostic Procedures

There are many kinds of dermatologic procedures, and many different procedures can be used to treat the same condition. For instance, a basal cell carcinoma may be treated successfully under certain conditions by any of the following, depending on its size and location and the skills of the clinician: elliptical excision, electrocautery and curettage, cryotherapy, laser therapy, radiation, or micrographic surgery (Mohs). It is the responsibility of the clinician to choose the procedure that combines the highest cure rate, the lowest morbidity rate, and the least expensive treatment.

Most dermatologic procedures are simple to perform and are not time-consuming, if the proper equipment is easily accessible. The procedures discussed in this chapter can be mastered by learning the proper indications for a particular procedure and the common pitfalls to an unsatisfactory outcome. The decision to perform or not perform a procedure depends on several factors, including the skill of the clinician, level of diagnostic uncertainty, acceptance of possible side effects, and patient consent.

Dermatologic procedures can be used to confirm a suspected diagnosis (e.g., scabies preparation), to differentiate between two diagnoses (e.g., potassium hydroxide [KOH] preparation to differentiate between fungal infection and dermatitis), and to give a definitive treatment for common dermatoses (e.g., cryosurgery for actinic keratoses).

In addition to having the proper equipment on hand before starting any procedure, good lighting is essential. Poor lighting places stress on the clinician. A magnifying hand lens may also be helpful in delineating the types of lesions present and deciding where to perform a procedure.

BOX 3–1.

Patient Guidelines in Preparation for Skin Surgery

1. Avoid all aspirin and aspirin-containing products (e.g., Ecotrin, Bufferin, Excedrin, Alka-Seltzer, BC Powders, Stanback, Goody's, Anacin, Ascriptin, Advil, Motrin) for 7 days before surgery. If necessary, take acetaminophen (e.g., Tylenol).
2. Let your physician know if you must take or have taken aspirin within several days of surgery. This does not mean that the surgery cannot be performed, but there may be more bleeding during the surgery and bruising afterward. Icepacks on the day of surgery will help to minimize any bleeding.
3. Avoid any alcoholic beverages (e.g., beer, wine, liquor) for 48 hours before surgery; they may increase bleeding.
4. Let your physician know if you take any blood thinners (e.g., warfarin [Coumadin], dipyridamole).
5. Let your physician know if you routinely take antibiotics before you undergo any procedures (e.g., before having your teeth cleaned).
6. Let your physician know if you are allergic to any antibiotics.
7. If you are having surgery near your eye, bring someone to drive you home.
8. If you are having surgery on your head, wear a button-up shirt so you do not have to pull the shirt back on over the dressing.

Although many dermatologic procedures are done at the initial visit, when the patient presents with a skin lesion, sometimes the clinician should reschedule the patient for a particular procedure, either because of time constraints or for medical reasons.

Rushing a dermatologic procedure is not helpful to the patient or to the physician and may result in a poor outcome. If the patient is being scheduled specifically for cutaneous surgery, suggested patient preoperative guidelines (Box 3–1) are useful.

When performing procedures such as cryosurgery, biopsies, and excisions, it is important to inform your patients of potential side effects,

such as scarring, and document this education appropriately in the medical record. Obtaining the patient's informed consent (Fig. 3–1) may not necessarily prevent a malpractice lawsuit, but is highly recommended nevertheless.

Finally, all clinicians should develop the habit of following universal precautions when performing dermatologic procedures. Such precautions include the use of gloves and masks or goggles when doing any procedure that involves contact with blood or mucous membranes. Clinicians and their office staff should not recap needles, because most office needle sticks occur in the process of recapping.

OFFICE SURGERY CONSENT FORM

Patient Name_____Chart # _____ Date_____

I consent to the following procedure(s): _____

This has been explained to me as: (e.g., numbing the area, cutting out the mole, and sewing it up)
_____
_____

I understand that there are risks to having procedures performed on the skin. These risks may include a scar where the skin was cut, bleeding, infection, recurrence of the lesion, need for further surgery, and allergic reaction to the numbing medicine.

I have had an opportunity to ask any and all questions about the procedure, and I understand it as it has been explained to me.

_____
Patient Signature

_____
Witness Signature

_____
Physician Signature

Fig. 3–1
Office surgery informed consent form.

ANESTHESIA

Purpose

Using an appropriate anesthetic agent is an important consideration for many dermatologic procedures. Clinicians should become very familiar with 2 to 3 different anesthetic preparations and techniques to optimize patient comfort, flexibility, and outcomes.

Indications

Anesthetic agents are useful for any medical procedure that has potential for causing pain and for which the use of an anesthetic agent can lead to a decrease in the overall amount of pain experienced during the procedure.

Equipment

The choice of an anesthetic agent depends on the type of procedure, the age and personality of the patient, the skill of the clinician, and the properties of the agent.

Choice of Anesthetic

- *Ice or ethyl chloride:* These simple topical agents are quite effective for superficial anesthesia of short (less than 5 seconds) duration (e.g., before snip excision of an acrochordon). These modalities may also be useful to lessen the pain of lidocaine injection.
- *Lidocaine 1% (without epinephrine):* For most dermatologic procedures, inject 1 to 5 ml (maximum 4.5 mg/kg) into lesion. *Lidocaine* is particularly useful for procedures requiring anesthesia of the fingers, toes, nose, penis, or earlobes.
- *Lidocaine 1%, (with epinephrine 1:100,000):* This is particularly useful for anesthesia in all procedures *except* those that involve the fingers, toes, nose, penis, or earlobes or in patients on nonselective beta-blockers.
- *0.9% Normal saline:* Benzyl alcohol, which is a preservative in this solution, acts as a superficial anesthetic agent. Normal saline is useful alone for superficial procedures, such as superficial shave or gradle excisions.
- *Lidocaine 2.5% and prilocaine 2.5% cream (EMLA, 5 g, 30 g):* This cream is applied generously to the affected area (not rubbed in), the area is occluded with plastic wrap for 1.5 to 2 hours before the scheduled procedure. The cream is an effective method for providing anesthesia for scheduled procedures to infants and children, to those with a needle phobia, or for superficial procedures, such as shave or gradle excisions.
- *Combinations:* In some patients, combinations of the above treatments are useful. For instance, when performing an excisional or punch biopsy, 2 hours after a patient has applied the *lidocaine/prilocaine* cream, the clinician can infiltrate the area with 0.9% normal saline and then inject 1% *lidocaine,* giving excellent overall anesthesia for the procedure but with little to no discomfort. Drawbacks to this kind of approach include the amount of patient education and advance preparation time needed to achieve such results.

POTASSIUM HYDROXIDE PREP

Purpose

Potassium hydroxide (KOH) can be used to microscopically identify fungus or yeast from epidermal skin scrapings. KOH dissolves epidermal keratinocytes, allowing for easier demonstration and identification of organisms.

Indications

Fungal infections (e.g., tinea pedis, manus, corporis, cruris, capitis; onychomycosis).
Yeast infections (e.g., tinea versicolor; candidiasis [oral, skin, nails]).

Equipment

- Alcohol preparations.
- No. 15 blade or glass slide for scraping.
- Glass slide and coverslip.
- KOH solution.
- Alcohol lamp.
- Microscope.
- Hemostats or 2 × 2 gauze for scalp lesions. Tongue blade for oral lesions. Nail clippers for nail lesions.

Technique

1. Clean the skin of any lotions or creams with an alcohol preparation.
2. Obtain a specimen:
   a. *Skin:* Use either a no. 15 blade or the side of a glass slide to scrape material loose from a leading edge. If there are pustules or vesicles, scrape the roof onto a glass slide.
   b. *Oral candidiasis:* Use a tongue blade to scrape white plaques onto a slide.
   c. *Nail infections:* Remove as much nail as possible with nail clippers to expose the most proximally involved area, then scrape the subungual debris onto a slide with a 1- to 2-mm curette or a no. 15 blade.
   d. *Hair infections:* Using a hemostat, pluck 5 to 10 hairs from an active scaling area and place them on a slide *or* rub a 2 × 2 gauze vigorously to an area of alopecia and scaling, placing the broken-off hairs onto a glass slide.
3. Apply 2 or 3 drops of KOH to the slide, then apply the coverslip.
4. Heat the slide gently over an alcohol lamp until the KOH just starts to boil.
5. Examine at 10× magnification, using the lowest light possible (lowering the condenser is helpful). Examine at 40× magnification if necessary to confirm the presence of hyphae in fungal infections and pseudohyphae or yeast forms for *Candida* or *Pityrosporum* infections (Figs. 3–2 through 3–4).

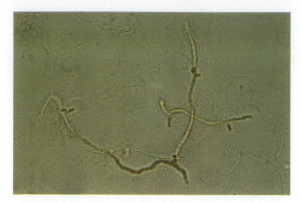

Fig. 3–2
KOH preparation from skin scrapings in a patient with tinea pedis. Note the dissolving epidermal cells with refractile hyphae (×40).

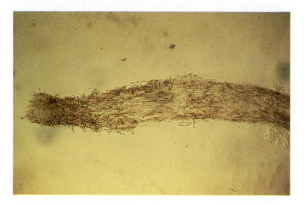

Fig. 3–3
KOH preparation of a hair, demonstrating hyphae and spores in a patient with tinea capitis (×10).

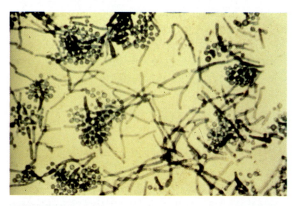

Fig. 3–4
Preparation from a patient with tinea versicolor, demonstrating pseudohyphae and spores in a "spaghetti and meatball" configuration.

Use the fine focus to help demonstrate refractile properties of organisms compared with epidermal cell walls.

6. For nail specimens, use KOH with dimethyl-sulfoxide (DMSO) or allow the preparation to sit for several hours, then reexamine it. This helps the thick keratin dissolve and aids in examination of fungal elements.

FUNGAL CULTURE

Purpose

Fungal cultures are used to help confirm the diagnosis of fungal or yeast infection when the KOH test is negative and to identify the particular fungal organism in resistant or special circumstances.

Indications

Fungal cultures are especially useful in hair or nail infections, because often the KOH test results are negative or, in the case of nail infections, may not be helpful in differentiating fungal from yeast infections. Such differentiation may influence therapy. For example, nail infections caused by molds will not respond to oral therapies but may respond to nail removal. Alternatively, fungal cultures are rarely needed to diagnose fungal or yeast infections of the skin.

Equipment

- Alcohol preparation.
- No. 15 blade or glass slide for scraping.
- Hemostats or gauze for scalp lesions. Tongue blade for oral lesions. Nail clippers for nail lesions.
- Dermatophyte Test Medium* for cultures.

Technique

1. Obtain a specimen:
   a. *Hair:* Remove 5 to 10 hairs from an involved, scaling area with one quick motion, using a hemostat, or rub a 2 × 2 gauze vigourously to an area of alopecia and scaling, placing the broken off hairs into the media. After placing the hairs in the culture medium, loosely recap the bottle and store it in a dark cabinet.
   b. *Nails:*
      i. Remove a portion of the involved nail with nail clippers to expose the most proximal involved area. Using a no. 15 blade or a curette, scrape the proximal subungual debris into the culture medium. Nail clippers can be used to remove the involved proximal areas, but cover the nail with 4 × 4 gauze to avoid having a specimen fly across the room.
      ii. After imbedding some of the specimen in the medium, apply the cap loosely and store in a dark cabinet.
2. Examine the specimen every 2 weeks for 4 to 8 weeks, looking for the phenol indicator in the test medium to turn from yellow to red (Fig. 3–5).

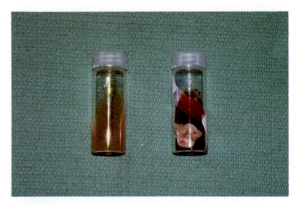

Fig. 3–5
Dermatophyte test medium. Note the positive culture from a toenail specimen on the right, as indicated by the color change from yellow to red. This culture took 3 weeks to become positive.

*Troy Biologicals, Inc., Troy, Mich.

3. Monomorphous colony growth indicates a dermatophyte infection. Yeast looks like creamy, discrete colonies. Be aware that bacterial contaminants and nonpathogenic molds may also grow. Referral of the specimen to a mycology laboratory may be necessary if the diagnosis still is in doubt.

SCABIES TEST

Purpose

The diagnosis of scabies can be confirmed by demonstrating microscopically the presence of the human mite or its eggs or feces. This will help to differentiate this intensely pruritic skin infestation from several other pruritic skin disorders (e.g., atopic dermatitis, insect bites).

Indications

To demonstrate *Sarcoptes scabiei* or its eggs or feces from a skin lesion.

Equipment

- Alcohol preparation.
- Mineral oil.
- Fountain pen.
- No. 15 blade.
- Glass slide and coverslip.
- Microscope.

Technique

1. The key to confirming the diagnosis of scabies with a microscope is to identify and scrape material from a burrow, the lesion most likely to yield an adult mite and its eggs or feces. There are approximately 10 or 11 adult mites per scabies infestation; therefore a diligent search for burrows is necessary. Even when the diagnosis is scabies, tests to demonstrate the mite may yield negative results. However, in Norwegian (disseminated) scabies, many lesions will be teeming with mites, and microscopic confirmation is made easily.

2. Areas most likely to yield mites are between the fingers, sides of the hands, wrists, elbows, axillae, groin, breasts, and feet.

3. Ink technique:
   a. Look for a nonexcoriated papule with a fine white to gray line across the top, and place 2 or 3 drops of ink over the papule. Leave the ink on for 5 to 10 seconds, then wipe the area clean with an alcohol prep. The ink will seep into the burrow, and a fine white to gray line will be evident.
   b. Place a drop of mineral oil on the skin, and either scrape the area with a no. 15 blade or pinch the area between the thumb and index finger, and superficially shave the top layer of skin. Anesthesia is not necessary.
   c. Place the specimen on a glass slide, apply the coverslip, and examine it under the microscope at 10× magnification to identify the female adult mite (0.4 mm long), the male (0.2 mm long), the eggs, or feces (see Fig. 6–3).
   d. Mite eggs are all the same size, whereas air bubbles are of several different sizes and change with compression of the slide.

TZANCK SMEAR

Purpose

To aid in diagnosis of certain vesicular viral skin infections.

Indications

Herpes infections: herpes simplex, varicella, zoster.

Equipment

- Alcohol preparation.
- No. 15 blade.
- Cotton swab.
- Glass slide and coverslip.
- Mineral oil.
- Microscope.
- For modified quick Tzanck: Cyto Prep spray fixative and Sedi Stain.
- For routine staining: 95% methanol, distilled water, and Giemsa, Wright's, or Hansel stain.
- Diff-Quick Stain Set.*

Technique

1. Clean an area with an intact vesicle for best results. If no intact vesicles are present, use the edge of the most recently appearing erosion or ulcer.
2. Remove a blister roof with a no. 15 blade, blot any excess blister fluid, then *scrape the base* of the vesicle, erosion, or ulcer with the scalpel blade, spreading a *thin* layer of the resultant material onto a glass slide.
3. For a modified Tzanck test:
   a. Immediately fix the slide with Cyto Prep, and air dry for 5 to 10 minutes.
   b. Flood the slide with Sedi-Stain for 30 to 60 seconds, rinse gently with tap water, and air dry.

*American Scientific Products, McGaw Park, Ill.

4. For routine staining:
   a. Fix the specimen by flooding the slide with 95% methanol for 5 seconds, then air dry for 1 to 2 minutes.
   b. Flood the slide with nuclear stain (Wright's, Giemsa, or Hansel stain) for 30 to 60 seconds.
   c. Add distilled water to the slide for 30 seconds, then flood it with distilled water to remove any remaining stain.
   d. Flood the slide again with 95% methanol for Hansel stain.
   e. Air dry without blotting.
5. Diff-Quick will stain in less than 1 minute, but unless several Tzanck smears are done every week, the expense to maintain a prepared set may not be worthwhile because of evaporation.
6. Observe the slide initially at 40× magnification to find areas where individual cells are best identified, that is, not clumped together because the cells are too thick. Then use oil immersion to identify multinucleated giant cells, where nuclei are molded together in giant epithelial cells (Fig. 3–6). Using microscope settings under high light and with the condenser up is most helpful.

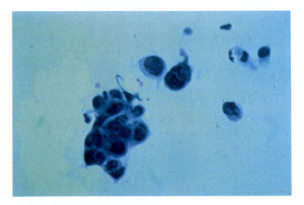

Fig. 3–6
Multinucleated giant cells consistent with herpes simplex infection. (Courtesy Paul Fischer, MD.)

WOOD'S LAMP EXAMINATION (BLACK LIGHT)

Purpose

To aid in the diagnosis of tinea capitis, erythrasma, and porphyria cutanea tarda. Certain specimens, when examined under a Wood's lamp, will fluoresce. Wood's light, with a wavelength of 365 nm, is passed through a Wood's filter.

Indications

Tinea capitis caused by *Microsporum canis* or *Microsporum audouinii* causes less than 20% of tinea capitis in the United States; therefore negative Wood's lamp findings on the scalp do not rule out tinea capitis. In erythrasma, the bacterium causing the inguinal scaling eruption, *Corynebacterium minutissimum,* produces a compound that fluoresces coral-red under a Wood's lamp. A presumptive diagnosis of porphyria cutanea tarda is possible if pink or orange-red fluorescence is seen in urine examined under a Wood's light.

Equipment

- Wood's light.
- Electrical source.
- Darkened room.

Technique

1. Examine the specimen under the Wood's lamp in a darkened room to optimally observe any fluorescence.
2. If the patient has recently bathed, fluorescence may be minimal.
3. Fibers, scale, and clothing also may fluoresce routinely.

ACNE SURGERY: COMEDO EXTRACTION

Purpose

Comedonal acne is often slow to respond to topical and oral acne therapies. Mechanical removal of open (blackheads) or closed (whiteheads) comedones is an important adjunct in the treatment of acne. Milia removal is achieved rapidly and effectively with the procedure.

Indications

To remove resistant comedones and milia. Pretreatment with tretinoin cream for 4 to 6 weeks often facilitates successful performance of the procedure.

Equipment

See Fig. 3–7.

- Alcohol preparation.
- 18-gauge needle or sterile lancet or no. 11 blade.
- Comedo extractor.

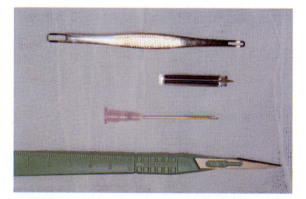

Fig. 3–7
Comedo extractor with lancet, 18-gauge needle, and no. 11 blade.

- *Lidocaine* 2.5% and *prilocaine* 2.5% cream (EMLA cream), if multiple lesions are to be treated in a single session.

Technique

1. Gently excise the roof or enlarge the opening of the comedo with an 18-gauge needle, a sterile lancet, or a no. 11 blade.

2. Gently but firmly apply pressure with the comedo extractor to the skin at a lateral angle to remove the keratin plug or milial cyst through the opening of the extractor.
3. If *lidocaine/prilocaine* cream is used, apply it generously for 1.5 to 2 hours before the procedure, occluding the involved area with plastic wrap.

CRYOSURGERY

Purpose

To rapidly, safely, and effectively treat many common skin lesions. Liquid nitrogen is the cryogen of choice, with a boiling point of 196° C. Cellular destruction occurs secondary to ice crystal formation, cellular dehydration, and subsequent protein and enzymatic denaturization. Destruction is more pronounced with rapid freezing and slow thawing cycles.

Indications

Removal of:

Benign lesions (e.g., warts, seborrheic keratoses).
Premalignant lesions (e.g., actinic keratoses).
Malignant skin tumors (rarely).

Equipment

- Storage tank.
- Liquid nitrogren.
- Thermos bottle with hole in lid and cotton-tipped swab or Cry-Ac Spray.*

Technique

1. It is always best to underfreeze than to overfreeze a lesion, to prevent complica-

*Brymill Corporation, P.O. Box 2392, Vernon, CT 06066; 860-875-2460, 800-777-2796.

tions (see p. 30); more can be frozen at a later date, if necessary.
2. Frozen areas of the skin will turn white immediately. This is referred to as the "freeze ball" or "iceball." The depth of freeze should be roughly equal to one and one half the radius of the freeze ball.
3. To treat small papules or thin, flat lesions, freeze the lesion for 5 to 10 seconds, leaving a rim of white 1 to 3 mm around the lesion.
4. For thicker warts or seborrheic keratoses, freeze for up to 40 seconds. This does not mean that the liquid nitrogen should be applied for 40 seconds but that the "iceball" should be maintained for 40 seconds. Repeat applications may be necessary for thicker lesions.
5. Often the skin will quickly become edematous and "urticarial" because freezing causes separation of the epidermis from the dermis, with resultant blister formation. A hemorrhagic area may develop if the lesion is frozen deeper than the epidermis (Fig. 3–8).
6. Liquid nitrogen often provides adequate anesthesia when using a curette to remove lesions. Such therapy is particularly useful for warts, acrochordons, or seborrheic keratoses, because often patients want the lesion removed before they leave the office. Subsequent use of aluminum chloride for

hemostasis, applied with a cotton swab, is often necessary when lesions are removed in this manner.

7. Treatment of a malignant tumor should be performed with a thermocouple, which allows for the temperature of a lesion to be monitored during treatment, to ensure adequate temperature for tumor necrosis. Local anesthesia with lidocaine 1% usually is required.

8. Patient education and documentation of explanations of potential complications are important.

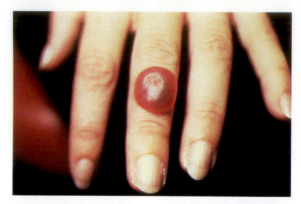

Fig. 3–8
Hemorrhagic bulla resulting from cryosurgery of a verruca.

Complications

Short-term

Pain is variable among individuals; however, be ready for vasovagal reactions. Do not use cryotherapy in small children. After freezing, lesions may be painful as a result of pressure from edema caused by the blister. Educate patients to use a sterile lancet, and "pop" the blister if this occurs.

Hemorrhage is common. Inform patients that formation of a "blood blister" is normal, especially when treating thick lesions, such as warts.

Infection is possible. Educate patients on proper wound care with dilute hydrogen peroxide and bacitracin or Polysporin until healing occurs.

Pyogenic granuloma occurs rarely with healing.

Long-term

Nerve damage is the most serious complication, and is especially likely where nerves are superficial, such as on the sides of fingers, the postauricular area, or the peroneal nerve.

Pigmentary changes are frequent and may be especially disfiguring in black patients.

Hypertrophic scar formation and *tissue defects* with delayed healing are possible when freezing thick lesions or if lesions are frozen too deeply.

Permanent nail dystrophy may occur if a periungual lesion is frozen too deeply.

Recurrence of a lesion, particularly warts, always is possible.

CURETTAGE AND ELECTRODESICCATION

Purpose

To provide removal or destruction of skin tumors, using a curette and electrical current to the affected area. This technique does not provide the best tissue sampling for pathologic diagnosis. If carcinoma is a strong consideration, consider performing a small shave biopsy before curettage to help provide the pathologist with adequate architecture for diagnosis.

Indications

Removal of:

Benign lesions (e.g., warts, seborrheic keratoses, pyogenic granuloma, acrochordons).
Malignant lesions (e.g., basal cell and squamous cell carcinomas, including squamous cell carcinoma in situ [Bowen's disease] and keratoacanthomas).

Avoid tumors that are fibrotic, scarlike (morpheaform), or located in areas of embryonic fusion lines (e.g., nasolabial folds, inner canthal region, posterior auricular folds).

Lesions extending into the subcutaneous fat should be removed by other means (e.g., excision).

Equipment

- Gloves, goggles, and mask.
- Alcohol prep, cotton swabs, and 4 × 4 gauze.
- Anesthesia: local anesthetic with 30-gauge needle.
- Aluminum chloride.
- Curettes: sizes 1 to 7 mm.
- Electrosurgical electrodesiccation instrument.*
- Antibiotic ointment.
- Telfa dressing and surgical tape.

Technique

1. For benign lesions, curettage and electrodesiccation are performed superficially, whereas for malignant lesions, the techniques are used more aggressively to destroy more tumor tissue. A small acrochordon may be quickly electrodesiccated, and the curette may then be used to simply scrape off the char.
2. Wipe the area(s) to be treated with an alcohol prep, and mark the site with a surgical marking pen if the lesion tends to "disappear" with anesthesia.
3. Anesthetize the area.
4. The smaller the lesion, the smaller should be the curette; 3-, 4-, and 5-mm curettes are used most commonly.
5. Using the sharp side of the curette, scrape the base of the lesion. When treating a carcinoma, scrape the base in several different directions until the underlying tissue feels firm. Cancer cells are not very adhesive and will feel "mushy."
6. Electrodesiccate the area. Most instruments will work only in a dry field. If necessary, apply aluminum chloride to the area using a cotton swab and rolling it very slowly to dry the area.
7. Benign lesions require only one treatment whereas malignant lesions should be curetted and dessicated 3 times.
8. After obtaining hemostasis, apply antibiotic ointment and a dressing. A pressure dressing may be required.
9. Educate patients about wound care (see Appendix Y).

Complications

Table 3–1 lists the potential complications of common dermatologic surgery.

SHAVE BIOPSY/EXCISION

Purpose

For therapeutic removal of superficial skin lesions or to biopsy superficial lesions as an aid in diagnosis. "Superficial" means epidermal and upper dermal lesions; therefore this procedure usually is not indicated for lesions extending down into the fat layer.

Indications

Removal/Biopsy of:

Benign lesions (e.g., moles, seborrheic keratoses).

Rashes of unknown etiology (e.g. ruling out vasculitis, drug eruption).

Malignant lesions (e.g., superficial basal cell, keratoacanthoma).

*E.g., Hyfrecator, Birtcher Corp., El Monte, Calif.

TABLE 3–1.

Potential Complications of Common Dermatologic Surgery

	Scar	Recurrence	Infection	Insufficient Tissue	Vital Structure Damage
Curettage/ electrodesiccation	++	++	++	+++	+
Shave biopsy	++	++	+	+	+
Punch biopsy	+	++	+	+	+
Elliptical excision	+++	+	+	+	+++
Cyst excision	+++	++	++	+	+++

Scar:	Warn patients that all skin surgery leaves some type of residual evidence. Ask if patient has a history of keloids.
Recurrence:	When removing carcinomas, remember that the recurrence rate for the initial treatment of skin cancers <2 cm in diameter (except morpheaform) is approximately 3%–7%. With a mole that has a hair protruding from it, it is important to remove any hair follicles that may extend into the subcutaneous fat, to prevent regrowth.
Infection:	Educate patients about wound care (see Appendix Y).
Insufficient tissue:	If a diagnosis of carcinoma is suggested, perform a shave biopsy before performing the surgery. If the deeper dermis or subcutaneous fat is required for diagnosis, punch biopsy or elliptical excision is necessary to provide adequate tissue for diagnosis.
Vital structures:	Be cautious of superficial vital structures such as nerves and arteries.
Suture spitting:	Extrusion of absorbable, buried suture, which dissolves in the skin, can be minimized by burying the knot. It is also easily remedied by removing the suture as it protrudes.
Pigmentation:	Hypopigmentation or hyperpigmentation may decrease over 6 months, but overall tends to be permanent.
Need for further treatment:	If margins are not clear, a wider excision may be indicated to fully treat carcinomas and prevent recurrence of atypical nevi, etc.

Equipment

- Gloves.
- Alcohol prep, 4 × 4 gauze, cotton swabs.
- Local anesthetic, using a 30-gauge needle.
- No. 15 blade scalpel or Gillette double-edged blade, broken in half horizontally.
- Aluminum chloride 30%, commercially prepared as 20% solution.*
- Formalin bottle.
- Antibiotic ointment and adhesive bandage.

Technique

1. Clean the skin site with an alcohol prep, and mark the area to be excised, if the lesion will be difficult to define after anesthesia.
2. Anesthetize the area: If the shave is very superficial, raising a wheal with normal saline solution is less painful than *lidocaine* and will provide adequate anesthesia; otherwise use *lidocaine* 1% to raise a wheal.
3. Stabilize the skin with one hand. Using either a no. 15 scalpel blade or bowing half of a double-edged razor blade between the thumb and index finger, gently saw the skin back and forth, keeping the blade parallel to the surface of the skin. Increasing the blade angle will aid in making deeper cuts but will also leave an indented scar.
4. Place the specimen in formalin solution.
5. Obtain hemostasis with aluminum chloride on a cotton swab.
6. Apply antibiotic ointment and an adhesive bandage.
7. Further treatment via a wider excision is indicated if the margins are not clear (e.g., atypical nevi, carcinomas, etc.).

*Drysol, by Person and Covey.

Complications

See Table 3–1.

SNIP EXCISION

Indication

The snip excision is especially useful for removing pedunculated nevi or acrochordons.

Equipment

- Gloves.
- Alcohol prep and cotton swabs.
- Gradle or iris scissors.
- Forceps.
- Local anesthesia for larger lesions, using a 30-gauge needle.
- Aluminum chloride 30%, commercially prepared as 20% solution.*
- Formalin for preserving lesions suspected of being carcinomas.
- Antibiotic ointment and adhesive bandage.

Technique

1. Wipe the area with an alcohol prep, anesthetizing if necessary.
2. Grasp the lesion with the forceps and snip it off at the base.
3. Apply aluminum chloride for hemostasis as needed.
4. Apply antibiotic ointment and an adhesive bandage.
5. When excising large lesions, electrocautery or suturing may be required for hemostasis, along with a pressure dressing.
6. Educate patients about the use of an ice pack to help stop any bleeding that may occur at home.

PUNCH BIOPSY/EXCISION

Indications

Punch biopsy/excision is used to remove all or part of a lesion and to provide a cylindrical tissue sample to aid in diagnosis.

Equipment

- Gloves.
- Alcohol prep, 4 × 4 gauze, and cotton swabs.
- Local anesthetic, using a 30-gauge needle.
- Disposable punches, 2 to 8 mm.†
- Iris or gradle scissors.
- Adson forceps.
- Needle holders.
- Sutures (Table 3–2).
- Formalin.
- Antibiotic ointment and adhesive bandage.

Technique

1. Clean the skin site with an alcohol prep, and mark it if the lesion will be difficult to define after anesthesia.
2. Anesthetize the area.
3. Using one hand, stretch the skin perpendicular to the normal skin lines, to get an oval (rather than circular) defect, which makes suturing easier and avoids "dog ears."
4. Use a punch of sufficient size (usually size 4) to provide adequate tissue for sampling. Circular defects larger than 6 mm are harder to repair than elliptical excisions, so use 8-mm punches cautiously, if at all.
5. Holding the punch between the thumb and shaft of the index finger:
   a. Twirl the punch back and forth until it "gives," using caution where the tissue is thin or vital structures are involved.
   b. Remove the punch, grasping the specimen at the very edge of the epidermis

*Drysol, by Person and Covey.
†Acuderm, Inc., Fort Lauderdale, Fla.; or Baker Cummins Dermatologics Inc., Miami, 1-800-842-6704.

with forceps and taking great care not to crush it.
c. Remove the specimen's remaining deep connections by cutting it with iris or gradle scissors.
6. Place the specimen in formalin.
7. Using simple interrupted sutures, close the punch site. Table 3–2 suggests which size suture is best for use on different body sites.
8. If the biopsy specimen is not taken from a cosmetically sensitive area, 2- to 3-mm punches may not require suturing, 4- to 5-mm punches usually require two sutures and 6-mm punches require three sutures.
9. Apply antibiotic ointment and dressing. If bleeding persists, use a pressure bandage.
10. Suture removal guidelines are given in Table 3–3.

TABLE 3–2.

Suture Materials for Punch Biopsy

Location	Size	Type	Trade Name
Face	5-0 or 6-0	Nonabsorbable	Ethilon, Prolene
Trunk	4-0	Nonabsorbable	Ethilon, Prolene
Extremities	3-0 or 4-0	Nonabsorbable	Ethilon, Prolene

TABLE 3–3.

Guidelines for Suture Removal

Face	4–7 days
Trunk	7–14 days
Extremities	7–14 days
Scalp	7–14 days

Complications

See Table 3–1.

ELLIPTICAL EXCISION

Purpose

Elliptical excisions are used to remove all portions of a visible lesion and provide complete tissue for pathologic evaluation.

Equipment

- Alcohol prep, 4 × 4 gauze, and cotton swabs.
- Surgical marking pen.
- Local anesthetic, using a 30-gauge needle.
- Hibiclens or equivalent preparation to sterilize skin surface.
- Two sterile towels and towel clamps.
- Sterile gloves, goggles, and mask.
- Needle holders of appropriate size for suture needle.
- No. 15 blade scalpel.
- Iris scissors, curved.
- Adson forceps.
- Hemostats.
- Skin hooks.
- Sutures (Table 3–4).
- Electrocoagulation unit.
- Formalin.
- Antibiotic ointment and adhesive bandage.

Technique

1. Define the best closure lines to coincide with the least tension on the final wound (Fig. 3–9).

TABLE 3–4.

Suture Materials for Ellipse Excision

Location	Size	Type	Trade Name
Deep layer closure			
Face	5-0, 6-0	Absorbable	PDS, Dexon, Vicryl
Trunk	3-0, 4-0, 5-0	Absorbable	PDS, Dexon, Vicryl
Extremities	3-0, 4-0	Absorbable	PDS, Dexon, Vicryl
Skin closure			
Face	5-0, 6-0	Nonabsorbable	Ethilon, Prolene
Trunk	4-0	Nonabsorbable	Ethilon, Prolene
Extremities	3-0, 4-0	Nonabsorbable	Ethilon, Prolene

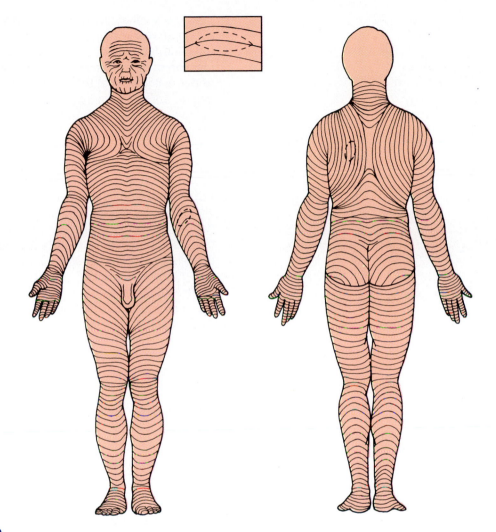

Fig. 3–9
Skin tension lines, with sample ellipse oriented for proper surgical excision.

2. Clean the skin site with an alcohol prep and mark the area to be excised.
3. Sterilize the skin, drape the area with sterile towels secured with towel clips, then anesthetize the area.
4. Stabilize the skin by stretching it with one hand in three-point traction, using pressure at three sites.
5. Perform an ellipse excision with a no. 15 scalpel blade, carrying the excision into the superficial subcutaneous fat. In the classic ellipse excision, the length of the ellipse is 2.5 to 3 times the width of the lesion. Excision angles should be approximately 30 degrees for proper skin closure (Fig. 3–10).
6. Using forceps, grasp one end of the ellipse and remove the undersurface with either the iris scissors or scalpel, taking care to remove an even amount of fat. This process is aided by keeping the scissors or scalpel blade as evenly horizontal as possible throughout specimen removal.

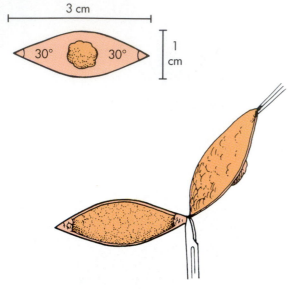

Fig. 3–10
Model for elliptical excision.

7. Place the specimen in formalin.
8. Obtain hemostasis with electrocoagulation, tying off any deep bleeding vessels.
9. Undermine the area. With a skin hook or gently with forceps, elevate one side of the wound and insert the iris scissors, spreading the scissors and cutting only fibrous tissue. The level of undermining is determined by the anatomic site, but is usually done in the superficial subcutaneous fat, at the junction of the dermis. Perform sufficient undermining so that the two wound edges can be approximated with minimal tension, using the skin hooks and forceps or by simply pinching the skin. Some areas may require little or no undermining.
10. Obtain any further hemostasis necessary before suturing.
11. Closing the wound in a layered fashion provides the best cosmetic result, but it may not be necessary in all cases. A layered closure is particularly important wherever there is significant stress on the wound. Suture materials for ellipse excisions are given in Table 3–4.
12. Apply antibiotic ointment and a pressure dressing.
13. Suture removal guidelines are given in Table 3–3.
14. Wound care: See Appendix Y.

Complications

See Table 3–1.

CYST EXCISION

Indication

Removal of cystic lesions.

Equipment

- Alcohol prep, 4 × 4 gauze, and cotton swabs.
- Surgical marking pen.
- Local anesthetic, using a 30-gauge needle.
- Hibiclens or equivalent preparation to sterilize skin surface.
- Two sterile towels and towel clamps.
- Sterile gloves.
- Needle holders of appropriate size for suture needle.
- No. 15 scalpel blade.
- Iris scissors, curved.
- Adson forceps.
- Hemostats.
- Skin hooks.
- Sutures (Table 3–4).
- Electrocoagulation unit.
- Formalin.
- Antibiotic ointment and adhesive bandage.

Technique

See Fig. 3–11.

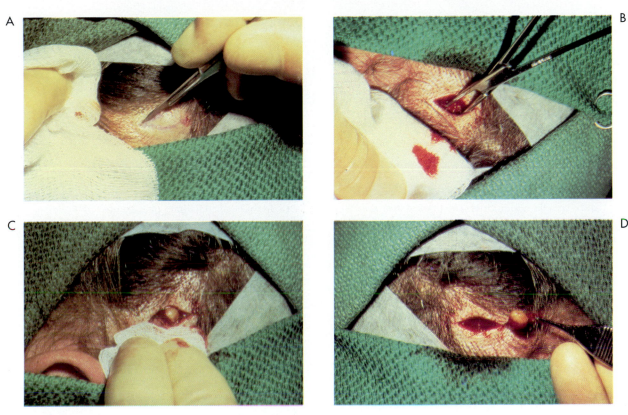

Fig. 3–11
Pilar cyst removal on scalp. **A,** Note elliptical excision into superficial dermis. **B,** Blunt dissection through the dermis and around the cyst. **C,** Note the isolated cyst. **D,** Intact cyst is removed. (Courtesy Department of Dermatology, University of North Carolina at Chapel Hill.)

1. Define the best closure lines to coincide with least tension on the final wound (see Fig. 3–9).
2. Clean the skin site with an alcohol prep, and mark the area to be excised.
3. Anesthetize the area, sterilize the skin, and drape the area with sterile towels, secured with towel clips.
4. Stabilize the skin with one hand by stretching it in three-point traction, using pressure at three sites.
5. Excise the ellipse with a no. 15 scalpel, carrying the excision into the superficial dermis only. If the lesion is very small, a punch may be used to remove the superficial skin, taking great care not to incise the cyst itself. Many cysts are very superficial.
6. Using forceps, grasp one end of the ellipse or punch, and with curved iris scissors, gently work into the dermis surrounding the cyst to shell it out. Continue shelling it out in all directions, taking care to avoid rupture.
7. Obtain hemostasis with either electrocoagulation or by tying off any bleeding vessels.
8. Close the wound in a layered fashion if there is any significant dead space. Layered closure also is important if significant stress is placed on the wound.

9. Apply antibiotic ointment and a pressure dressing.
10. Suture removal guidelines are given in Table 3–3.
11. Wound care: see Appendix Y.

Complications

See Table 3–1.

SUGGESTED READING

Addison LA, Fischer PM: *The office laboratory,* New York, 1980, Appleton and Lange.

Cohen PR: Tests for detecting herpes simplex virus and varicella-zoster virus infections, *Dermatol Clin* 12:51–68, 1994.

Drake LA et al: Guidelines of care for local and regional anesthesia in cutaneous surgery, *J Am Acad Dermatol* 33:504–509, 1995.

Grande DJ, Neuburg M: Instrumentation for the dermatologic surgeon, *J Dermatol Surg Oncol* 15:288–297, 1989.

Haas AF, Grekin RC: Antibiotic prophylaxis in dermatologic surgery, *J Am Acad Dermatol* 32:155–176, 1995.

Kuflik EG: Cryosurgery updated, *J Am Acad Dermatol* 31:925–944, 1994.

Matarasso SL, Geisse JK: Dermatologic surgery, *Semin Dermatol* 13:1–63, 1994.

Nahass GT, Goldstein BA, Zhu WY et al: Comparison of Tzanck smears, viral cultures, and DNA diagnostic methods in detection of herpes simplex and varicella-zoster infection, *JAMA* 268: 2541–2544, 1992.

Pfenninger JL, Fowler GC: *Procedures for primary care physicians,* St Louis, 1994, Mosby.

Sebben JE: Sterile technique and the prevention of wound infection in office surgery, *J Dermatol Surg Oncol* 15:38–48, 1989.

Telfer NR, Moy RL: Wound care after office procedures, *J Dermatol Surg Oncol* 19:722–731, 1993.

CHAPTER 4

Preventive Dermatology

Preventive dermatology is vastly underused and underappreciated as an essential and growing component of dermatologic care. With over 800,000 new cases of skin cancer in the U.S. each year and approximately 10,000 deaths annually, skin cancer alone makes a provocative case for increased prevention efforts. *Primary prevention* in dermatology is most readily appreciated by the prevention of skin cancer through avoidance of prolonged cumulative sun exposure and the use of sunscreens. *Secondary prevention* is equally important, as shown by the emphasis on teaching patients to be aware of the signs and symptoms of abnormal moles and melanoma. Finally, clinicians can practice *tertiary prevention* daily by teaching patients the proper use of dermatologic therapeutics and medications, thereby avoiding the morbidity or side effects associated with common skin diseases such as eczema and scabies.

The shift to managed care that is occurring throughtout the health care system increases the need and incentive for clinicians to prevent severe skin disease at all opportunities. Increasingly, clinicians are expected to take a community-oriented, epidemiologic approach to the diagnosis and management of skin diseases. This chapter describes both basic and more advanced mechanisms for clinicians to extend their involvement with preventive dermatology, ranging from traditional patient encounters to population-based approaches.

OCCUPATIONAL DERMATITIS

Dermatologic diseases are the second most common form of occupational disability, with contact dermatitis the most common diagnosis. The specific treatment of a known contact dermatitis is described fully in Chapter 14; however, several points are specific to occupational dermatitis, not the least of which is the financial implication to the patient or employer for a condition deemed to be occupationally related. *The majority of occupational dermatitis is due to direct trauma to the epidermis*, from harsh dusts (e.g., glass wool, brick, stone) or from acid, alkali, or solvent irritants (e.g., carbon tetrachloride, paint by-products, turpentine, gasoline).

The two most important components of occupational dermatology are identifying individuals prone to dermatitis and establishing the specific occupational cause for the dermatitis. Predisposed individuals include those with underlying eczematous dermatoses, especially atopic dermatitis. Some individuals may never have had hand eczema, but exposure to harsh chemicals or to sensitizers such as rubber products, cement products, or hair dyes may cause manifestation of the disease. Rarely the problem becomes unrelenting, possibly requiring a change in occupation. Proper identification of a causative agent, treatment of the dermatitis, use of protective clothing (e.g., gloves, long sleeves), and avoiding exposure are essential.

Proof of an occupational cause for a dermatitis may be difficult. In such cases a history of the lesions improving over a weekend or over holidays is helpful. Occasionally time away from work will help to define the relationship if there is still a question.

Some specific occupations place an employee at a greater risk for skin diseases (Table 4–1).

Those whose work requires prolonged time outdoors, with intense exposure to ultraviolet rays, should be educated about the use of protective clothing, hats, and sunscreens to help prevent sun-related dermatoses, such as actinic keratoses and skin cancers. In addition, all health care workers should become aware of the increasing incidence of occupational sensitivity to latex gloves, which may cause hypersensitivity asthma as well as skin dermatitis.

For more information about occupational dermatitis, contact the National Institute for Occupational Safety and Health, the Environmental Protection Agency, or the Occupational Safety and Health Administration.

TABLE 4–1.

Occupational Causes of Allergic, Irritant, or Infectious Dermatitis

Occupation	Cause
Bakers	Spices, garlic, onion, citrus, and dough exposure, along with frequent hand washing, cause hand dermatitis and monilial infections of the nails
Cement workers	Chromate exposure causes contact dermatitis
Dairy cow workers	"Milker's nodules," an infectious pox virus transmitted from cow's udders, causes a hand dermatitis; cases usually resolve in a month
Electronics workers	Chemical burns and hand dermatitis are caused by exposure to metals, acids, solder, and solvents
Farmers, industrial workers	Pesticides (insecticides, fungicides, herbicides, etc.) cause many kinds of allergic and irritant contact dermatitis, urticaria, folliculitis, and pigmentary changes
Forestry or paper workers	Chemicals, such as formaldehyde, may cause a paper dermatitis
Florists/gardeners	Contact or infectious dermatitis caused by plant exposures (e.g., furocoumarin, fennel, celery, chrysanthemum, poison ivy, or sporotrichosis from working with thorned plants [roses])
Health care workers	Risks associated with latex allergy and frequent hand washing
Painters	Allergic contact dermatitis caused by paint thinner or preservatives such as chloracetamide and merthiolate
Photographers	Derivatives of paraphenylenediamine or aniline causing lichen planus-like eruptions, vitiligo caused by hydroquinone, or hand eczema caused by developers, toners, etc.
Printing industry	Acrylate-based compounds and other caustic materials, such as alkali, grease, solvent, etc., found in ink, printers presses, printing plates
Sheep workers/butchers	"Orf," an infectious dermatitis caused by a pox virus, common in lambs and transmitted to humans by handling infected animals; resolves spontaneously
Skin/hair care workers	Caused by paraphenylenediamine (hair dye), glycerol, thioglycolate (hair straightener), formaldehyde (shampoo), and nickel sulfate (instruments)
Textile workers	Dyes cause skin pigmentary changes and formaldehyde causes purpuric lesions

ENVIRONMENTAL DERMATOLOGY

The main environmental issue of concern for the control and prevention of dermatologic disease is the relationship between increasing exposure to ultraviolet rays and the decline in the earth's ozone layer (Fig. 4–1). Such relationship is more extensive than previously thought. In 1995 alone, more than 600,000 new basal cell carcinomas and more than 200,000 new squamous cell carcinomas were diagnosed. The great majority of these skin cancers were on sun-exposed body parts.

The continued increase in incidence of all types of skin cancers is epidemiologically related to increased exposure to ultraviolet rays, with ultraviolet B the most strongly implicated. Although clouds reduce the amount of ultraviolet B that reaches the earth's surface, even on a cloudy day, substantial amounts remain. Reductions in the ozone layer will result in increased amounts of ultraviolet B reaching the earth's surface.

It has been estimated that for every 5% to 10% reduction in the ozone layer there will be a 30% to 50% increase in superficial skin carcinomas. Although chronic sun exposure has been most strongly linked to basal cell and squamous cell carcinomas, blistering childhood sunburns also are associated with increased risk for melanoma. Therefore, for every 1% decrease in ozone, melanoma mortality will likely increase 1% to 2%.

Current research places the atmospheric decline in the northern hemisphere ozone layer at 2% to 4%. This ozone decline results from the release of manmade substances into the atmosphere, particularly chlorofluorocarbons, carbon

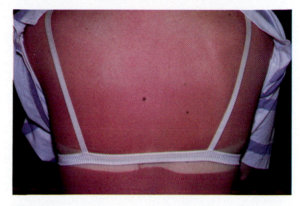

Fig. 4–1
Severe sunburn in an adolescent as a result of unprotected sun exposure. Such sunburns may occur even on a cloudy day.

tetrachloride, and methyl chloroform. The Montreal Protocol, an international group of major producers and consumers of such substances, outlined a proposal that eliminated the use of chlorofluorocarbon products in the United States by the end of 1995. However, it is likely that ozone levels will continue to decline, although at a slower rate, for at least the next 10 to 15 years.

Given these findings, health care clinicians should advocate regional, national, and international efforts to strengthen environmental regulations. Continued protection from ultraviolet rays, especially for individuals with fair skin and light-colored eyes, will remain essential. A clinical message must emphasize prevention and protection.

PREVENTION IN THE OFFICE

Clinicians should take full advantage of the many creative possibilities to incorporate preventive dermatologic techniques in the office setting. All patients should be counseled to:

- Limit cumulative sun exposure
- Reduce sun exposure during peak ultraviolet intensity time (10:00 AM to 3:00 PM)
- Use protective clothing, including hats

- Use sunscreens with a broad spectrum (UVA/UVB) and a high sun protection factor (greater than 15)
- Dispense health education pamphlets to patients

Other opportunities for prevention include displaying posters on skin cancer prevention, the signs and symptoms of melanoma, the hazards of tanning parlors, etc., in waiting rooms and patient examination rooms; having a personalized newsletter on skin diseases in the waiting room; encouraging office staff to model good health behaviors by avoiding sunburns; sending reminders to patients with previous skin cancers about regular follow-up; and using a behavioral prescription by writing down preventive dermatology actions on a prescription pad for patients. With every office visit of elderly patients, perform a quick screen for skin cancers by asking the patient if they have any new or changing skin lesions or any lesions that are failing to

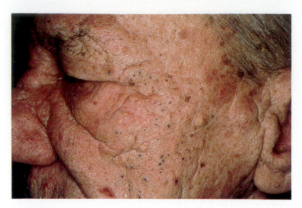

Fig. 4–2
Solar elastosis, lentigos, and comedone formation caused by prolonged exposure to ultraviolet radiation in an elderly man. This patient is at high risk for skin carcinoma. (Courtesy Department of Dermatology, Medical College of Georgia.)

heal. Pay particular attention to all new facial lesions (Fig. 4–2), and lesions on the backs of male patients and the legs of female patients.

COMMUNITY PREVENTION

Preventive dermatology can make a large contribution in educating the public about how to avoid serious skin disease. Look for creative opportunities to educate the community. For instance, community leaders and businesses can be encouraged to plant more shade trees for more structural protection against ultraviolet exposure.

Screening Programs

Clinicians can participate in public education campaigns through health screenings at malls, county fairs, gymnasiums, worksites, etc. Community outreach may help those patients who would not readily come into the office. Unlike high blood pressure or cholesterol screening, skin screens rarely provoke high levels of anxiety, and most patients appreciate the free opportunity to ask questions.

Although there is little definitive data on the long-term outcome of skin screening programs, many public policy organizations, including the U.S Preventive Services Task Force, the American Adacemy of Dermatology, and the American Cancer Institute, recommend skin cancer screening for high-risk individuals. Skin cancer screening programs may be effective in secondary prevention efforts because skin cancer is highly prevalent and serious; if left untreated, the disease worsens; early treatment prevents later consequences; and the screening test is inexpensive. Screening programs will hopefully increase the detection and treatment of serious skin cancers, particularly melanoma. Current research suggests that one melanoma will be detected for every 350 to 600 people screened.

Schools

The classroom presents another opportunity for community prevention efforts. Adolescents, like many adults, are preoccupied with the way they look. Their value system often places disproportionate importance on the worth of a suntan, and they may not know about the potential harm of tanning parlors. The difference between sunscreens and suntan oils often is not readily appreciated. Efforts to educate schoolchildren about preventing skin disease, particulary skin cancers, must begin in elementary school and continue throughout a child's education. Slide sets, videos, and brochures are available from the Skin Cancer Foundation.* Local chapters of the American Cancer Society also have videotapes and brochures that can be used to supplement presentations.

School administrators also need education and encouragement. For instance, athletic events may be scheduled at "non-peak" sun exposure hours. When prolonged outdoor exposure is anticipated, coaches can encourage the use of hats and sunblock.

Tanning Parlors

Despite well-recognized dangers and warnings from physicians, tanning parlors are a $1 billion plus business in the United States. Owners of such parlors state that they are safe because the ultraviolet source is predominantly ultraviolet A rather than ultraviolet B. With up to 1 million clients a day using tanning parlors in the United States, the perceived benefits of a "suntan" have thus far outweighed the perceived risks of exposure for many people.

However, the medical evidence indicates that tanning rays obtained from tanning parlors have acute and chronic effects and are carcinogenic.

*245 Fifth Ave., Ste., 1403, New York, NY 10016; 212-725-5176, 800-SKIN-490.

In some epidemiologic studies, tanning parlor cumulative exposure has been associated with a statistically significant increased risk of melanoma and basal cell carcinoma. Patients with lupus, porphyria, and rosacea may have disease exacerbation with ultraviolet A exposure. Up to 40% of ultraviolet-induced corneal burns result from exposure in tanning parlors. Severe generalized burns, although infrequent, also occur. The acute effects of ultraviolet A exposure through tanning parlors include:

- Pruritus (30%)
- Erythema (22%)
- Skin dryness (15%)
- Photodrug reactions (10%)
- Nausea (4%)

Clinicians can thus offer advice to individual patients or through media sources, such as newspapers and radio talk shows, about the potential dangers of tanning parlors. (See Appendix P.) In addition, clinicians can petition local and statewide professional organizations to establish and lobby for stronger standards and policy positions.

The public should understand that tanning parlors are not a "safe" way to get a suntan, and for some individuals they are actually dangerous. There is no national standard or oversight for tanning parlor operation; standards vary by state. Therefore parlors may not comply with adequate screening criteria that restrict patients with a history of photosensitivity or those taking a potentially photosensitive medication. *All individuals must wear goggles* while receiving tanning parlor rays, to prevent corneal damage. Unless a parlor posts its rules, the chances that it follows other safety concerns is doubtful. For more information, contact the Food and Drug Administration.*

*HFE-88, Rockville, MD 20857, HHS Publication No. (FDA)87-8270.

SUGGESTED READING

Bergfeld WF et al: *Proceedings of October 15–16, 1992, first national conference on environmental hazards to the skin*, 1994, American Academy of Dermatology.

Beyth R, Hunnicutt M, Alguire PC: Tanning salons: an area survey of proprietors' knowledge of risks and precautions, *J Am Acad Dermatol* 24:277–282, 1991.

Kripke ML: Impact of ozone depletion on skin cancers, *J Dermatol Surg Oncol* 14:853–857, 1988.

Mathias CGT: Contact dermatitis and worker's compensation: criteria for establishing occupational causation and aggravation, *J Am Acad Dermatol* 20:842–848, 1989.

Mathias CGT: Occupational dermatoses, *J Am Acad Dermatol* 19:1107–1114, 1988.

Patel NP, Highton A, Moy RL: Properties of topical sunscreen formulations, *J Dermatol Surg Oncol* 18:316–320, 1992.

Pathak MA: Sunscreens and their use in the preventive treatment of sunlight-induced skin damage, *J Dermatol Surg Oncol* 13:739–749, 1987.

Rietschel RL, Fowler JE: *Contact dermatitis,* Baltimore, 1995, Williams & Wilkins.

Rhodes AR et al: Risk factors for cutaneous melanoma: a practical method of recognizing predisposed individuals, *JAMA* 258:3146–3154, 1987.

Stern RS, Weinstein MC, Baker SG: Risk reduction for nonmelanoma skin cancer with childhood sunscreen use, *Arch Dermatol* 122:547–554, 1986.

Spencer JM, Amonette RA: Indoor tanning: risks, benefits, and future needs, *J Am Acad Dermatol* 33:288–298, 1995.

PART TWO

Common Skin Dermatoses

CHAPTER 5

Acne and Related Disorders

ACNE VULGARIS ICD-9 (706.1)

Acne vulgaris, or "acne" as it is known to millions of patients, is the most common dermatologic disease treated by physicians. The disease can lead to both physical and psychologic scarring, primarily as a result of inadequate or inappropriate treatment. Effective treatments exist for even the severest acne. The "art" of acne treatment involves:

- Use of multiple long-term medications
- Increasing compliance with therapy
- Understanding the natural history of the disease
- Dealing with underlying emotional issues

Acne is caused by a combined hormonal (androgen) and bacterial *(Proprionibacterium acnes)* disorder of the pilosebaceous units. The pilosebaceous unit is the "end organ" of androgens in the skin. Increased end organ sensitivity to androgens is thought to lead to follicular hyperkeratosis in combination with increased sebaceous gland activity. This follicular hyperkeratosis leads to accumulation of keratinous debris in follicular canals and subsequent occlusion of follicles. Bacteria multiply and break down the sebaceous material into irritating substances that subsequently cause an inflammatory response. *Comedones,* commonly known as blackheads *(open comedone)* and whiteheads *(closed comedone),* are simply lesions with the accumulated material within the follicle.

Left untreated, in some patients, acne may produce severe scarring when lesions are chronic, inflammatory, or deep-seated, such as nodules and cysts. The onset of acne usually is in adolescence, but it may occur into or even initially in adulthood. Seventy percent of women experience premenstrual flares. The diagnosis is made on the basis of clinical findings.

I. CLASSIC DESCRIPTION
Distribution: Predominantly face, back, shoulders, chest
Primary: Open (blackheads) or closed (whiteheads) comedones; papules, pustules, nodules, cysts
Secondary: Erythema, scar, excoriation

II. DIFFERENTIAL DIAGNOSIS (Table 5–1)
Severe acne in female patients with hirsutism and/or irregular menses may be an indication of androgen excess (e.g., polycystic ovary disease, androgen-secreting tumor). Diagnostic tests for this condition include free testosterone, dehydroepiandrosterone sulfate (DHEAS), androstenedione, follicle-stimulating hormone (FSH), and luteinizing hormone (LH) determinations.

III. TREATMENT
The treatment goal is to prevent new lesions and scarring, both physical and psychologic. Initial treatment may not eliminate existing lesions, but these usually resolve within 4 to 6 weeks with routine skin

TABLE 5–1.

Differential Diagnosis of Acne

Disease	Key Features	Population	Location
Acne rosacea	Significant erythematous component, no comedones, telangiectasia	Adults	Central face
Acne vulgaris	Papules, comedones, nodules, cysts; lesions at varying stages	Adolescents, adults	Face, back, shoulders, chest
Folliculitis	Look for hair protruding from individual lesions	All ages	Hair-bearing areas, especially trunk, extremities
Hidradenitis suppurativa	Comedones, nodules, cysts, sinus tracts, scarring	Usually appears after puberty	Axilla, inframammary, inguinal
Keratosis pilaris	Follicular-based papules and pustules	All ages	Lateral checks in children; posterolateral upper arms, trunk
Perioral dermatitis	Erythematous papulovesicles; may be associated with topical steroid use. Responds to PO tetracycline and/or clindamycin lotion bid	All ages, especially women 20–35 years	Perioral; may also be paranasal
Senile comedones (Favre-Racouchot syndrome)	Comedones and cysts in actinically damaged skin; responds to tretinoin or comedonal extraction	Older adults	Face, posterior neck
Steroid-induced	All lesions at same stage; no comedones	All ages	Diffuse or confined to site of topical steroid

turnover. Therapy often requires an individualized approach. Remember that counseling, mild treatment, and compliance with therapy work well for most patients. Inquire how the acne has affected the patient's life.

Acne in adolescent patients may be both physically disfiguring and psychologically traumatic. Barriers to successful treatment in these patients include noncompliance with therapy, emotional immaturity, stress, and cost of medications. Consider using the simplest possible treatment regimen.

Acne may be exacerbated by iodides, bromides, androgenics, corticosteroids, lithium, hydantoin, chlorinated hydrocarbons, occluding topical preparations (e.g., oil, tar, certain cosmetics, moisturizers), vigorous and extensive washing, and mechanical occlusion (e.g., leaning on hands, chin straps).

For women with acne who are also using birth control pills, consider prescribing a pill that has very low androgenic potential, such as Orthocyclen, Desogen, Brevicon, or Demulen-35.

A. Mild acne: Small papules and comedones; no nodules or cysts (Fig. 5–1): Choose one of the following, applying a thin layer to the entire face or affected area once a day, not just to individual lesions; spare the eyes.

1. *Topical antibiotics:* Use daily after washing, in combination with either benzoyl peroxide or tretinoin.

a. *Erythromycin 2%:* Available as pledgettes (boxes of 60), pads (boxes of 60), gel (30 g), solution (60 ml), ointment (25 g). Choose the delivery system the patient prefers. Ointment is useful in patients with dry skin.

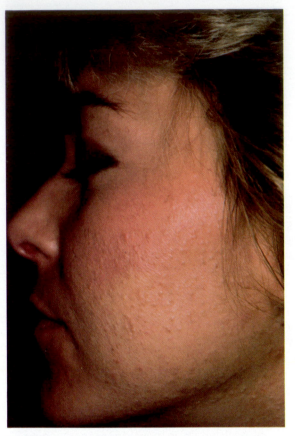

Fig. 5–1
Comedonal acne. Note predominance of closed comedones. (Courtesy Department of Dermatology, Medical College of Georgia.)

b. *Clindamycin:* Solution (30, 60 ml), gel (30 g), lotion (60 ml). Use lotion on more sensitive or dry skin, although some patients prefer the gel formulation.

c. *Meclocycline:* Cream (20, 45 g). Good option in patients whose skin tends to get very dry with acne therapy. Emphasize using only a very thin layer.

d. *Sodium sulfacetamide 10% and sulfur 5%:* Lotion (Sulfacet R—tinted, 25 g); (Novacet—untinted, 30 g). Useful if a lotion-based topi-

cal antibiotic is preferred and clindamycin or erythromycin are not working or well tolerated. Tinted formulas may cover areas of redness.

2. *Benzoyl peroxide:* 2.5%, 5%, 10%: If acne is very mild, benzoyl peroxide may be used as a single agent, or it may be used daily in combination with topical antibiotics or tretinoin. Warn patients that benzoyl peroxide may bleach clothing.

a. Apply a thin layer once or twice a day, after washing, to the entire affected area, starting with 2.5% to 5% strength, unless the patient has very oily skin. With oily skin and a large comedonal component, use benzoyl peroxide with tretinoin.

b. *Available in many vehicles (60 to 90 g):* Water-based preparations (Clear by Design 5%, OTC; Benzac AC gel 2.5%, 5%, 10%; Desquam E gel 2.5%, 5%, 10%; Panoxyl AQ 2.5%, 5%, 10%) are milder, less drying, and potentially less irritating than alcohol or acetone-based preparations (Persa-gel 5%, 10%, OTC; Benzagel 5%, 10%; Brevoxyl gel 4%; Panoxyl gel or soap 5%, 10%; Desquam X gel 2.5%, 5%, 10%). Alcohol and acetone-based preparations may be more useful in patients with very oily skin.

c. *Washes and soaps* 5% to 10%: (4 oz, 8 oz). Washes: Desquam E, Benzac AC, Brevoxyl 4%, Desquam X; soaps: Desquam X 10%, Panoxyl 5%, 10%. A good option for acne involving the chest, shoulders, and back. Patients use it like soap in a shower, applying it once daily to affected areas for 1 to 2 minutes, then rinsing.

d. *Benzamycin Gel* (23.3 g): Combination product of erythromycin and benzoyl peroxide. Apply a thin layer to the affected area once or twice a day. Must be kept refrigerated.

3. *Tretinoin* (Retin-A): 0.025%, 0.05%, 0.1% cream (20, 45 g) for dry or sensitive skin; 0.01%, 0.025% gel (15, 45 g) for oily skin; 0.05% liquid (28 ml) for very oily skin or large areas on chest or back.
    a. Especially good for comedonal (blackheads and whiteheads) or papular acne. Use very small amount (i.e., size of a pea for entire face); apply 30 minutes after cleansing with a mild soap *at bedtime*. Begin use with lower doses (0.025% or 0.05%); apply 3 times per week for 2 weeks, then daily if tolerated.
    b. Increases photosensitivity. Apply sunscreen daily in the morning for any sun exposure. May cause pigmentary changes in black patients.
    c. Educate patients that the drug may initially cause a flare reaction, with scaling and redness. If burning is experienced, decrease treatment schedule or strength or both.
4. *Salicylic Acid 2%* (SalAC wash OTC, Neutrogena oil-free wash OTC): May use in conjunction with tretinoin or topical antibiotics, especially for patients with mild acne.
5. *Azelaic acid* (Azelex) 20%: cream (30 g) qd-bid for facial acne. Useful for patients intolerant of tretinoin or allergic to benzoyl peroxide.
6. *Compliance and follow-up:*
    a. Use these agents individually or in combination. No more than two products should be used initially (e.g., topical antibiotic and tretinoin, benzoyl peroxide and tretinoin). Each product should be used at separate times of the day.
    b. Judge effectiveness only after 6 to 8 weeks of therapy. Acne may worsen before it starts improving. If the acne is not improving, is still mild, and the skin is not too irritated, consider increasing the strength or number of topical preparations.
    c. If compliance with therapy is suspect, have patients bring in their bottles and/or tubes, (e.g., one tube of tretinoin should last 3 to 4 months, 60 g of benzoyl peroxide should last 4 to 6 months, etc.).
    d. Typical monthly costs for medication range from $10 to $25.
B. **Moderate acne:** Papules predominate, with few nodules and rare cysts (Fig. 5–2). In addition to the above regimen:
    1. *Oral antibiotics:* Choose one:
        a. *Tetracycline* 500 mg bid or *doxycycline* 50 to 100 mg/day.
        b. *Erythromycin* 500 mg bid or 333 mg bid to tid.
        c. If these are not effective after 2 to 4 months, use *minocycline* 50 to 100 mg/day or *trimethoprim-sulfamethoxazole* double strength qd to bid.

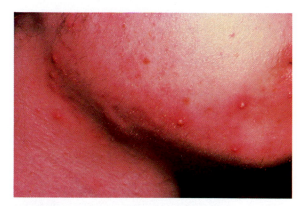

Fig. 5–2
Moderate acne. Note papules, pustules, and nodules with secondary erythema. (Courtesy Department of Dermatology, University of North Carolina at Chapel Hill.)

2. *Comedo Removal:* (See the discussion of comedo removal procedures in Chapter 3.) Comedo removal with an extractor may be useful as a short-term, adjuvant treatment for resistant comedones and in the prevention of deeper lesions. It is most useful to extract sebaceous material from open or closed comedones.

3. *Compliance and follow-up:*
   a. Nausea and gastrointestinal upset may interfere with antibiotic use.
   b. Avoid tetracycline derivatives in pregnant women and children younger than 12 years. Warn patients about possible photosensitivity and allergic reactions.
   c. Once acne is under control, taper the antibiotic dosage slowly over several months (e.g., decrease tetracycline by 250 mg q6wk).
   d. Follow up at 6 to 8 weeks initially, then every 3 to 4 months.
   e. Typical monthly costs for medication may range from $25 to $75.

C. **Severe acne:** Nodules and cysts predominate (Fig. 5–3). Follow moderate regimen above for 2 to 4 months. If response is inadequate, consider using *isotretinoin* (Accutane).

1. *Isotretinoin:* (Use in consultation with a dermatologist.)
   a. 1.0 to 2.0 mg/kg/day for 16 to 20 weeks is effective in "curing" or at least getting lesions to respond to conventional therapy in 80% of patients, although some may require a second course.
   b. Side effects, which are relatively frequent and usually dose-related, include xerosis, nosebleed, arthralgias, myalgias, photosensitivity, headache, elevated triglyceride and liver enzyme levels, and, less frequently, pseudotumor cerebri.

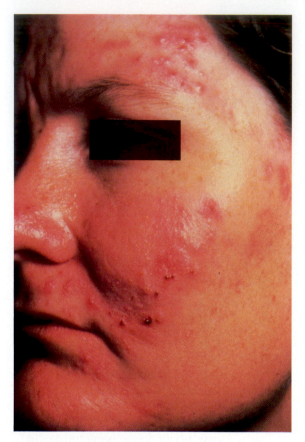

Fig. 5–3
Severe acne with predominance of nodules, cysts, excoriations, and secondary erythema. (Courtesy Marshall Guill, MD.)

   c. Laboratory monitoring must be frequent and includes serum pregnancy test within 1 week before starting course, then monthly; complete blood cell count before starting course; liver function tests, alanine aminotransferase (ALT, SGPT), aspartate aminotransferase (AST, SGOT), γ-glutamyl transpeptidase (GGT), lactic dehydrogenase, and fasting triglycerides and cholesterol levels before starting course, at 2 weeks after starting course, then monthly, until response to medication is established.

d. *Very teratogenic.* Strict criteria for use in female patients. Exposure of fetus to drug has resulted in major central nervous system, structural, and cardiovascular abnormalities. Two forms of birth control are recommended during the course of treatment and 1 month after the last dose.

e. Typical monthly costs for medications and laboratory work may range from $200 to $400. Roche has an indigent patient care program that will provide free medication to eligible patients.*

2. ***Corticosteroid injections:*** Intralesional injections are useful for more rapid resolution of (few or isolated) nodular or cystic lesions.

a. *Triamcinolone acetonide*: 10 mg/ml, diluted with sterile saline or *lidocaine* 1% to a concentration of 2.5 to 3.0 mg/ml. Inject 0.05 to 0.2 ml into well-defined, acutely inflamed cyst that is 24 to 72 hours old.

b. Such treatment may hasten healing but also can produce atrophy or hypopigmentation.

3. ***Consultation and/or referral:***

a. Sudden worsening of inflammatory acne previously controlled by oral antibiotics may herald gram-negative folliculitis. Consider referral for trial of *isotretinoin,* or culture pustules and treat based on sensitivities.

b. Consultation and/or referral with a dermatologist are indicated if the patient has a history of progressive acne scarring. Acne scarring can be treated by various methods (e.g., dermabrasion, collagen injection, punch excision).

IV. **PATIENT EDUCATION**
See Appendix A.

A. Emphasize that the patient likely will not see improvement for at least 6 to 8 weeks because treatment only prevents new lesions from developing.

B. Once the acne improves, it may be possible to decrease, but not discontinue, the regimen.

C. Advise use of mild soap and water for cleansing, and avoidance of scrubbing agents, pads, and vigorous rubbing.

D. Keep the regimen simple, with two or three medications.

E. If an adolescent patient fails to improve, investigate compliance with therapy.

F. Moisturizers that are "oil-free" and that include sunblock (e.g., Purpose, Neutrogena Moisture SPF 15, Oil of Olay Daily UV Protectant) are useful for patients with dry or sensitive skin or who are on photosensitizing medications, such as tretinoin cream.

ACNE ROSACEA ICD-9 (695.3)

Rosacea is derived from the Latin word for *rosy.* Acne rosacea is a chronic acneiform disorder of middle-age and older adults, characterized by vascular dilation of the central face: nose, cheek, eyelids, and forehead (Fig. 5–4).

*1-800-526-6367.

The spectrum of disease may range from mild erythema to severe sebaceous gland hyperplasia accompanied by papules, pustules, cysts, nodules, and telangiectasia. Eye involvement may include blepharitis, keratitis, conjunctivitis, and episcleritis. Rhinophyma is hyperplasia of the soft tissues of the nose and is seen in middle-age men with rosacea.

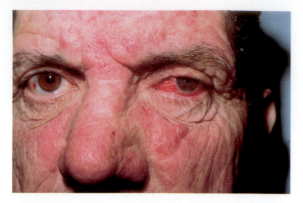

Fig. 5–4
Acne rosacea. Note erythematous papules and plaques on the central face. (Courtesy Department of Dermatology, University of North Carolina at Chapel Hill.)

Periodic facial flushing can be a significant feature, especially after increases in skin temperature from agents such as sunlight, hot or spicy foods, or alcohol ingestion. *Diagnosis is made on clinical findings. The key to diagnosis is the absence of comedones.* The cause of rosacea is unknown, and the disease most often is chronic, with remissions and exacerbations.

I. CLASSIC DESCRIPTION

Distribution: Central facial area: nose, cheeks, forehead, chin, eyelids
Primary: Papules, pustules, nodules, cysts, telangiectasia
Secondary: Erythema, scarring

II. DIFFERENTIAL DIAGNOSIS

Acne rosacea is distinguished from *acne vulgaris* by the latter's propensity for the younger patient, presence of comedones, lack of flushing, and lack of significant background erythema. *Seborrheic dermatitis* lacks acneiform lesions, despite scales around the nose, eyebrows, ears, and scalp. The flushing seen in *carcinoid syndrome* is transient, whereas that of rosacea persists; in carcinoid syndrome there is increased urinary 5-hydroxyindoleacetic acid (5-HIAA). With *systemic lupus erythematosus* there is an absence of papules and pustules in the presence of systemic complaints.

III. TREATMENT

The key to treating rosacea is the knowledge of the treatment goal, which often is control rather than cure of the disease.

A. Topical antibiotics and benzoyl peroxide: For papular and pustular lesions, apply a thin layer of one of the following to the entire involved area, not just to individual lesions, once or twice daily.

1. *Metronidazole cream or gel:* 0.75% (28.4, 45 g) bid.
2. *Sodium sulfacetamide* 10%/sulfur 5% lotion; *clindamycin* 1% solution, gel, or lotion; and *erythromycin* 2% solution are useful (bid) but somewhat less effective than metronidazole.
3. *Benzoyl peroxide* 2.5%; may increase up to 5% or 10% if the patient does not complain too much of dry skin. Use 2.5% in patients with a history of sensitive skin. Use once or twice daily.
4. Use for at least 4 to 6 weeks before assessing effectiveness.

B. Tretinoin: 0.025%, 0.05%, 0.1% cream (20, 45 g).

1. Useful for papular or pustular lesions that are unresponsive. Always start with 0.025%, 2 to 3 times a week at bedtime, gradually increasing to nightly use.
2. May be used in combination with topical antibiotics.

C. Oral antibiotics: Especially useful if nodular lesions are present.

1. *Tetracycline* 250 to 500 mg PO bid or *doxycycline* 50 mg PO qd to bid.
2. After 1 to 2 months of control, attempt to gradually taper the dosage over 1 to 2 months to the minimum that will control the disease. Long-term therapy may be required.
3. *Erythromycin* and *minocycline* are alternative oral antibiotics.

D. Referral:

1. Consider referral for surgical intervention if patient has rhinophyma unre-

sponsive to topical or oral therapy. Options include electrosurgery, surgical steel resculpturing, dermabrasion, or carbon dioxide laser treatment.

2. In severe nodulocystic rosacea, if there has been no response to the above therapeutic regimens after 3 to 4 months, refer for trial of *isotretinoin.*

3. Pulsed dye vascular laser therapy is useful for resistant telangiectasias and recalcitrant disease.

IV. PATIENT EDUCATION

A. Control, not cure, is the usual management goal.

B. Avoid excessive sunlight, temperature extremes, hot or spicy foods, and alcohol, if these agents are exacerbating factors.

C. Medications should be used long-term, not just for flare-ups of the condition, and should be tapered to the lowest dose of oral medications.

D. "Flares" may require higher doses of antibiotics for several weeks on a prn basis.

E. For more information, contact the National Rosacea Society.*

HIDRADENITIS SUPPURATIVA ICD-9 (705.83)

Hidradenitis suppurativa is a severe, chronic, scarring, inflammatory disease in the apocrine gland–bearing areas (axilla, areola, anogenital region). First described more than 150 years ago, the condition is characterized by recurrent abscess formation. The pathophysiology involves keratin plugging of the distal follicle, leading to dilatation and severe inflammatory changes. Bacterial multiplication and rupture of the follicle lead to spread of the inflammation, infection, and involvement of the apocrine glands. Subsequent healing involves fibrous scarring and sinus tract formation.

Although the cause of hidradenitis is unknown, the disease is seen only after puberty, and more frequently in obese patients and those with acne vulgaris. *The diagnosis is made by the clinical finding of recurrent abscess formation in apocrine gland regions.*

I. CLASSIC DESCRIPTION (Fig. 5–5)

Distribution: Axilla, areola, anogenital skin, including inguinal folds

Primary: Nodules, cysts, occasional comedones

Secondary: Erythema, exudate, scar, sinus tract, edema, ulceration

II. DIFFERENTIAL DIAGNOSIS

Initially, an *infected inclusion cyst* or a *car-*

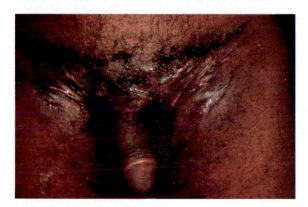

Fig. 5–5

Hidradenitis suppurativa. Note acutely inflamed inguinal nodules and cysts with secondary fistula formation and scarring. (Courtesy Marshall Guill, MD.)

buncle may mimic hidradenitis, but these lesions usually are solitary and are not confined to apocrine gland–bearing areas. In patients with anogenital ulceration, consideration of other *fistula- or sinus-forming diseases* (e.g., lymphogranuloma venereum [LGV], granuloma inguinale, Crohn's disease, tuberculosis) is appropriate. Hidra-

*800 S. Northwest Hwy, Ste. 200, Barrington, IL 60010; 847-382-8971; Web site: http://www.rosacea.org; e-mail: rosacea s @ aol.com

denitis can occur as part of a rare *follicular occlusion triad,* which includes acne conglobata (severe nodulocystic acne with draining sinuses) and dissecting cellulitis of the scalp.

III. TREATMENT

The treatment goal is to prevent scarring insofar as possible. For this reason, avoid multiple, repeat, piecemeal incision and drainage of the lesions.

A. **Systemic antibiotics:** Long-term therapy is indicated to prevent further scarring.
   1. *Erythromycin* 1.0 g/day; *cephalexin* 1.0 to 1.5 g/day; *tetracycline* 1.0 g/day; *sulfamethoxasole/trimethoprim* double strength qd to bid.
   2. Bacterial cultures and sensitivity tests may be used to direct antibiotic therapy if lesions become resistant to prior therapy (e.g., *Staphylococcus aureus* resistant to erythromycin).
   3. Use systemic antibacterial therapy for a minimum of 2 weeks; then try tapering to the lowest dosage of antibiotic that controls the disease.

B. **Intralesional injection:** *Triamcinolone acetonide* 5 to 10 mg/ml, intralesionally, if lesions are nonfluctuant and acute. Inject sufficient volume directly into the cyst so that the lesion blanches.

C. **Topical antibiotics:** *Clindamycin* 1% or *erythromycin* 2% solution; use as deodorant once or twice a day.

D. **Incision and drainage:** Drain lesions only if fluctuant.

E. **Referral:**
   1. Surgical excision is recommended for localized, chronic lesions; sinus tract involvement; or, if extensive, for all involved apocrine gland–bearing skin.
   2. *Isotretinoin* may be effective in some cases, particularly if it is used before extensive scarring develops.

IV. PATIENT EDUCATION

A. Avoid tight clothing.

B. Avoid shaving affected areas and using chemical depilatories.

C. Antibacterial soaps (e.g., Hibiclens, Dial, Lever 2000) may be used.

D. Weight reduction in overweight patients may improve the disease.

SUGGESTED READING

Acne: new perspectives, *J Am Acad Dermatol (Suppl)* 32:S1–S56, 1995.

Banerjee AK: Surgical treatment of hidradenitis suppurativa, *Br J Surg* 79:863–866, 1992.

Drake LA et al: Guidelines of care for acne vulgaris, *J Am Acad Dermatol* 22:676–680, 1990.

Ertl GA, Levine N, Kligman AM: A comparison of the efficacy of topical tretinoin and low-dose oral isotretinoin in rosacea, *Arch Dermatol* 130:319–324, 1994.

Highet AS, Warren RE, Weekes AJ: Bacteriology and antibiotic treatment of perineal suppurative hidradenitis, *Arch Dermatol* 124:1047–1051, 1988.

Pochi PE et al: Report of the consensus conference on acne classification, *J Am Acad Dermatol* 24:495–500, 1991.

Wilken JK: Rosacea: pathophysiology and treatment, *Arch Dermatol* 130:359–362, 1994.

Yu CC, Cook MG: Hidradenitis suppurativa: disease of follicular epithelium rather than apocrine glands, *Br J Dermatol* 122:763, 1990.

CHAPTER 6

Arthropods

SCABIES ICD-9 (133.0)

Scabies (from the French *scabo,* to scratch) is a contagious disease caused by the mite *Sarcoptes scabiei* var. *hominis* (0.3 mm diameter). *The hallmark of scabies is severe pruritus.* The mite life cycle begins as the female burrows into the most superficial layer of the skin, where she lives for up to 30 days. Each female mite deposits on average two to three eggs per day, which mature in 14 to 17 days, then repeat the cycle. The average infestation consists of only 10 or 11 adult mites.

The intense pruritus is due to a hypersensitivity reaction to the mite and its feces, which accounts also for the generalized eruption. The itching is classically worse at night. Symptoms usually occur 3 to 6 weeks after the primary infestation, and other household members or close contacts also may have symptoms. Transmission most often occurs with direct skin-to-skin contact. The adult mite does not live long on fomites (e.g., bedding or clothing).

Norwegian scabies is a rare but highly contagious infestation usually found in mentally impaired, institutionalized, or immunocompromised patients (see Fig. 16–13). Manifestations of the disease include asymptomatic crusting with hyperkeratotic plaques, especially on the hands and feet, and even under the nails in long-standing cases.

I. CLASSIC DESCRIPTION
Distribution: Fingerwebs, wrists, sides of hands and feet, axilla, groin, areola, extensor surface of elbows and knees; spares the face in adults but can involve the face in younger infants (Fig. 6–1).
Primary: Burrows are 0.5 to 1.0 mm long linear or wavy ridges where the adult mite has burrowed into the top layer of skin; papules, pustules, vesicles, nodules.
Secondary: Erythema, crust, excoriation, scale (Fig. 6–2).
Primary lesions may not be readily appreciated and burrows not seen if the secondary lesions are extensive or in patients with meticulous hygiene.

II. DIAGNOSIS
A. Scabies preparation:
1. To find a burrow, look closely at fingerwebs, wrists, groin, and the sides of the hands and feet. Consider performing a "felt-tip pen" test to help identify burrows; a burrow track takes up the ink and is subsequently notable as a dark line in the skin.
2. Use a no. 15 scalpel blade to scrape the burrow to its base; this may cause bleeding.
3. After placing all of the material on a glass slide and covering it with either mineral oil or potassium hydroxide, try to demonstrate mites, mite eggs, or mite feces microscopically (Fig. 6–3).

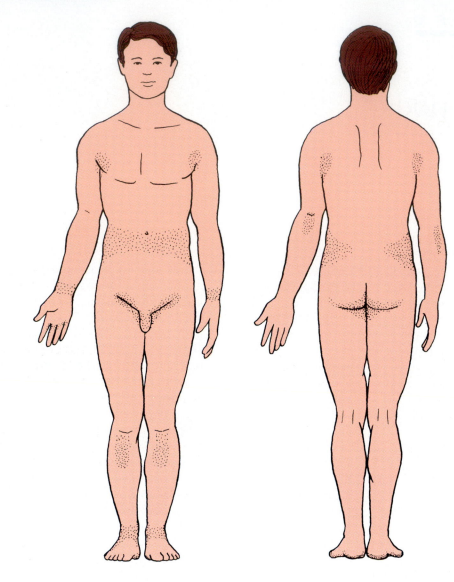

Fig. 6–1
Characteristic distribution of scabies lesions.

B. The diagnosis may be difficult because the mite, even if present, may not be demonstrated. Therefore if the lesions have the characteristic distribution, the patient complains of intensifying pruritus, and other family members or close contacts have similar symptoms, diagnosis and treatment on clinical grounds is appropriate.

III. DIFFERENTIAL DIAGNOSIS

A. Papular urticaria/insect bites: The distribution differs from scabies; it is usually confined to exposed areas, and there are no burrows.

B. Eczema: The distribution is different, close contacts are not affected, and eczema will resolve with topical corticosteroid therapy.

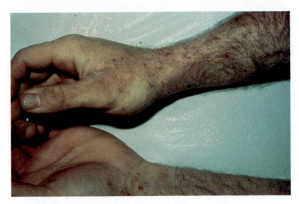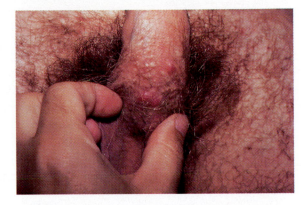

Fig. 6–2
Scabies. Note excoriations on wrists and erythematous papules on the penis. (Courtesy Department of Dermatology, University of North Carolina at Chapel Hill.)

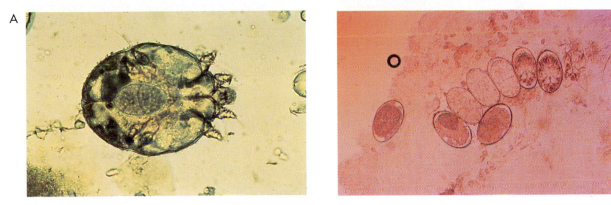

Fig. 6–3
A, Adult mite with ova. **B,** Ova with and without larva. (**A** and **B,** potassium hydroxide; original magnification × 10.) (Courtesy Marshall Guill, MD.)

IV. TREATMENT (Table 6–1)

A. **Topical medications:** Use one of the following, all of which are available by prescription only:

1. *Permethrin* 5% (Elimite): cream (60-g tube).
   a. The drug of choice for treating most cases of scabies; one 30-g application per adult is curative in 91% of patients.
   b. The cream is safe for use in children older than 2 months.
2. *Lindane* 1%: cream, lotion, shampoo (2 oz, 8 oz, 1 gal).
   a. Two applications (1 oz per application), 1 week apart, are necessary to kill any remaining larva that may have hatched since the initial treatment; such applications are curative in 87% of patients, although increasing resistance has been reported.
   b. Use with precaution when there are large areas of excoriation, in cases of immunosuppression, or in patients with a history of seizures caused by systemic absorption of potentially neurotoxic substances.

TABLE 6–1.

Treatment of Scabies

Population	Preferred Treatment	Alternatives
Adults	Permethrin 5%	Lindane 1%, crotamiton
Children > 2 months	Permethrin 5%	Lindane 1%, crotamiton
Children < 2 months	Precipitated sulfur	Permethrin 5%
Pregnancy	Precipitated sulfur	
Immunocom- promised	Multiple sequential	Ivermectin
Nursing home	Permethrin 5%	Lindane 1%, crotamiton

    c. Less expensive than permethrin 5%.
3. *Crotamiton* 10% (Eurax); cream (60-g tube); lotion (2, 16 oz).
    a. Repeat nightly for 3 to 5 nights.
    b. Safety profile in children and pregnancy not well-established.
    c. Cure rates in children less than with permethrin 5%.
4. *Precipitated sulfur* 6% in petrolatum (90 g).
    a. Leave on for full 24 hours, then bathe and reapply for next 24-hour period.
    b. Apply for a total of three applications in 3 days.
    c. Useful in pregnant or nursing women and neonates, although it is messy and has an unpleasant odor.
5. *Ivermectin* (6-mg tablets): Meinking et al[1] found the use of ivermectin, 200 μ/kg, particularly useful (recommended in combination with a topical scabicide and environmental measures) to treat scabies in HIV-positive individuals.

B. **Procedure:**
1. Apply one of the above treatments to dry skin, treating the entire skin surface from the neck down (adults very rarely have infection above the neck). *Tell patients to pay special attention to the groin, fingerwebs, toewebs, and under the fingernails* (because of scratching).
2. Using approximately 30 g per application in adult patients, leave the medication on overnight and wash off with soap and water the following morning (except for precipitated sulfur).
3. Treat any underlying secondary infection.

C. **Environmental measures:**
1. All close contacts and household members should be treated, even if asymptomatic.
2. Wash all bed linens, towels, and clothes that were worn in the 2 days before each application. Use hot water, and dry on hot cycle (or dry clean); hanging clothes to dry will not effectively kill the mites. No other environmental treatment is indicated.

D. **Special considerations:**
1. Infants may have infestation of the temple, forehead, and scalp, in addition to the rest of the body. Therefore advise topical treatment to these areas, avoiding the eyes and mucous membranes.
2. Nursing home infestations may be difficult to treat, requiring treatment of the entire nursing home staff, patients, and any frequent visitors, including family members.
3. Immunosuppressed patients may require multiple sequential treatments, and application may need to include the scalp, temples, and forehead.

E. **Adjuncts to therapy:**
1. Oral antihistamines for relief of itching: *Hydroxyzine hydrochloride:* adults, 10 to 50 mg q4 to 8h prn; children, 2 mg/kg/day divided q6h, 10 mg/5 ml.
2. Topical corticosteroids for relief of pru-

ritic papules or nodules; hypersensitivity reaction: in adults, use *triamcinolone* cream or ointment 0.1% bid to tid; in children, use *hydrocortisone* cream 1% to 2.5% bid to tid or *hydrocortisone valerate* 0.2% bid to tid. Avoid use in groin and axillae because of potential for steroid atrophy.

3. Systemic corticosteroids, tapered over 7 to 10 days, are indicated for relief of pruritus when the hypersensitivity reaction is severe or prolonged.

V. PATIENT EDUCATION
See Appendix L.
A. Emphasize that medications *must* be used correctly to eradicate the infestation and to avoid further harm.
B. Explain that *itching and a few new lesions may occur for several weeks after treatment* because of an allergic reaction, but eventually the condition will improve.
C. Review all necessary environmental measures.
D. Dispel stereotypes about the disease: e.g., reassure the patient and family members that the disease affects all ages and all socioeconomic groups.
E. Have the patient return for follow-up if the rash has not improved after 10 days.

PEDICULOSIS

Pediculosis Capitis ICD-9 (132.0)

Pediculosis, or head lice, has been a common infestation for thousands of years, and is still a significant source of disability and concern for many patients. Pediculosis capitis is an infestation by the head louse, *Pediculus humanus capitis,* and most commonly occurs in school-age children. The adult louse is approximately 2 mm in diameter (Fig. 6–4). The eggs and their casings, known as nits, are attached to the hair shaft (Fig. 6–5), and the eggs hatch in approximately 10 days. Transmission occurs via head-to-head contact or through sharing of infested combs, brushes, or hats. Pediculosis capitis is characterized by severe pruritus, usually of the sides and back of the scalp and may be complicated by secondary bacterial infection.

I. CLASSIC DESCRIPTION
Distribution: Scalp, especially sides and

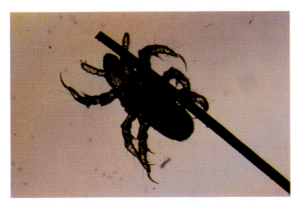

Fig. 6–4
Dry mount slide of pediculosis capitis attached to hair shaft. (Courtesy Department of Dermatology, Medical College of Georgia.)

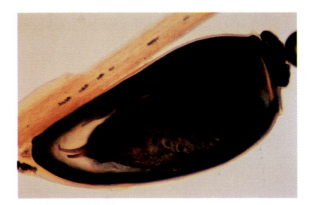

Fig. 6–5
Pediculosis capitis nit with larva attached to hair shaft. (Courtesy Department of Dermatology, Medical College of Georgia.)

posterior aspects; more rarely posterior neck

Primary: Papules

Secondary: Excoriations, erythema, crust There may be enlargement of the cervical lymph nodes if the lesions are infected secondarily.

II. DIAGNOSIS

The key to diagnosis is careful observation of the scalp. Although lice may actually be seen, it is more common to see *nits attached to the hair shaft*. Nits can be distinguished from other hair debris because the nit has an intact shell casing totally surrounding it, allowing it to slide up and down along the hair shaft when combed or examined.

III. DIFFERENTIAL DIAGNOSIS

A. Seborrheic dermatitis: Nits are absent in seborrheic dermatitis. The scales are easily scraped, but the nits are firmly attached to the hair shaft and are not easily removed.

B. Folliculitis: With scalp folliculitis, pustules and crusting are scattered throughout the scalp, and nits or lice are absent. If pediculosis becomes secondarily infected, it may appear similar to folliculitis.

IV. TREATMENT (See Table 6–2)

A. Pediculocides:

1. *Permethrin* 1% (Nix Creme Rinse, OTC): 2-oz bottle.
   a. Use to treat *head* lice only (not approved for use in pubic lice).
   b. Shampoo hair with regular shampoo, then towel dry. Apply sufficient amount of permethrin to saturate the scalp and hair. Leave on for 10 minutes, then rinse thoroughly.
   c. A second treatment is indicated only if live lice (not nits alone) are seen 7 to 10 days after the first application. Such treatments are required in fewer than 1% of patients.
   d. Use a nit comb to remove dead lice and nits.

2. *Pyrethrin* 0.33%: for use with head or pubic lice.
   a. *RID Lice Shampoo* (pyrethrin 0.3%, piperonyl butoxide 3%; 2.4, 8 oz):
      (1.) Apply enough shampoo to dry scalp or infected area to wet completely. Leave on for 10 minutes, then apply a small amount of water to lather. Rinse thoroughly and towel dry. Use a nit comb to help remove dead lice and eggs.
      (2.) Repeat the procedure in 7 to 10 days.
      (3.) Contraindicated if patient is allergic to ragweed.
   b. *A-200 Lice Control Spray and Kit:* shampoo (4 oz), nit comb, and environmental spray to kill lice and eggs on bedding and furniture.

3. *Lindane* 1% shampoo: for use with head or pubic lice.
   a. Apply to dry hair, enough to wet the entire area. Leave on for 4 minutes, then add enough water to lather. Rinse thoroughly, and towel dry. Remove nits and dead lice.
   b. Increased nit resistance to this treatment has been reported.

4. *Eyebrow/eyelash involvement:* If the eyebrow or eyelash is infected, look for *pubic,* not scalp, involvement.
   a. Vaseline to the affected area 3 times a day for 5 days is curative,

TABLE 6–2.

Treatment of Pediculosis

Location	Preferred Treatment	Alternatives
Head/scalp	Permethrin 1%	Pyrethrin 0.33%, lindane 1%
Pubic	Pyrethrin 0.33%	Lindane 1%
Eyebrows/ eyelash	Vaseline	Fluorescein dye
Resistance	Permethrin 5%	

OTC: Permethrin 1%, pyrethrin 0.33%
Rx: Lindane 1%, permethrin 5%

along with appropriate treatment of pubic lice.

   b. Fluorescein dye applied to the affected area produces an immediate toxic reaction in the lice.

B. Nit removal:

   1. *Step 2:* Over-the-counter product that contains 8% formic acid as a cream rinse.

   2. Vinegar is useful in helping to remove nits with a nit comb.

   3. Nit combs are provided in most treatment kits.

C. Environmental measures:

   1. Disinfect all personal headgear, scarfs, coats, stuffed animals, towels, and bed linens by machine washing in hot water, then drying using the hot cycle. Dry cleaning of articles also is acceptable, as is sealing items in a plastic bag for 2 to 4 weeks after spraying them with a pediculocide. Combs and brushes should be soaked in hot water for 5 to 10 minutes. Furniture and rugs should be vacuumed.

   2. Family members and schoolmates must be treated. Alert school teachers or nurses when an index case is identified.

D. Treat any secondary infection.

V. PATIENT EDUCATION

See Appendix J.

A. Encourage compliance with therapy, particularly nit removal.

B. Follow environmental measures strictly, including care of hair items and treatment of family members.

C. If the patient is a child, have the parents inform all playmates, schoolmates, and teachers of the diagnosis.

D. Reassure parents that the disease affects children of all socioeconomic levels.

Pediculosis Pubis (Phthiriasis) ICD-9 (132.2)

Pediculosis pubis, also known as *crabs,* is an infestation by *Phthirus pubis,* occurring most commonly in young, sexually active adults. The disease is characterized by severe itching in the pubic area, with eczematization and possibly secondary infection. Pediculosis pubis is highly contagious and often associated with other sexually transmitted diseases; therefore, after taking a thorough sexual history, screening for other sexually transmitted diseases may be appropriate.

I. CLASSIC DESCRIPTION

   Distribution: Pubic region, less often axillary hair or eyelashes

   Primary: Papules, macules

   Secondary: Blue-gray pigmentation, excoriations, erythema, crust

   Bite sites may show blue-gray macules *(maculae ceruleae).* Nits are less obvious than in head lice (Fig. 6–6). Eyelashes and axillary hair should be examined for involvement.

II. DIAGNOSIS

   Lice may appear as small moving freckles, and brown specks on underwear are mite feces. The adult lice may be seen, but more often nits are seen attached to hair shafts.

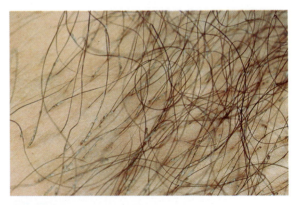

Fig. 6–6

Pediculosis pubis with nits attached to pubic hair. (Courtesy Department of Dermatology, Medical College of Georgia.)

A hand lens is helpful in identifying lice obscured by thick pubic hair.

III. TREATMENT

A. **Pediculocides:** (See Table 6–2)
1. *Pyrethrin* 0.33%:
   a. *RID Lice Shampoo* (pyrethrin 0.3%, piperonyl butoxide 3%; 2.4, 8 oz):
      (1.) Apply shampoo to infected area, using enough shampoo to wet the hair. Leave on for 10 minutes, then apply a small amount of water to lather. Rinse thoroughly, and towel dry. Use a nit comb to help remove dead lice and eggs.
      (2.) Repeat the procedure in 7 to 10 days.
      (3.) Contraindicated if patient is allergic to ragweed.
   b. *A-200 Lice Control Spray and Kit:* shampoo (4 oz), nit comb, and environmental spray to kill lice and eggs on bedding and furniture.
2. *Lindane* 1% shampoo:
   a. Apply to dry hair, enough to wet the entire area. Leave on for 4 minutes, then add enough water to lather. Rinse thoroughly, and towel dry.

Remove nits and dead lice.
      b. Increased nit resistance to this treatment has been reported.
B. **Nit removal:**
1. *Step 2:* Over-the-counter product that contains 8% formic acid as a cream rinse.
2. Vinegar is useful in helping to remove nits with a nit comb.
3. Nit combs are provided in most treatment kits.
C. **Evaluate for other sexually transmitted diseases.**
D. **Treat close contacts,** particularly sexual partners.
E. **Environmental measures:** Underclothing, linens, and towels must be laundered in hot water and put through a hot dryer cycle or dry-cleaned.

IV. PATIENT EDUCATION

A. Encourage compliance with therapy, particularly nit removal.
B. Remind patients that a second treatment is necessary.
C. Recommend to patients that they be screened for sexually transmitted diseases (HIV, RPR, etc.).
D. Encourage patients to tell their partners to be treated.

TICK BITES

Tick bites are concerning to many patients and physicians, despite the fact that the great majority of such bites cause no disease. Tick bites usually are painless, but they may become symptomatic as a result of a significant foreign body reaction. The major concern is that ticks are vectors for several infectious agents, some fatal if left untreated (Table 6–3). Tick bites occur most typically in summer. Although many patients may not remember the presence of a tick, clinicians must keep tick bites in the differential diagnosis for a variety of dermatoses.

Lyme Disease ICD-9 (088.81)

Lyme disease gets its name from the community where it was first identified, Old Lyme, Connecticut. The initial skin manifestation, known as *erythema migrans,* is seen in 60% to 80% of people with Lyme disease. The rash is characterized by an expanding erythematous macule or patch, with central clearing at the site of a tick bite (Fig. 6–7). Secondary areas of annular erythema may erupt remote from the tick bite, resulting from hematogenous spread of spirochetes. Erythema migrans usually attains a *diameter exceeding 5*

TABLE 6–3.

Tick-Borne Diseases in the United States

Disease	Etiology	Tick Vector
Lyme Disease	*Borrelia burgdorferi*	*Ixodes*
Babesiosis	*Babesia microti*	*Ixodes*
Rocky Mountain spotted fever	*Rickettsia rickettsii*	*Dermacentor*
Tularemia	*Francisella tularensis*	*Dermacentor, Amblyomma*
Tick paralysis	Neurotoxin	*Dermacentor, Amblyomma*
Ehrlichiosis	*Ehrlichia chaffeensis*	*Dermacentor, Amblyomma*
Colorado tick fever	Coltivirus	*Dermacentor*
Relapsing fever	*Borrelia* sps.	*Ornithodoros*

cm, lasts several weeks, and resolves spontaneously. Lesions smaller than 5 cm that persist for less than 7 days probably represent harmless dermal reactions to tick salivary antigens. Symptoms of flu-like illness often accompany the skin lesions for a few days to 6 weeks (typical incubation 7 to 10 days) after a tick bite infected with *Borrelia burgdorferi.*

Less than 50% of patients will recall an antecedent tick bite. Because some patients may not notice even large bulls-eye rashes, particularly those located on the back or legs, careful examination of the entire skin, including the scalp, is necessary.

I. CLASSIC DESCRIPTION
Distribution: Anywhere on the body

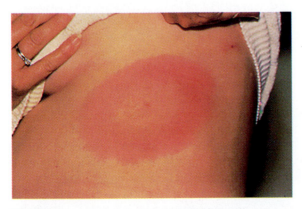

Fig. 6–7
Erythema migrans. Note expanding erythematous lesion with central clearing on trunk. (Courtesy John Cook, MD.)

Primary: Macules and plaques; rarely papules and wheals
Secondary: Erythema, central ulceration

II. DIAGNOSIS
Understanding the early manifestations of Lyme disease is the key to making a correct diagnosis, possibly avoiding more serious sequelae of the later stages of Lyme disease (Table 6–4).

A presumptive diagnosis is made for patients with a history of a recent tick bite who reside in an endemic area and exhibit erythema migrans appearing within 1 to 2 months of the tick bite. In areas with a high prevalence of Lyme disease, patients may develop flu-like illnesses during the summer months, without knowledge of a tick bite but with definite tick exposure from activities such as camping, hunting, or hiking. Over 90% of U.S. cases occur in a belt from Virginia to Massachusetts, along with an increased incidence in northeast Wisconsin, Minnesota, and California.

Serologic tests usually yield negative results if performed when erythema migrans is present, and early treatment with antibiotics may blunt the serologic response. Enzyme-linked immunosorbent assay (ELISA) may show an immunoglobulin M (IgM) antibody response in untreated patients 3 to 4 weeks after initial infection, and immunoglobulin G (IgG) may be detectable after 4 to 6 weeks of ongoing infection. Western immunoblot may be useful to clarify

TABLE 6–4.

Manifestations and Treatment of Lyme Disease

	Symptoms	Treatment	Comment
Stage 1 (3 days–4 wk after tick bite)	Constitutional flu-like symptoms, erythema migrans at bite site, persistent fatigue	Doxycycline 100 mg bid x 10–21 days, amoxicillin 500 mg tid (25–50 kg/day children) x 10–21 days, azithromycin 500 mg/day then 250 mg qd days 3–10; cefuroxime 500 mg bid (250 mg bid children) x 21 days; clarithromycin 500 mg bid x 21 days.	Treat for 14-21 days, except azithromycin. Treatment of early disease usually shortens duration of rash and flu symptoms and prevents progression to later stages; however, progression can occur despite early therapy.
Stage 2 (weeks to months)	Skin: Secondary erythema migrans lesions	Treat as in early disease	Treat for 30 days.
	Joints: Brief periarticular arthritis	Doxycycline 100 mg bid Amoxicillin 500 mg tid (50 mg/kg/day–children)	Tends to recur, particularly in the knees.
	Cardiac: Carditis, heart block: 1st-degree AVB*<0.3 msec, 1st-degree AVB*>0.3 msec, 2nd- or 3rd-degree AVB*	Treat as in early disease Hospitalize; give ceftriaxone 2 g IV qd (75–100 mg/kg/day–children) or cefotaxime 2 g q4h Penicillin G 20–24 million U/day IV (300,000 U/kg/day children	Treat for 14–21 days. Cardiology consultation and/or a temporary pacemaker may be necessary.
	Neurologic: Bell's palsy, cranial or peripheral neuropathies, meningitis, encephalitis	For facial nerve paralysis, ceftriaxone 2 g/day IV (75–100 mg/kg/day–children) penicillin G 20–24 million U/day IV (3000 U/kg/day) or cefotaxime 2 g q8h IV	Treat for 14–21 days. Many patients may experience exceedingly debilitating fatigue and recurrent headache.
Stage 3 (weeks to months to years)	Arthritis: Chronic joint pain, particularly in the knees, but also arthralgias and muscle aches	Doxycycline 100 mg bid 30 day or amoxicillin 500 mg tid (25–50 mg/kg/day–children) Ceftriaxone 2 g IV or Penicillin G 20–24 million U/day IV 14 days	Treat for 30 days orally. Treat for 14–21 days IV. Optimal treatment not well established; rheumatology consultation.
	Neurologic syndromes: Profound fatigue and atrophic skin lesions; subacute encephalopathy/axonal polyneuropathy		

*AVB = atrioventricular block

questionable ELISA results. In seropositive patients, the serum may remain positive for months to years, even after successful treatment. Current tests still have high variability, and given the poor sensitivity/specificity of the tests, false negative/positive results are not uncommon. Although isolation of the organism from an erythema migrans lesion remains the most specific test, the special media required is not widely available. For further information on both diagnostic testing and updated treatment recommendations, contact the Centers for Disease Control and Prevention.*

*Centers for Disease Control and Prevention: 404-332-4555.

III. DIFFERENTIAL DIAGNOSIS

A. **Normal tick bites:** Lesions usually do not exceed 5 cm in diameter and last less than 7 days.

B. **Cellulitis:** There is no history of endemic exposure, tenderness is localized, and there is no central clearing.

C. **Contact dermatitis:** Pruritus predominates, along with progression to vesiculation; systemic complaints are absent.

D. **Tinea corporis:** Potassium hydroxide prep from scale of the leading edge will demonstrate hyphae. Systemic complaints are absent.

E. **Spider bite:** Pain and ulceration at the site of bite are acute. Central clearing is usually not seen.

F. **Erythema multiforme:** Lesions are not necessarily 5 cm in diameter, the appearance is targetoid, and there is a predilection for mucous membranes and acral areas; look for a recent herpes outbreak.

G. **Pityriasis rosea:** Herald patch may resemble erythema migrans initially, but there is no history of endemic exposure; look for the appearance of multiple oval, scaling pink papules and plaques.

H. **Annular urticaria:** Individual lesions should last less than 24 hours, and pruritus is major symptom.

IV. TREATMENT

A. **Systemic antibiotics for Lyme disease:** (See Table 6–4). A recent decision analysis suggests that if the probability of infection with Lyme disease after a tick bite in an area is 3.6% or higher, then presumptive empirical therapy is indicated, whereas if it is 1% or less, antibiotics should be withheld, pending confirmation of the diagnosis.

B. **Environmental measures**
   1. *Removing ticks:* Lightly grasp the tick near its attachment site with a pair of tweezers, and attempt to remove it with a gentle, constant pulling motion, without twisting. Hot matchheads or fingernail polish are ineffective and potentially dangerous.
   2. *Tick nodules:*
      a. Residual tick mouth parts may cause a foreign body reaction, with a resultant nodule that may have to be excised in order for resolution to occur.
      b. An alternative to excision is to inject the nodule intralesionally with *triamcinolone* 10 to 25 mg/ml (0.5 to 1.0 ml).

C. **Skin and clothing repellent:**
   1. *DEET* 20% to 30% (available OTC as Deep Woods Off Spray, Cutter, Repel). Apply no greater than 30% concentration *to exposed skin.*
   2. *Permethrin* 0.5% (Permanone OTC). The repellent, sprayed *on clothing,* lasts 2 days per application, killing ticks on contact.
   3. Concentrated lotions and liquids containing DEET over 30% may be toxic in infants, children, and pregnant women.

V. PATIENT EDUCATION

See Appendix Q.

A. Inform patients that using hats; light-colored, long-sleeved shirts; and pants tucked in at the cuffs will provide protection when there is anticipated significant outdoor exposure in endemic areas.

B. Instruct patients about using tick repellent, performing a head-to-toe skin search within 24 hours after significant outdoor exposures in endemic areas, and promptly removing any imbedded ticks.

C. Emphasize compliance with treatment. Explain that some patients may experience a *Jarisch-Herxheimer* type of reaction, in which the rash and "flu" may worsen for the first 48 hours of therapy.

D. Explain that fatigue may remain for several weeks after successful treatment.

E. Advise the patient that a tick bite is

probably harmless if erythema migrans and/or "summer flu" fail to develop in the 4 to 6 weeks following a bite.

Rocky Mountain Spotted Fever ICD-9 (082.0)

Rocky Mountain spotted fever (RMSF) is a tick-borne Rickettsial disease. Despite its name, the disease occurs most commonly in Oklahoma and the southern Atlantic states. The most common age group affected is 5- to 9-year-old children, with most cases occurring between April and late September. Within 2 to 14 days after the tick bite, systemic manifestations appear, as the result of vascular wall involvement. Fever (99%), severe headache (90%), myalgias (80%), and emesis (60%) are frequently seen. The rash (83%) appears usually on the fourth day after tick exposure. Multiorgan infection may lead to extensive central nervous system, gastrointestinal, and pulmonary sequelae. If left untreated, the mortality rate is 70%.

I. **CLASSIC DESCRIPTION** (Figs. 6-8, 6-9)
   Distribution: Initially wrists and ankles; spreads to trunk, face, palms, and soles
   Primary: Macules initially, then papules and petechiae

Secondary: Blanchable erythema that become purpuric
The rash may be difficult to see in patients with dark pigmentation.

II. **DIAGNOSIS**
The diagnosis is based on the clinical syndrome of headache, fever, sometimes the eruption, and, possibly, exposure to ticks or travel to an endemic area. Several antibody tests (indirect hemagglutination and indirect immunofluorescent) may be confirmatory 7 to 10 days after the onset of disease; however, early treatment may blunt or delay any increase in antibody titers. A highly specific test to diagnose RMSF in the early stages involves direct immunofluorescent examination of skin biopsy tissue for *R. rickettsii* antigen. The test is available through the Centers for Disease Control and Prevention and may be available through some major medical centers. For further information on both diagnostic testing and updated treatment rec-

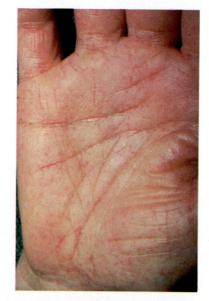

Fig. 6–9
Multiple petechiae on the hand in a patient with Rocky Mountain spotted fever. (Courtesy Department of Dermatology, University of North Carolina at Chapel Hill.)

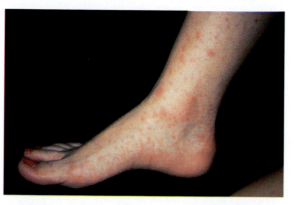

Fig. 6–8
Rocky Mountain spotted fever with nonblanching, erythematous lesions of the ankle. (Courtesy Department of Medical College of Georgia, Department of Dermatology.)

ommendations, contact the Centers for Disease Control and Prevention.*

III. DIFFERENTIAL DIAGNOSIS
  A. Neisseria meningitidis: The rash is similar, but usually appears earlier than in RMSF, there is no history of endemic exposure, and organisms may be demonstrable by Gram stain from an unroofed lesion.
  B. Ehrlichiosis: A petechial rash is not frequently found.
  C. Viral infections: With infections such as enterovirus, measles, hepatitis, or rubella, petechiae are uncommon, and there is no endemic exposure.

IV. TREATMENT
  Clinicians should empirically treat individuals presenting with the triad of fever, myalgias, and headache (with or without a suspicious rash) and with a history of travel to an endemic area during the summer months.
  A. Antibiotics:
    1. Adults: Choose either:
      a. *Doxycycline* 100 mg PO bid, or 4.4 mg/kg IV, up to 200 mg/day, in divided doses, or
      b. *Tetracycline* 500 mg PO qid, or 15 mg/kg IV loading dose, then 15 mg/kg/day divided q6h.
    2. Children younger than age 8 and in pregnancy: *Chloramphenicol,* 50 mg/kg loading dose, then 50 mg/kg/day divided in four doses.
  B. Supportive therapy: Maintain appropriate hydration, and monitor for complications, such as disseminated intravascular coagulation.

V. PATIENT EDUCATION
  See Appendix Q.
  A. Teach patients with a history of a recent tick bite from an endemic area to seek treatment immediately if they develop combinations of fever, headache, myalgias, and rash.
  B. Inform patients that using hats; light-colored, long-sleeved shirts; and pants tucked in at the cuffs will provide protection when there is anticipated significant outdoor exposure in endemic areas.
  C. Instruct patients to use tick repellent, to perform a head-to-toe skin search within 24 hours after significant outdoor exposures in endemic areas, and to promptly remove any imbedded ticks.

PAPULAR URTICARIA/INSECT BITES ICD-9 (919.4)

Insects such as mosquitoes, chiggers, fleas, or flies commonly bite humans, resulting in pruritic lesions. Some people react to these bites with marked edema and erythema. In addition, an allergic-type reaction known as *papular urticaria* may develop, in which typical lesions of acute bites are seen, along with reactivation of papules from previous bites. Such lesions may persist for many months, and old lesions may flare on reexposure. Papular urticaria is more common during warm months, especially in children playing outdoors.

*Centers for Disease Control and Prevention: 404-332-4555.

I. CLASSIC DESCRIPTION (Fig. 6–10)
  Distribution: Exposed surfaces, grouped irregularly
  Primary: Papules with central punctum; if severely reactive, vesicles or bullae
  Secondary: Erythema, excoriation, crust

II. DIAGNOSIS
  Diagnosis is based on the presence of irregularly grouped pruritic papules, occurring predominantly on exposed surfaces, along with a history of flare-up of old lesions on reexposure.

III. DIFFERENTIAL DIAGNOSIS
  Scabies: Papular urticaria typically involves

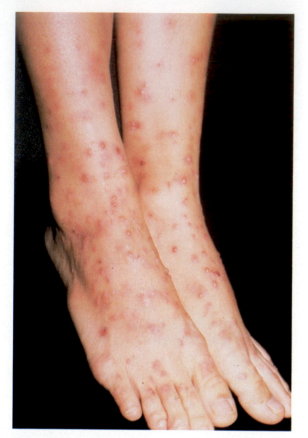

Fig. 6–10
Papular urticaria with multiple papules and excoriations on lower legs. (Courtesy Department of Dermatology, University of North Carolina at Chapel Hill.)

exposed extremities, whereas scabies usually involves not only extremities but also the axilla, waist area, and groin.

IV. TREATMENT

A. Pruritus relief

1. *Hydroxyzine hydrochloride* 10 to 50 mg q4 to 8h prn; children, 2 mg/kg/day q6h prn.

2. Prescription preparations with menthol, phenol, camphor, or pramoxine, such as Cetaphil with ½% menthol and ½% phenol, or nonprescription preparations, such as Sarna or Prax, may be used prn for pruritus.

B. Topical Steroids

1. Children: Apply topical corticosteroids such as *hydrocortisone valerate* or *desoximetasone* to affected areas 3 times a day, avoiding the face, axillae, and groin.

2. Adults: Use *triamcinolone* cream or ointment 0.1% tid prn; resistant lesions may require *betamethasone dipropionate* 0.05% bid, but for only 2 weeks at a time.

C. Oral Steroids: Extensive or resistant cases may require short courses of oral *prednisone,* tapered over 14 to 21 days (0.5 to 1.0 mg/kg/day).

D. Reexposure prevention: (See discussion under Patient Education.)

V. PATIENT EDUCATION

A. Teach patients that prevention of reexposure is essential for successful treatment.

B. Trace the source of bites (e.g., examine all pets, especially dogs and cats, for fleas).

C. Use insect repellents (particularly for flying insects), such as long-acting *DEET* cream or lotion (e.g., Ultrathon) or Skeedaddle, OFF Skintastic, Hour Guard by Amway.

SPIDER BITES ICD-9 (989.5)

Among the several thousand species of spiders, 50 bite humans, and only two, the black widow spider and the brown recluse spider, cause the majority of spider-related problems.

The black widow spider (*Latrodectus mactans)* has a black, gray, or brown abdomen, with ventral red hourglass abdominal markings (Fig. 6–11). It is found throughout the United States, and mature females are up to 4 cm long. The actual bite may be painless, with no initial symptoms other than urticaria or erythema and two red puncta at the bite site. However, minutes to

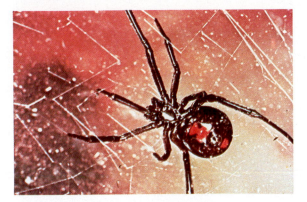

Fig. 6–11
Black widow spider with characteristic ventral red hourglass abdominal marking. (Courtesy Entomological Society of America/Ries Memorial Slide Collection.)

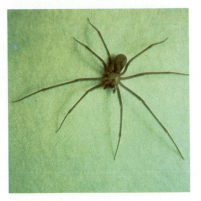

Fig. 6–12
Brown recluse spider with yellow-brown body and violin-shaped dark brown mark on abdomen. (Courtesy Entomological Society of America/Ries Memorial Slide Collection.)

hours later, severe muscle cramping usually ensues, as a result of neurotoxin. Symptoms may include severe abdominal pain, fever, paralysis, and, rarely, death, particularly in very young or very old people. Severe symptoms usually resolve over 2 to 3 days, but some neurologic symptoms may linger (rarely) for weeks to months.

The brown recluse spider *(Loxosceles reclusa)* is found most commonly in the central and south central United States. Named because it prefers dark, secluded places, it is small (1 to 2 cm) and has a yellow-brown body with a violin-shaped dark brown marking on its abdomen (Fig. 6–12). Initial symptoms from a bite may be minimal or absent, but within hours patients may have severe local pain, peaking 2 to 8 hours after the bite. Initial symptoms, when present, include swelling and erythema. Purpura with subsequent extensive necrosis may ensue, because of a necrolytic toxin (Fig. 6–13). A hemolytic toxin also is present, which may cause hemolytic anemia and systemic symptoms, such as fever, nausea, and vomiting.

I. CLASSIC DESCRIPTION
Distribution: Most common on extremities, but can occur anywhere; black widow spider bites often are found on buttocks or genitalia, secondary to outdoor toilet use

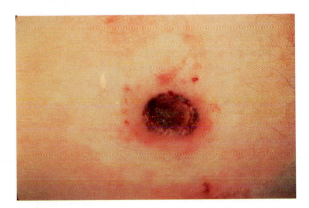

Fig. 6–13
Brown recluse spider bite. Note necrotic ulcer and erythema. (Courtesy Marshall Guill, MD.)

Primary: Expanding wheal with two central puncta (black widow)
Secondary: Edema, erythema, blister, ulceration; generalized macular erythema may occur

II. DIAGNOSIS
The diagnosis usually is not difficult in a patient with a recent spider bite and the characteristic symptoms. Occasionally the patient may not see or feel the spider and its bite. In such cases, presenting symptoms may be confused with other acute respiratory, cardiac, and abdominal symptoms. Save the spider if it can be located.

III. TREATMENT

A. Black widow spider bite:

1. Close clinical observation with ice packs to the affected area.
2. Muscle relaxants: *Calcium gluconate:* 10 to 20 ml 10% solution given IV may relieve muscle cramping, although *methocarbamol* (Robaxin) or *diazepam* (Valium) may also be effective.
3. Antivenom antiserum: from horse serum, 1 vial 2.5 ml IM, neutralizes effects of the venom, but is indicated only in severe cases (i.e., younger than age 16 or older than age 60, pregnancy, marked hypertension, respiratory distress, or severe symptoms not responding to other measures) because of side effects (e.g., serum sickness).
4. Pain control is necessary if the above steps are ineffective. Use morphine cautiously because of associated corespiratory depression.

5. Give tetanus toxoid.

B. Brown recluse spider bite:
Treatment remains controversial because there is *no proven benefit* to current treatments. Local excision or intralesional corticosteroids are no longer recommended.

1. Ice pack on affected area; avoid heat.
2. Treatment and prevention of secondary infection with oral antibiotics (e.g., erythromycin).
3. Pain control.
4. Tetanus toxoid.
5. Consider *dapsone* 50 mg bid for 10 days, avoiding in G6PD-deficient individuals.
6. Because systemic reactions may occur in minor-appearing wounds and not be apparent for 2 to 3 days, observe cases closely for signs of renal failure or coagulation disorders, such as disseminated intravascular coagulopathy or hemolysis. Prednisone 1 mg/kg/day may be indicated for such severe cases.

SUGGESTED READING

Brown S, Becher J, Brady W: Treatment of ectoparasitic infections: review of the English language literature, 1982–1992, *Clin Infect Dis* 20S:S104–109, 1995.

Franz TJ et al: Comparative percutaneous absorption of lindane and permethrin, *Arch Dermatol* 132:901–905, 1996.

Inger A et al: Morbidity of brown recluse spider bites. Clinical picture, treatment, and prognosis, *Acta Derm Venereol* 71:337–340, 1991.

Miller TA: Lactrodectism: bite of the black widow spider, *Am Fam Physician* 45:181–187, 1992.

Rahn DW, Malawista SE: Lyme disease: recommendations for diagnosis and treatment, *Ann Int Med* 114:472–481, 1991.

Reisman RE: Insect stings, *N Engl J Med* 331:523–527, 1994.

Schultz MW et al: Comparative study of 5% permethrin cream and 1% lindane lotion for the treatment of scabies, *Arch Dermatol* 126:167–170, 1990.

Spach DH et al: Tick-borne diseases in the United States, *N Engl J Med* 329:936–947, 1993.

Taplin D et al: Comparison of crotamiton 10% cream (Eurax) and permethrin 5% cream (Elimite) for the treatment of scabies in children, *Pediatr Dermatol* 7:67–73, 1990.

Treatment of Lyme disease, *Med Let Drugs Ther* 34:95–97, 1992.

Vander stichele RH, Dezeure EM, Bogaert MG: Systemic review of clinical efficacy of topical treatments for head lice, *Brit Med J* 311:604–608, 1995.

Wong RC, Hughes SE, Voorhees JJ: Spider bites, *Arch Dermatol* 123:98–104, 1987.

REFERENCES

1. Meinking et al: The treatment of scabies with ivermectin, *N Engl J Med* 33:26–30, 1995.

CHAPTER 7

Bacterial Diseases

IMPETIGO ICD-9 (684)

Impetigo is a contagious, acute, purulent infection most commonly seen in preschool-age children and teenagers. Named after the French and Latin words meaning *a scabby eruption that attacks,* this superficial skin infection is primarily caused by *Staphylococcus aureus* (Figs. 7–1 and 7–2). Mixed infection, with *S. aureus* and group A β-hemolytic *Streptococcus,* also occurs, but pure streptococcal infections are rare. Predisposing factors include warm, moist climates and underlying excoriated skin conditions (e.g., bug bites, excoriated eczema, scabies, varicella). Poststreptococcal glomerulonephritis (but not rheumatic heart disease) occurs rarely (usually in infants) after impetigo with certain streptococcal strains, and treatment does not necessarily prevent the complication.

I. CLASSIC DESCRIPTION

Distribution: Face, arms, and legs typically, but may be anywhere
Primary: Vesicles, pustules
Secondary: Yellow/honey-colored crust, erythema, erosions
Lesions typically are vesicular before crusting. Adenopathy may be present.

II. DIAGNOSIS

The diagnosis is usually clinically made in the setting of a young infant or child with

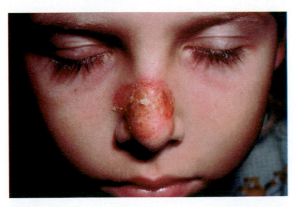

Fig. 7–1
Impetigo with honey-colored crusts. (Courtesy Department of Dermatology, University of North Carolina at Chapel Hill.)

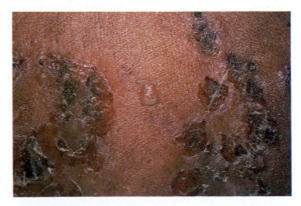

Fig. 7–2
Bullous impetigo with flaccid bulla, superficial erosions, and crusting. (Courtesy Department of Dermatology, University of North Carolina at Chapel Hill.)

honey-colored crusted lesions. If doubtful, a Gram's stain of the vesicles or pustules will demonstrate gram-positive cocci in clusters (staphylococcal infections) or in chains (streptococcal infections).

III. DIFFERENTIAL DIAGNOSIS.

A. Tinea: With impetigo, the KOH test is negative, there is no central clearing, and there is no response to antifungal agents.

B. Varicella: Varicella produces discrete, small vesicles on an erythematous base, and the lesions are in various stages. However, varicella may become secondarily infected through "impetiginization."

C. Herpes simplex virus (HSV): HSV is characterized by isolated distribution, prodromal illness, and a positive Tzanck test for multinucleated giant cells. As in varicella, HSV may become secondarily infected through "impetiginization".

D. Pemphigus vulgaris and **bullous pemphigoid** occur in older populations, are recurrent, and do not respond rapidly to antibiotics.

E. Ecthyma: (Fig.7–3) An ulcerative bacterial infection caused by group A β-hemolytic streptococci, the infection commonly occurs on the legs of children and young adults. The infection is often a consequence of excoriated lesions from pruritic conditions, such as insect bites,

A 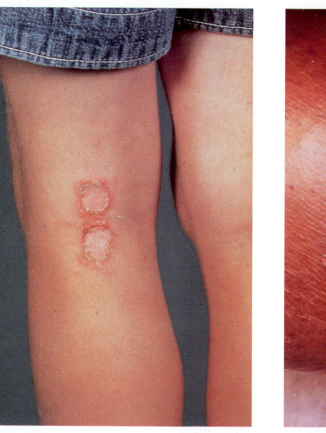 B

Fig. 7–3
Ecthyma. (Courtesy Department of Dermatology, University of North Carolina at Chapel Hill.)

and from lesions of neglect, such as minor trauma. Treat ecthyma with oxacillin or erythromycin for 2 to 3 weeks.

F. **Allergic contact dermatitis:** Pruritus is usually marked, and lesions are usually sharply demarcated. Impetigo may occur secondarily because of excoriation.

IV. **TREATMENT**

A. **Oral antibiotics:** Preferred therapy for multiple lesions.
1. *Cephalexin* 30 to 40 mg/kg/day divided in two doses in children, 1 to 2 g/day divided in two or three doses in adults.
2. *Oxacillin* 50 to 100 mg/kg/day divided in four doses in children less than 20 kg, 1 to 2 g/day divided in four doses in children more than 20 kg.
3. *Erythromycin* 30 to 50 mg/kg/day divided in four doses in children, 250 mg qid in adults. Resistance to erythromycin has been reported.

B. **Topical ointments:** Preferred therapy for limited disease and in patients unable to tolerate oral antibiotics.
1. *Mupirocin:* (Bactroban) ointment 15 and 30 g, by prescription.
   a. Apply to affected areas 3 times a day for 7 to 10 days or until all lesions have cleared.
   b. This is the only topical ointment approved for treating impetigo.
2. OTC (over-the-counter) antibacterial ointments may be used in conjunction with oral antibiotics, but will not work alone.

C. **Supportive measures:**
1. Remove crusts with warm compresses before applying topical antibiotic therapy.
2. Use a mild antibacterial soap (e.g., Lever 2000) for body cleansing.
3. Treat close contacts if they have symptoms or signs of infection.

D. **Cultures:** Cultures are indicated if the infection is resistant to therapy or if it is recurrent. For recurrent infection, consider culture, with typing of infected individual and household members for nasal carriage of *Staphylococcus.*

E. **Follow-up:** Follow-up is indicated for resistant or recurrent cases and for any cases with signs of kidney disease (e.g., hematuria or other urinary tract involvement).

V. **PATIENT EDUCATION**

See Appendix I.

A. Emphasize compliance with medications by writing down instructions and having the patient or parent repeat them.

B. Instruct patients about antibacterial soaps and to clean off crusted lesions with warm water before applying topical therapies.

C. Educate patients that lesions are likely to be contagious for up to 24 hours after initial treatment. Therefore strict hygiene measures (e.g., thorough hand-washing and avoiding direct lesion contact with those unaffected) need to be followed, and affected children should remain out of school for 1 or 2 days, until lesions show signs of healing.

D. Inform patients that postinflammatory pigmentary skin changes may persist for several months after the initial infection has cleared.

ERYSIPELAS ICD-9 (035)

Erysipelas literally means "red skin," and is an acute, well-demarcated infection of the superficial layers of the skin and associated cutaneous lymphatics (Fig. 7–4). The disease is most often caused by group A β-hemolytic *Streptococcus,* but sometimes is caused by group B, C, or G

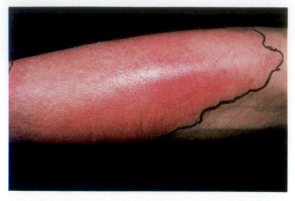

Fig. 7–4
Erysipelas. Note well-demarcated erythematous plaque on arm. (Courtesy Department of Dermatology, University of North Carolina at Chapel Hill.)

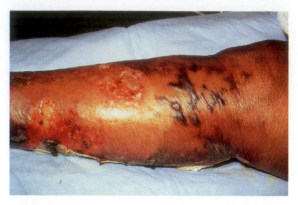

Fig. 7–5
Necrotizing cellulitis. (Courtesy Department of Dermatology, University of North Carolina at Chapel Hill.)

Streptococcus or by *S. Aureus*. It most commonly occurs in infants, young children, and older adults. Erysipelas typically arises from small inapparent breaks in the skin, such as sites of chronic edema, tinea pedis, or skin permanently scarred from burns or previous surgery. Predisposing conditions include IV drug use, nephrotic syndrome, alcoholism, dysgammaglobulinemia, diabetes mellitus, stasis dermatitis, lymphedema, and possibly a recent upper respiratory infection with group A strep.

Cellulitis implies a deeper infection, at least into the subcutaneous tissues, with poorer skin demarcation. Systemic signs and symptoms range greatly, from mild to severe, and include chills, headache, fever, tachycardia, confusion, and hypotension. Some group A strep infections produce toxins, causing generalized rashes, such as that found in *scarlet fever*. Fever, hypotension, and shock may be seen in *streptococcal toxic shock-like syndrome*. *Perianal streptococcal cellulitis* can also occur, especially in young boys, with pruritus, maceration, exudate, and tenderness, and it may be confused with candidiasis.

Necrotizing cellulitis (Fig. 7–5) is rapidly invasive and usually heralded by pain out of proportion to physical findings. The disease can cause severe local destruction, septicemia, and possibly death. Diagnosis is critical and time-

dependent, because surgery and IV antibiotics are essential. Imaging techniques, such as MRI or CT scan, may be helpful in determining extent of disease.

I. CLASSIC DESCRIPTION
Distribution: Sites of chronic edema, old scars, extremities, face
Primary: Plaque
Secondary: Marginated erythema, edema Vesicles, bullae, and cutaneous hemorrhage may occur in the presence of severe edema.

II. DIAGNOSIS
The diagnosis is usually made from the clinical findings of sharply marginated erythema, edema, and/or streaking, sometimes associated with systemic complaints of fever, chills, malaise, and localized pain. Needle aspiration cultures of the leading edge and skin biopsies for culture are often negative. Infants with perianal cellulitis usually are not systemically ill, and cultures of exudative lesions may confirm the diagnosis.

III. DIFFERENTIAL DIAGNOSIS
A. Facial cellulitis: Found most often in children age 6 months to 3 years and caused by *Haemophilus* influenza type B; initial differentiation may be difficult. Look for signs of otitis media, and watch

carefully for any signs of meningitis. Cefuroxime is the treatment of choice.

B. Periorbital cellulitis: Usually caused by *H. influenzae* in children, and by *Staphylococcus* or *Streptococcus* in adults; it is critical to differentiate between periorbital and orbital cellulitis.

C. Pseudomonal, mycobacterium, and other atypical cellulitis: Usually found in patients with burns, in those hospitalized, or in those immunocompromised from other medical conditions.

D. Erysipeloid: Found most often on hands of patients who have a history of working with meat, bones, or fish. The rash usually is dull, with erythematous plaques, has less margination, follows a less aggressive course, and responds readily to penicillin or erythromycin.

E. Herpes zoster: Pain usually precedes the onset of herpes zoster, and Tzanck smears of vesicles demonstrate multinucleated giant cells; cultures or direct viral antigen smears are positive.

F. Contact dermatitis: Pruritus is more common than pain, and few systemic complaints are reported.

G. Necrotizing cellulitis: Consider in any case of cellulitis in which the pain is out of proportion to the physical findings.

IV. TREATMENT

A. Oral antibiotics: For uncomplicated cases, choose one of the following and treat for 10 to 14 days.

1. *Oxacillin* 50 to 100 mg/kg/day divided in four doses in children less than 20 kg, 1 to 2 g/day divided in four doses in children more than 20 kg, 500 mg qid in adults.
2. *Cephalexin* 25 to 100 mg/kg/day q6h in children, 500 mg tid to qid in adults.
3. *Erythromycin* if penicillin-allergic, 30 to 50 mg/kg/day divided in four doses in children, 250 mg qid in adults.
4. *Azithromycin* 500 mg on day 1, then 250 mg days 2 to 5.

B. IV Antibiotics: Indicated for toxic, debilitated, and elderly patients, or in children with facial involvement.

C. Supportive measures: Use warm compresses to the affected area for 20 minutes 3 to 4 times a day, along with adequate pain control.

D. Recurrent episodes: Consider long-term suppressive therapy with oral antibiotics.

V. PATIENT EDUCATION

A. Instruct patients to remain at bed rest if they are febrile or if the infection involves the lower extremity.

B. Remind patients to elevate an affected leg or arm above the level of the heart to assist in drainage.

C. Educate patients that other family members should follow strict hygiene measures (e.g., handwashing) to help avoid transferring causative agents to a susceptible host.

FOLLICULITIS ICD-9 (704.8)

Folliculitis describes an array of pustular infections that involve the hair follicle. Folliculitis may be limited to the superficial area of the hair follicle or may progress to involve the deep follicle (Fig. 7–6). The most common organism identified in either type of folliculitis is *S. aureus*. Two types of lesions typically are described with deep folliculitis: *furuncle,* which is a deep inflammatory nodule, and *carbuncle,* which is an aggregation of furuncles. *Folliculitis may occur as a secondary infection in excoriated lesions from scabies, insect bites, and eczema.* Systemic factors predisposing to folliculitis include diabetes mellitus, obesity, malnutrition, immunodeficiency states, and chronic staphylococcal carriage. Complications from folliculitis may include lymphangitis, septicemia, and cavernous sinus thrombosis when there is facial involvement.

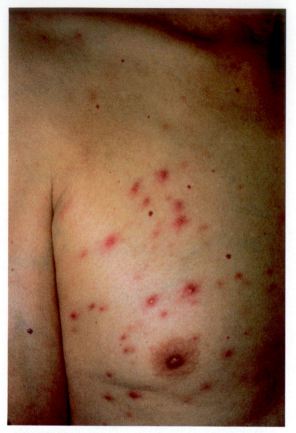

Fig. 7–6
Folliculitis of trunk with erythematous papules and pustules. (Courtesy Beverly Sanders, MD.)

I. CLASSIC DESCRIPTION
SUPERFICIAL FOLLICULITIS:
Distribution: Scalp and extremities, most commonly, but may occur on any hair-bearing area
Primary: Pustule pierced by a hair
Secondary: Erythema, crust
DEEP FOLLICULITIS:
Distribution: Any hair-bearing area; most common in sites of friction (e.g., buttocks, groin)
Primary: Nodule
Secondary: Erythema, edema, exudate, draining sinuses

II. DIAGNOSIS
The diagnosis of superficial folliculitis is based on finding a pustule pierced by a hair. Carbuncles and furuncles are diagnosed by the presence of an erythematous nodule, with fluctuance in advanced lesions. If folliculitis is resistant, recurrent, found in an immunocompromised patient, or associated with systemic involvement, consider culturing a pustule or exudate for causative organisms and antibiotic sensitivities.

III. DIFFERENTIAL DIAGNOSIS
A. **Tinea barbae:** These highly inflamed, KOH-positive fungal lesions are located in the beard area, with combinations of pustules, nodules, and exudates, rather than discrete pustules.
B. **Pseudofolliculitis barbae:** Lesions are found most commonly in the beard area of black men, where curved hair pierces normal skin.
C. **Keratosis pilaris:** This chronic nonbacterial follicular inflammation is distributed symmetrically on the postero-lateral upper arms, anterior thighs, and buttocks, often in atopic individuals. Patients may have a history of wearing tight-fitting clothing.
D. **Hidradenitis suppurativa:** The disease is limited to apocrine gland distribution (e.g., axillae, groin), is recurrent, and has a tendency to scar.
E. **Ruptured epidermal inclusion cyst:** Such patients often have a history of a long-standing cyst with recent enlargement and tenderness, but there are no piercing hairs.
F. **Pseudomonal folliculitis:** Associated with contaminated hot tubs, this infection is self-limited.
G. **Pityrosporum folliculitis:** Found more frequently during the summertime, consider the diagnosis when the folliculitis is resistant to antibiotics, and the KOH prep identifies multiple budding yeasts.

IV. TREATMENT

A. Warm compresses: Such compresses, 20 to 30 minutes 3 or 4 times a day, are frequently sufficient in mild superficial cases.

B. Oral antibiotics: For adult cases of deep folliculitis, choose either: *cephalexin* 500 mg PO tid to qid; *cloxacillin* 250 to 500 mg q6h; *erythromycin,* if penicillin-allergic, 250 mg qid, for 7 days; or *azithromycin* 250 mg PO two pills on day 1, followed by 250 mg qd days 2 to 5.

C. Incision and drainage: Consider draining lesions that are pointed and have a head, after anesthetizing with 1% *lidocaine.* If a significant cavity is present (representing dead space), pack the cavity with iodoform gauze to allow drainage for 24 to 48 hours.

D. Recurrent lesions:

1. Consider culturing specimens from the nose, groin, and beneath the nails for *S. aureus.*
2. Consider obtaining culture specimens from family members.
3. Check for underlying diabetes mellitus.
4. For chronic lesions, use an antibacterial soap (e.g., pHisoDerm or Lever 2000).

V. PATIENT EDUCATION

A. Emphasize the importance of local care measures, such as warm compresses.

B. Educate patients that deep-seated lesions may have continued drainage for several days.

C. Educate patients about the signs and symptoms of systemic involvement (e.g., high fever, red streaking).

SUGGESTED READING

A compendium of cellulitis pathogens, *Fitzpatrick's J of Clin Dermatol* 2:16–23, 1994.

Bisno AL, Stevens DL: Streptococcal infections of skin and soft tissues, *N Engl J Med* 334:240–245, 1996.

Breneman, DL: Use of mupirocin ointment in the treatment of secondarily infected dermatitis, *J Am Acad Dermatol* 22:886–892, 1990.

Feingold DS: Staphlococcal and streptococcal pyodermas, *Semin Dermatol* 12:331–335, 1993.

McLinn S: A bacteriologically controlled, randomized study comparing the efficacy of 2% mupirocin ointment (Bactroban) with oral erythromycin in the treatment of patients with impetigo, *J Am Acad Dermatol* 22:883–885, 1990.

Rice TD, Duggan AL, DeAngelis C: Cost-effectiveness of erythromycin versus mupirocin for the treatment of impetigo in children, *Pediatrics* 89:210–214, 1992.

The choice of antibacterial drugs. *The Medical Letter* 36:53–60, 1994.

CHAPTER 8

Bullous Diseases

PEMPHIGUS VULGARIS ICD-9 (694.4)

Pemphigus vulgaris is a chronic, potentially fatal, vesiculobullous disease of the mucous membranes and skin. The term *pemphigus* (from the Greek *pemphix,* bubble) was used to describe most bullous diseases until the twentieth century; *vulgaris* refers to the vulgar, or common, form of the disease. The incidence of pemphigus vulgaris is approximately 1 in 100,000, and it usually occurs in middle-age and older people. Before the introduction of systemic corticosteroids, this disease was associated with a high mortality rate. The current mortality rate is 5%, usually as a result of steroid-induced complications and sepsis. A more superficial form of pemphigus may be related to use of D-penicillamine and, rarely, captopril.

Classically, pemphigus is characterized by autoantibodies, usually immunoglobulin G, that bind to desmoglein-3, an adhesion molecule, thereby interfering with the intercellular cement that holds epidermal cells together.

This results in *intraepidermal blister formation,* caused by loss of cohesion. Secondary problems include bacterial infection of open denuded areas and the side effects of prolonged use of immunosuppressive agents required to control the disease. The oral mucosa is almost always involved, frequently as the initial site (Fig. 8–1). Severe oral involvement may impair oral intake. Long-term follow up is the rule, and some patients require years of or lifelong suppressive therapy.

Although the cause of pemphigus vulgaris is unknown, certain autoimmune-type diseases, including myasthenia gravis, thymoma, and possibly lymphoreticular malignancies, occur more frequently in patients with pemphigus. Paraneoplastic pemphigus is a rare, distinct entity, with its own clinical and histopathologic presentation.

I. CLASSIC DESCRIPTION
Distribution: Localized (e.g., mouth) or generalized, with predilection for scalp, face, chest, axillae, groin
Primary: Bullae

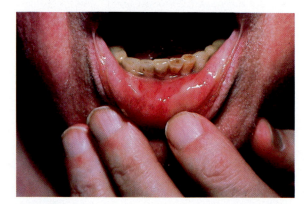

Fig. 8–1
Pemphigus vulgaris with oral erosions and no intact bullae. (Courtesy Department of Dermatology, University of North Carolina at Chapel Hill.)

TABLE 8–1.

Differentiation of Pemphigus Vulgaris and Bullous Pemphigoid

Characteristics	Pemphigus Vulgaris	Bullous Pemphigoid
Age	$\geq$ 50 years	$\geq$ 60 years
Site	Oral mucosa, face, chest, groin	Flexural areas, groin, axilla, less often oral
Findings	Flaccid bullae, intraepidermal blisters, IgG autoantibodies	Intact bullae, subepidermal blisters, IgG and complement autoantibodies
Treatment	Prednisone 40–60 mg/day, immunosuppressant agents; often chronically steroid-dependent	Prednisone 1 mg/kg/day or higher initially; taper over months to years
Prognosis	> 90% respond; steroid side effects significant	> 90% respond; remissions and recurrences common

Secondary: Erosions, erythema

Flaccid bullae occurring on normal skin rupture easily, so that *the patient often presents with only erosions and no intact bullae.* Such presentation is usually the case with mucous membrane involvement.

II. DIAGNOSIS

The diagnosis is confirmed by (1) performing a deep shave or 4-mm punch biopsy specimen for routine light microscopy from an early, small bulla or from the edge of a new erosion and (2) taking a biopsy of a section of normal skin a few millimeters from an involved area and performing direct immunofluorescence, looking for deposits of IgG between epidermal cells.

Performing serum analysis for the presence of circulating autoantibodies, directed to the intercellular cement substance, correlates loosely with clinical activity and may be useful to gauge disease activity in some patients.

III. DIFFERENTIAL DIAGNOSIS (Table 8–1)

A. If mouth erosions predominate: Consider herpes simplex virus, aphthae, lichen planus, or erythema multiforme.

B. If widespread erosions predominate: Consider pyoderma, impetigo, or other bullous diseases (e.g., bullous pemphigoid, bullous drug eruptions).

IV. TREATMENT

A. Systemic steroids: *Prednisone* 1 mg/kg/day may be required to initially control the disease.

B. Immunosuppressant agents: *Azathioprine, methotrexate,* and *cyclophosphamide* are often used as steroid-sparing agents.

C. Referral: Patients should be referred to a dermatologist for initial consultation, management, and control of the disease. Long-term use of and complications from medications often are the rule.

BULLOUS PEMPHIGOID

Bullous pemphigoid is a chronic, blistering autoimmune disease of unknown cause that most commonly affects people 60 years or older and occurs twice as often as pemphigus vulgaris. Pemphigoid refers to a pemphigus-like blistering disease, but pemphigoid is less aggressive than pemphigus vulgaris and usually not life-threatening. However, bullous pemphigoid also requires long-term use of immunosuppressant agents.

The disease is characterized by deposits of polyclonal autoantibodies, usually IgG and complement, in a linear pattern at the junction of the dermis and epidermis (i.e., the basement membrane zone). These deposits are thought to cause the release of various proteolytic enzymes via the complement cascade, which then cause blister formation. Therefore *blisters occur subepidermally,* deeper than those seen with pemphigus vulgaris. *A common presentation is a widespread blistering eruption in a middle-age or elderly patient who is taking multiple medications.* Proper diagnosis is especially important to determine if the bullae are the result of bullous pemphigoid or are drug-induced, so that the etiologic agent may be identified and removed. The mortality rate is low, but death may occur in some elderly or debilitated patients. Recurrent disease is common.

I. CLASSIC DESCRIPTION (Fig. 8–2)

Distribution: Flexural areas, especially the groin, axillae; oral involvement occurs in approximately one third of cases but is rarely the presenting feature

Primary: Bullae, urticarial plaques

Secondary: Erosions, erythema

II. DIAGNOSIS

Perform a deep shave or 4-mm punch biopsy specimen for routine light microscopy from an intact bulla to reveal a subepidermal blister. The diagnosis is confirmed by direct immunofluorescence of an additional biopsy specimen of normal skin taken a few millimeters from an involved area. Deposits of IgG, complement, and other immunoglobulins are seen in a linear pattern along the basement membrane zone, where the blister occurs. Seventy percent of patients will have demonstrable circulating autoantibodies directed to the basement membrane zone, although titers do not correlate with clinical activity.

III. DIFFERENTIAL DIAGNOSIS

A. Pemphigus vulgaris: In pemphigus vulgaris, mucous membrane involvement is more common and intact bullae are rare.

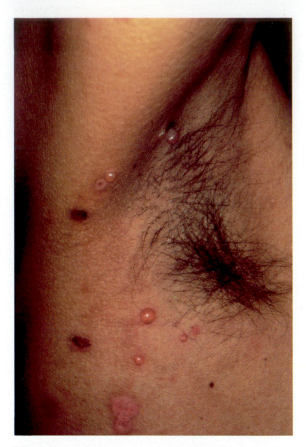

Fig. 8–2
Bullous pemphigoid. Note intact bullae with erosions in a flexural distribution. (Courtesy Marshall Guill, MD.)

Skin biopsy for routine and direct immunofluorescence is needed to differentiate from bullous pemphigoid (see Table 8–1).

B. Bullous drug eruptions: The onset of bullous drug eruptions may correlate with the addition of new medications or with use of long-standing ones (e.g., furosemide, sulfonamides). Routine and direct immunofluorescence studies of skin biopsy specimens usually differentiate these disorders.

C. Bullous lupus erythematosus: This disease is very rare, and other signs and symptoms of lupus erythematosus (e.g., positive antinuclear antibody, anemia) usually are present.

D. **Dermatitis herpetiformis:** Vesicles are grouped in dermatitis herpetiformis. Usually only excoriated lesions are present, with extensor rather than flexural distribution.

E. **Bullous erythema multiforme:** In bullous erythema multiforme, lesions are targetoid, linear IgG immunofluorescence is negative, and usually there is a history of an antecedent infection or drug ingestion.

F. **Linear IgA disease, cicatricial pemphigoid, and epidermolysis bullosa acquisita** are infrequent causes of bullous disease.

IV. TREATMENT

A. **Acute phase:**
1. *Prednisone* 1 mg/kg/day or higher may be necessary to control development of new lesions.
2. With extensive involvement, management is similar to that in a burn patient, with management of fluid loss and good topical care as primary concerns. Hospitalization is required only if there are significant concerns about denuding of skin, fluid balance, temperature control, or septicemia.
3. Localized involvement may be treated with high-potency topical steroids (e.g., *clobetasol propionate* cream 0.05% bid).

B. **Maintenance:**
1. The treatment goal is to achieve the lowest maintenance dosage of prednisone that will prevent new lesions and allow alternate-day therapy.
2. *Azathioprine* or *methotrexate* may be used as a steroid-sparing agent.
3. Complications often occur from prolonged use of immunosuppressants.

C. **Follow-up:** Pemphigoid often is self-limiting, and treatment usually can be tapered gradually within 1 to 2 years. Tapering of prednisone can occur much faster in drug-induced bullous eruptions, whereas rapid tapering of prednisone in pemphigus vulgaris or non–drug-induced bullous pemphigoid may cause a severe outbreak in a patient with otherwise well-controlled disease.

D. **Pruritus:** For control of pruritus, use *hydroxyzine* 10 to 50 mg q4 to 6h.

E. **Referral:** Patients should be referred for dermatologic consultation in diagnosis, treatment, and long-term management.

PORPHYRIA CUTANEA TARDA ICD-9 (277.1)

The porphyrias are a group of photosensitive disorders characterized by recurrent skin fragility and blisters (Fig. 8–3). Abnormalities in heme biosynthesis result in accumulation of abnormal metabolites of porphyrins. *Porphyria cutanea tarda (PCT)* is the most common porphyria and is the result of a deficiency of uroporphyrin decarboxylase. PCT is either familial or sporadic and is precipitated by exposure to chemicals toxic to the liver (e.g., alcohol, hexachlorobenzene), infections (hepatitis), or by drugs metabolized in the liver (e.g., estrogens). Diabetes mellitus can be found in as many as 25% of patients with PCT. Other associated findings include

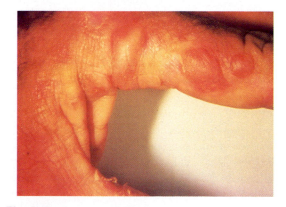

Fig. 8–3
Porphyria cutanea tarda presenting with intact bullae and erosions on the hand. (Courtesy Beverly Sanders, MD.)

increased liver iron stores, elevated serum iron levels, and, very rarely, hepatoma.

I. CLASSIC DESCRIPTION

Distribution: Sun-exposed areas, especially the dorsa of the hands

Primary: Bullae, vesicles

Secondary: Erosions, crusts, scars, milia, facial hypertrichosis, mottled hyperpigmentation

Typically, the patient is a 30- to 40-year-old man who complains of fragile, photosensitive skin that is easily traumatized.

II. DIAGNOSIS

Urine from patients with PCT may appear red-orange or brown. Spot urinalysis will demonstrate elevated porphyrin levels, but a 24-hour urine collection is needed to fully characterize the disease, looking for elevated uroporphyrins and coproporphyrins in a ratio of approximately 3:1.

III. DIFFERENTIAL DIAGNOSIS

A. **Variegate porphyria:** Skin findings of PCT are seen, along with the abdominal pain and neurologic findings of acute intermittent porphyria.

B. **Pseudoporphyria cutanea tarda:** Caused by sulfonamides, furosemide, tetracyclines, maintenance hemodialysis, nalidixic acid, and tanning bed use; urine porphyrin levels will not be elevated.

C. **Hepatoerythropoietic porphyria:** Patients present in childhood with photo-

sensitivity and increased levels of zinc protoporphyrin in red blood cells.

D. **Epidermolysis bullosa acquisita:** The disease is often similar to PCT in that both affect the hands and heal with scarring and milia. With epidermolysis bullosa, there is no history of photosensitivity, the distribution involves areas of trauma, often there is mucosal involvement, and urinalysis is negative for porphyrins.

E. **Bullous lupus erythematosus:** Although there is photosensitivity and blistering, the urinalysis is negative for porphyrins.

IV. TREATMENT

A. **Referral** to a dermatologist is helpful to initially confirm the diagnosis and coordinate treatment.

B. **Eliminate all hepatotoxins.**

C. **Phlebotomy** 500 ml/wk or bimonthly, until hemoglobin is 10 to 11 g/dL, to deplete excessive iron stores. Remission for 1 to 8 years may occur after phlebotomy.

D. **Antimalarial agents** (e.g., low-dose *chloroquine*). Use in consultation with a clinician experienced with such drugs.

E. **Erythropoietin** may be useful for dialysis-induced PCT.

F. **Hepatitis and HIV serologies** are indicated, especially if the family history is negative.

DERMATITIS HERPETIFORMIS ICD-9 (694.0)

Dermatitis herpetiformis is a chronic, recurrent, symmetric vesicular eruption (Fig. 8–4). The term *herpetiformis* refers to herpetiform, or grouped, vesicles, although this disease is not a viral infection and is not related to herpes simplex virus. The disease is thought to be related to gluten or other diet-related antigens that may cause the development of circulating immune complexes and their subsequent deposition in the skin. It most commonly occurs in the 20- to 40-year age group, with men affected more often than women.

The disease is characterized by deposition of IgA in a granular pattern along the tips of the dermal papillae. Eighty percent of patients have blunting and flattening of the small bowel villi, which may lead to steatorrhea and a gluten-sensitive enteropathy but usually is asympto-

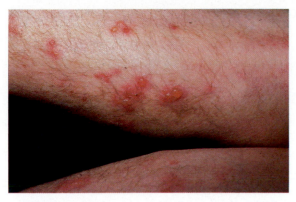

Fig. 8–4
Dermatitis herpetiformis. Grouped vesicles with erythema on an extensor surface. (Courtesy Department of Dermatology, University of North Carolina at Chapel Hill.)

matic. Rarely, anemia, atrophic gastritis, thyroid disease, and small bowel lymphomas are associated with the disease.

I. CLASSIC DESCRIPTION

Distribution: Extensor surfaces (e.g., sacrum, elbows, knees, lower back, shoulders)

Primary: Vesicles, papules, urticarial plaques

Secondary: Excoriations, erythema

Because of the intensely pruritic nature of the disease, often only excoriations in the characteristic distribution are seen, with no intact primary lesions.

II. DIAGNOSIS

If the clinical eruption is characterized by severe itching, burning, or stinging and is in the characteristic extensor distribution, consider obtaining a specimen by deep shave or 4-mm punch biopsy for routine light microscopy. The specimen should be obtained from an early, small, intact vesicle. Biopsy tissue will demonstrate eosinophils, microabscesses of polymorphonuclear leukocytes in the dermal papillae, and subepidermal blister formation. The diagnosis is confirmed with direct immunofluorescence of normal skin, obtained several millimeters from an involved area. Deposits of IgA and complement are seen within the dermal papillae.

III. DIFFERENTIAL DIAGNOSIS

A. **Scabies:** Distribution of scabies involves the wrists, sides of the hands, fingerwebs, feet, axillae, areola, and groin. Family members may have symptoms. Mites and mite feces are found in scrapings.

B. **Excoriated eczema:** The distribution of eczema in adults does not follow the extensor pattern of dermatitis herpetiformis, and eczema responds to topical corticosteroids.

C. **Insect bites:** Usually bites have an asymmetric distribution on exposed surfaces.

IV. TREATMENT

A. **Dapsone**
   1. 100 to 200 mg/day, with gradual reduction to 25 to 50 mg/day, may be required indefinitely.
   2. Obtain glucose-6-phosphate dehydrogenase levels before treatment, because dapsone may precipitate severe hemolytic anemia in patients deficient for this enzyme.
   3. Obtain complete blood cell counts weekly for 1 month, then every 6 to 8 weeks, to monitor for anemia.
   4. Other dapsone side effects include dose-related hemolysis and peripheral neuropathy.

B. **Gluten-free diet:**
   1. Such a diet may decrease the risk of small bowel lymphoma and avoid long-term dapsone use.
   2. 4 to 8 months may be required before any response is seen.
   3. Contact the Celiac Society* or the American Celiac Society.*

C. **Consultation** with a dermatologist is recommended to confirm the diagnosis and to help with management.

*Celiac Society, P.O. Box 31700, Omaha, NE 68131-0700; American Celiac Society, 58 Musano Ct., West Orange, NJ 07052.

ERYTHEMA MULTIFORME AND TOXIC EPIDERMAL NECROLYSIS ICD-9 (695.1)

Erythema multiforme is the general name for a diverse group of skin reactions to many different causal exposures. The common underlying pathway is thought to represent an immunologic reaction in the skin, possibly triggered by circulating immune complexes. Many agents have been implicated, including common drugs and infections, especially herpes simplex virus (Box 8–1). When the cause is linked to recurrent herpes simplex, the infection usually precedes erythema multiforme by a few days to a week or more. Despite these associations, the cause may remain idiopathic in many cases. Erythema multiforme is seen more commonly in older children and adults and may be recurrent.

The term *multiforme* indicates the wide variety of lesions, which vary from plaques to blisters and target lesions. *Stevens-Johnson syndrome (SJS)* is severe erythema multiforme, with extensive mucosal erosions, target-like lesions, and occasional skin blisters, with erosions that cover less than 10% of the body surface area. Often there are associated complaints of fever and malaise. Eye involvement can lead to permanent scarring, corneal ulcers, anterior uveitis, and panophthalmitis.

When more than 10% of the body surface area is involved, with sheetlike loss of the epidermis, the condition is called *toxic epidermal necrolysis (TEN)*. Mortality of 20% to 30% is seen, usually as a result of sepsis. Although the use of certain agents increases the risk of TEN and SJS (sulfonamides, anticonvulsant agents, oxicam-derived nonsteroidal antiinflammatory agents, allopurinol, chlormezanone, and oral corticosteroids), the rate does not exceed 5 cases per million users per week.

I. CLASSIC DESCRIPTION

Mild disease: Nonbullous, lasting 2 to 6 weeks (Fig. 8–5)
Distribution: Symmetric, with predilection for extremities and genital area
Primary: Papules, plaques
Secondary: Erythema; lesions typically are target-like, and blanch with pressure

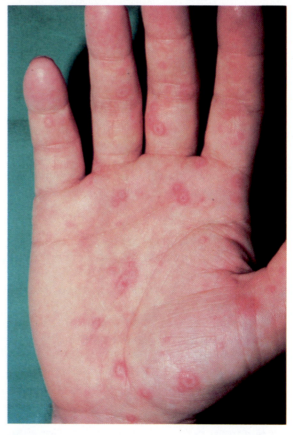

Fig. 8–5
Mild erythema multiforme. Note target lesions and no bullae. (Courtesy Department of Dermatology, University of North Carolina at Chapel Hill.)

BOX 8–1.

Causes of Erythema Multiforme

Drugs
   Penicillins, sulfonamides, barbiturates, hydantoins, nonsteroidal antiinflammatory agents, sulfonylureas, sulindac
Viral infections
   Herpes simplex, hepatitis A and B
Bacterial infections
   Streptococcus, dental abscess
Fungal infection
   Coccidiodomycosis
Mycoplasma infections
Pregnancy
Malignancy/radiotherapy
Idiopathic

Widespread disease: (Fig. 8–6)
Distribution: Widespread, with mucosal involvement including the tracheobronchial tree and genitalia
Primary: Plaques, bullae, vesicles
Secondary: Erythema, erosions

II. DIAGNOSIS

The diagnosis usually is made clinically in patients with typical target-like lesions. Punch biopsies of active lesions will confirm the diagnosis. If possible, define the inciting agent by taking a thorough oral medication history and by obtaining evidence of a recent herpes simplex or respiratory tract infection.

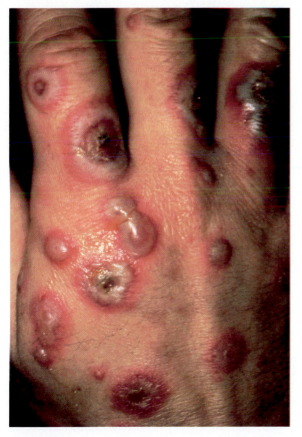

Fig. 8–6
Bullous erythema multiforme with multiple erosions secondary to recent herpes simplex infection. (Courtesy Department of Dermatology, Medical College of Georgia.)

III. DIFFERENTIAL DIAGNOSIS

A. Mild disease:

1. *Urticaria:* Urticarial lesions last less than 24 hours and usually are not target-like, although initially differentiation may be difficult.
2. *Viral exanthems:* Lesions typically are monomorphic, confluent, and central.

B. Severe disease:

1. *Staphylococcal scalded skin syndrome (SSSS):* The disease is characterized by diffuse erythema and superficial blistering; mucous membrane involvement is limited to the conjunctiva, there are no target-like lesions, and there is little oozing from erosions.
2. *Pemphigus vulgaris:* Intact bullae are rarely seen in pemphigus vulgaris, and there are no target-like erythematous lesions. Biopsy may be necessary for differentiation, especially if mucous membrane involvement predominates.
3. *Bullous pemphigoid:* Although both conditions involve subepidermal blistering diseases, distribution of bullous pemphigoid typically is flexural, and target-like lesions are absent. Biopsy will differentiate the two.
4. *Other bullous diseases:* Differentiate by obtaining a biopsy specimen from an early, intact bulla for routine and direct immunofluorescence. Sections may be sent for frozen section on an urgent basis to confirm a diagnosis of TEN.

IV. TREATMENT

A. Identify and treat precipitating causes.

B. Remove any suspected drugs.

C. Potent topical corticosteroids:

1. *Betamethasone dipropionate* 0.05% or *clobetasol propionate* 0.05% bid for up to 2 weeks.

2. May be useful in patients with few lesions.
3. Avoid use on the face and groin.
D. **Systemic corticosteroids:** Use is controversial and no controlled studies have demonstrated effectiveness. With children, systemic steroids may only increase the risk of infection and prolong healing, although adults with limited skin involvement may have symptomatic improvement.
E. **Chronic and/or recurrent infection**:
1. Rule out sources of chronic infection, neoplasia, or connective tissue disease.
2. Consider chronic viral suppression therapy for recurrent herpes simplex viral infections associated with erythema multiforme.

F. **Stevens-Johnson syndrome.**
1. Restore fluid losses. Oral intake may be inhibited because of painful oral lesions. Hospitalize if necessary.
2. Viscous *lidocaine* may be used for relief of pain from oral lesions.
3. Ophthalmology consultation is useful to help prevent conjunctival scarring.
4. Use Burow's solution as compresses for topical therapy for denuded body lesions.
5. Monitor closely for and treat any secondary infections.
G. **Referral:** Consultation is indicated for chronic or recurrent cases of erythema multiforme. Severe cases are best managed in a burn unit.

STAPHYLOCOCCAL SCALDED SKIN SYNDROME ICD-9 (695.1)

Staphylococcal scalded skin syndrome (SSSS) is a superficial blistering disease that occurs secondary to cutaneous response to a circulating toxin. Some staphylococcal infections release a toxin (exfoliatin) that causes a split high in the epidermis, with subsequent superficial blistering and peeling of skin. Cultures of the superficial peeling skin will be negative because the circulating toxin is responsible for the damage. The localized staphylococcal infection may be distant from the involved skin (e.g., in conjunctivitis, sinusitis, external otitis, cutaneous abscess). SSSS most commonly occurs in previously healthy children younger than 6 years. Although the disease usually resolves over 7 to 10 days, mortality may approach 2% to 3% or higher in adults, particularly in immunocompromised adults or those with renal failure. Treatment of any underlying staphylococcal infection is essential.

I. CLASSIC DESCRIPTION

Distribution: Face, neck, axillae, and groin are involved first, usually with sparing of mucous membranes

Primary: Superficial bullae
Secondary: Scale, desquamation, erythema
Characteristic skin findings include generalized tender erythema, often with a sandpapery feel, and postinflammatory desquamation (Fig. 8–7).

II. DIAGNOSIS

Perform staphylococcal cultures from any suspicious sites (e.g., nose, eyes, ears, throat, vagina). *Cultures from skin bullae usually are negative.*

III. DIFFERENTIAL DIAGNOSIS

A. **Toxic epidermal necrolysis (TEN):** Often caused by drugs or a viral infection, the blisters in TEN are deeper (in the dermoepidermal junction) and the level of blister formation can be confirmed on frozen or routine skin biopsy.
B. **Perianal streptococcal cellulitis:** Desquamation is confined to the perianal region, and bacterial cultures are positive for *Streptococcus.*

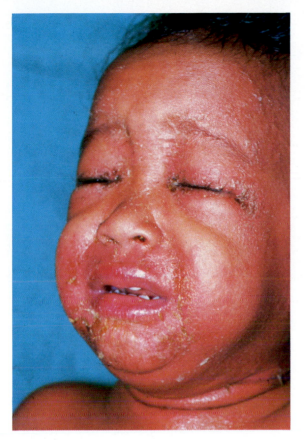

Fig. 8–7
Staphylococcal scalded skin syndrome with diffuse superficial scaling and desquamation. (Courtesy Department of Dermatology, Medical College of Georgia.)

C. Kawasaki syndrome: Desquamation is not generalized, there is no evidence of a staphylococcal infection, and persistent fever and mucous membrane involvement are characteristic.

IV. TREATMENT

A. Penicillinase-resistant antistaphylococcal antibiotics: Choose one of the following.

1. *Cloxacillin*
   a. Less than 20 kg: 50 to 100 mg/kg/day in four divided doses.
   b. More than 20 kg: 1 to 2 g/day, not to exceed 4 g/day.
2. *Dicloxacillin*
   a. Less than 40 kg: 25 to 75 mg/kg/day in four divided doses.
   b. Adults: 125 to 500 mg q6h.

B. Hospitalization: In severe cases, the patient may require hospitalization for intravenous antibiotic therapy (e.g., methicillin, nafcillin, oxacillin) and for hydration.

SUGGESTED READING

Anhalt GJ et al: Paraneoplastic pemphigus: an autoimmune mucocutaneous disease associated with neoplasia, *N Engl J Med* 323:1729–1730, 1990.

Assier H et al: Erythema multiforme with mucous membrane involvement and Stevens-Johnson syndrome are clinically different disorders with distinct causes, *Arch Dermatol* 131:539–543, 1995.

Avakian R et al: Toxic epidermal necrolysis: a review, *J Am Acad Dermatol* 25:69–77, 1991.

Beers B, Wilson B: Adult staphylococcal scalded skin syndrome, *Int J Dermatol* 29:428–429, 1990.

Elder GH: The cutaneous porphyrias, *Semin Dermatol* 9:63–69, 1990.

Fine JD: Management of acquired bullous skin diseases, *N Engl J Med* 333:1475–1484, 1995.

Garioch JJ et al: Twenty-five years' experience of a gluten free diet in the treatment of dermatitis herpetiformis, *Br J Dermatol* 131:541–545, 1994.

Green D, Law E, Still JM: An approach to the management of toxic epidermal necrolysis in a burn center, *Burns* 19:411–414, 1993.

Hall RP: The pathogenesis of dermatitis herpetiformis: recent advances, *J Am Acad Dermatol* 16:1129–1144, 1987.

Kauppinen R, Timonen K, Mustajoki P: Treatment of the porphyrias, *Ann Med* 26:31–38, 1994.

Korman N: Bullous pemphigoid, *J Am Acad Dermatol* 16:907–924, 1987.

Korman N: Pemphigus, *J Am Acad Dermatol* 18:1219–1238, 1988.

Roujeau JC, Stern RS: Severe adverse cutaneous reactions to drugs, *N Engl J Med* 331:1272–1285, 1994.

Roujeau JC, Kelly JP, Naldi L: Medication use and the risk of Stevens-Johnson syndrome or toxic epidermal necrolysis, *N Engl J Med* 333:1600–1607, 1995.

CHAPTER 9

Drug Reactions

Although many drugs can cause a cutaneous eruption, clinicians often fail to appreciate the scope of potential drug reactions, which can occur in 1% to 3% of all hospitalized patients. Reactions range from mild pruritus, with no skin lesions, to generalized erythroderma and skin sloughing. Drug reactions usually are considered in the differential diagnosis of most skin diseases, including toxic epidermal necrolysis, purpura, urticaria, erythema multiforme, erythema nodosum, and morbilliform eruptions.

One way of classifying drug eruptions is by nonimmunologic vs. immunologic response. Many patients will experience a nonimmunologic or nonallergic reaction if they take enough of a drug for a long enough time. For example, hyperpigmentation may occur secondary to prolonged use of certain phenothiazines. Immunologic or allergic reactions occur less often, after lower doses, and usually after a latent period, allowing for some type of sensitization to develop.

The etiologic agent in a drug eruption usually is the most recently prescribed drug; how-ever, it is important to remember that some medications may be tolerated without problem for weeks to years, but once sensitization occurs, reactions may develop within minutes to hours of reexposure to the drug. Chemically related compounds (e.g., furosemide and sulfonylureas or NSAIDs and aspirin) also may produce a cross-reaction.

The key to diagnosing and treating most drug reactions involves taking a careful history, with consideration of all medications, including nonprescription and homeopathic drugs. Drug eruptions may persist for several weeks, but usually lessen within days of removing the drug. *A hallmark of most drug reactions is symmetric distribution of lesions.*

When a drug reaction seems likely, it is prudent to discontinue the offending agent, particularly if there is associated urticaria, blisters, mucous membrane involvement, facial edema, ulcers, palpable or extensive purpura, fever, or adenopathy.

Information on cutaneous drug reactions may be obtained on the World Wide Web.*

MORBILLIFORM DRUG ERUPTION ICD-9 (995.2)

Morbilliform drug eruptions are diffuse eruptions characterized by blanching, erythematous papules and macules that occur in response to a drug (Fig. 9–1). Approximately 45% of drug eruptions fit this category. The morphologic characteristics are identical to those of many viral exanthems, making clinical distinction sometimes impossible. The most common pre-

*gopher://gopher.dartmouth.edu/1/Research/BioSci/CDRD

89

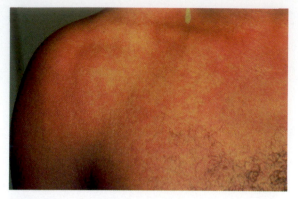

Fig. 9–1
Morbilliform drug eruption secondary to sulfa medications. Note discrete and confluent areas of blanching erythema. (Courtesy John Cook, MD.)

TABLE 9–1.
Common Drugs That Cause Morbilliform Eruptions

Allopurinol	Phenytoin/other anticonvulsant drugs
Barbiturates	Phenothiazines
Gentamicin	Quinidine
Gold	Sulfonamides
Isoniazid	Sulfonylurea compounds
Penicillin and related compounds	Thiazides

cipitating agents for drug-induced morbilliform eruptions are listed in Table 9–1. These eruptions usually occur 7 to 10 days after starting the responsible drug but may not appear until 2 weeks after the drug has been stopped, especially in the case of penicillin and related compounds.

A common presentation is a patient with infectious mononucleosis who develops a generalized eruption while taking ampicillin. The immune mechanism is probably the result of a type II or III immune response, involving damage to small vessels, with resultant vasodilation. Therefore *a morbilliform drug eruption does not necessarily put a patient at risk for a type I, or anaphylactic, reaction on reexposure to that drug.*

Rashes associated with anticonvulsant therapy, particularly phenytoin and carbamazepine, may, rarely, herald a severe hypersensitivity syndrome. Be alert to the possibility of developing pseudolymphoma (and, even more rarely, lymphoma) if the rash (1) is associated with facial edema, generalized exfoliation, purpura, bullae, adenopathy, arthralgia, or fever; (2) is associated with laboratory abnormalities, such as lymphocytosis, hepatitis, or eosinophilia; or (3) develops 2 weeks into therapy. Most cases resolve spontaneously.

I. CLASSIC DESCRIPTION
Distribution: Symmetric; usually begins on the upper trunk, then spreads to the neck, face, and distally to the extremities; it may involve the palms or soles, but usually spares the mucous membranes
Primary: Macules, papules
Secondary: Blanching erythema
Lesions initially are discrete, but may become confluent.

II. DIAGNOSIS
The diagnosis is based on the clinical appearance of lesions in a patient who has taken a medication within the previous 2 weeks or in a patient taking a longstanding medication that is a common culprit of morbilliform drug eruptions. In immunosuppressed or seriously ill patients, an extensive search for any underlying infection is necessary.

III. DIFFERENTIAL DIAGNOSIS
A. **Infectious causes** include rubella, rubeola, scarlatina, infectious mononucleosis, roseola, echovirus, coxsackievirus, toxic shock syndrome, and Kawasaki syndrome. A 4-mm punch biopsy specimen from two or three representative areas only rarely aids in identifying a possible infectious cause by demonstrating a typical histologic picture specific for infection or by demonstrating organisms in tissue with special stains or on culture.
B. **Secondary syphylis:** The palms, soles, and mucous membranes are preferentially involved, with scaling papules and

plaques on the trunk. The rapid plasma reagin (RPR) is positive.

C. **Pityriasis rosea:** Look for a herald patch. Papules and plaques should have classic centripetal scale.

IV. TREATMENT

A. **Taking a drug history:**
   1. Take a thorough drug history to identify any possible inciting agents taken within the previous 2 weeks.
   2. In the case of penicillins, patients may have finished the drug more than 2 weeks before eruption of lesions.
   3. Emphasize the possibility of prescription, as well as nonprescription, medications as exposure sources.

B. **Medication discontinuation:** Remove any possible inciting agent, noting any improvement after drug withdrawal. In some cases it may take several days to weeks to observe significant improvement.

C. **Rule out infection:** Workup is determined by taking into consideration the clinical appearance of the patient.

D. **Itching:**
   1. Pills: Antihistamines, such as *hydroxyzine hydrochloride* 10 to 50 mg q4 to 8h prn or *cetrizine* (Zyrtec) 10 mg qd.
   2. Lotions: *Cetaphil* with 0.25% menthol by prescription, or *Sarna* lotion by nonprescription prn.
   3. Topical corticosteroids: Mild to moderate strength is useful in treating pruri-

tus, but because the area to be covered often is extensive, use generic compounds to reduce expense.
   a. *Hydrocortisone* cream 1%, 120 g bid to tid in children and for use on the face, groin, and axillae in adults.
   b. *Triamcinolone* cream 0.1%, 120 to 240 g bid to tid in adults; avoid the face, groin, and axillae.

E. **Penicillin allergy:** If there is sufficient concern about penicillin allergy, testing for reaction to major and minor determinants may be indicated.

F. **Consultation** with a dermatologist or an allergist may be useful in guiding the workup of the most likely causes in nonspecific eruptions.

G. **Systemic involvement:** If the patient presents with arthralgia, malaise, or other such symptoms, consider ruling out systemic involvement, such as signs of vasculitis. The most typically involved organ systems are hematopoietic, kidney, and liver. Appropriate screening tests include a complete blood cell count with differential, platelets, liver profile, and urinalysis.

V. PATIENT EDUCATION

A. Explain that an eruption may take several weeks to entirely clear, even after the appropriate medication has been withdrawn.

B. Explain the potential problems of taking cross-reacting medications, which can cause similar eruptions.

FIXED DRUG ERUPTION ICD-9 (995.2)

Fixed drug eruptions are poorly understood, recurrent reactions thought to be the result of a hypersensitivity reaction to a particular compound. Reactions will occur in an asymmetric pattern at the same sites with each challenge of the drug. It is unclear why the reaction is localized. An itching or burning sensation often precedes an outbreak. The drugs most commonly associated with a fixed eruption are phenolphthalein (found in many over-the-counter laxatives), trimethoprim, barbiturates, sulfonamides, quinidine, salicylates, tetracycline, gold, and, rarely, acetaminophen.

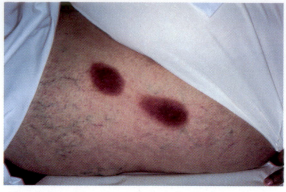

Fig. 9–2
Fixed drug eruption. Note macules with secondary, well-circumscribed hyperpigmentation on the lower extremity. (Courtesy Department of Dermatology, Medical College of Georgia.)

I. **CLASSIC DESCRIPTION** (Fig. 9–2)
Distribution: Extremities, glans penis, mucous membranes
Primary: Macules, plaques, bullae
Secondary: Erythema, purplish hue, erosion, hyperpigmentation
Lesions are round and discrete and range from small, localized, recurring erythematous areas to large bullae. Only erosions may be seen if bullae have ruptured. Lesions usually heal as a persistent, hyperpigmented macule.

II. **DIAGNOSIS**
The diagnosis is based on the characteristic skin lesions along with *a history of recurring lesions at the same site each time a drug is taken.* Carefully review all medications, with close attention to nonprescription drugs, to determine the causative compound.

III. **DIFFERENTIAL DIAGNOSIS**
  A. **Erythema multiforme** usually is symmetric in distribution, and lesions do not recur in the same location.
  B. **Postinflammatory hyperpigmentation** is usually associated with a previous skin eruption, including a fixed drug eruption.
  C. **Suction blisters** are associated with trauma.
  D. **Herpes simplex** occurs as grouped blisters on an erythematous base and is confined to one site. The Tzanck smear is positive, and the history is negative for a possible inciting drug.

IV. **TREATMENT**
  A. **Identify and eliminate causative agents** and their related compounds.
  B. **For symptom relief** apply Burow's solution cool soaks to eroded areas for 20 minutes 2 or 3 times daily.
  C. **Topical corticosteroid creams**: Class II or III steroid creams, such as *betamethasone dipropionate* 0.05% or *valerate* 0.1% bid, help with pruritus relief; avoid use on face and groin.

V. **PATIENT EDUCATION**
  A. Emphasize complete avoidance of the offending agent and related compounds, including over-the-counter medications.
  B. Educate patients that postinflammatory hyperpigmentation may last for several weeks after removal of the offending agent.

PHOTOALLERGIC AND PHOTOTOXIC DRUG ERUPTIONS ICD-9 (692.72)

Photoallergic and phototoxic drug eruptions result from the interaction of ultraviolet radiation and certain drugs. Common photosensitizing agents are listed in Table 9–2.

Phototoxic reactions are more common than photoallergic reactions and occur as a result of a particular drug's ability to enhance the skin's reaction to ordinary light. They are characterized

TABLE 9–2.
Some Photosensitizing Drugs

Photoallergens	Phototoxins
Benzodiazepine	Amiodarone
Benzophenones	Antibiotics (esp. tetracyclines, sulfonamides)
Diuretics (thiazides)	Antineoplastic agents
Fragrances	Coal tar
Methoxycinnamate	Diltiazem
NSAIDs	Diuretics
Nifedipine	Griseofulvin
PABA	NSAIDs
Phenothiazines	Phenothiazines
Quinidine	Psoralens
Quinine	Quinidine
Retinoids	Quinine
	Retinoids

by erythema resembling a sunburn that occurs within 24 hours after ultraviolet radiation exposure, with the eruption confined to light-exposed areas (Fig. 9–3). Phototoxic reactions are also related to a drug's total body concentration. Although they may occur after first administration of a drug, often they occur only after a sufficient concentration has accumulated in the body. Phototoxicity may exist along with photoallergic eruptions.

Photoallergic reactions are less common, may spread to areas not exposed to the sun, are not dose-related, and usually occur 48 hours after ultraviolet exposure. These reactions require a period of allergic sensitization. The responsible drug reacts with sunlight, and the reaction products are allergenic. Therefore repeated exposure is required; a reaction will not occur with the first drug dose. Photoallergic reactions are eczematous, similar to contact dermatitis. Rarely, sunscreens may cause photoallergic reactions, especially sunscreens that are cinnamate-derived.

I. CLASSIC DESCRIPTION
Distribution: Sun-exposed areas (e.g., face, distal arms, V of neck, and chest); sparing in shaded areas (e.g., philtrum of nose, beneath lower lip, behind ears, superior aspect of neck); may extend beyond exposed areas

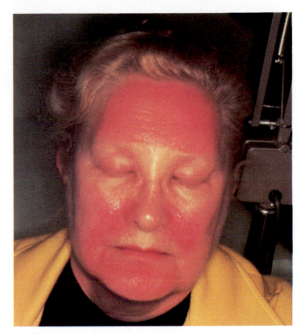

Fig. 9–3 Phototoxic drug eruption. Note sparing of eyes secondary to use of sunglasses and of the philtrum secondary to shading by the nose. (Courtesy Marshall Guill, MD.)

Primary: Plaque; may see vesicles and bullae in photoallergic reactions
Secondary: Erythema, edema, scale, hyperpigmentation

II. DIAGNOSIS
The diagnosis is based on the clinical photodistribution, a history of exposure to a photosensitizing compound, and a history of exacerbation with sun exposure.

III. DIFFERENTIAL DIAGNOSIS
A. **Allergic contact dermatitis, particularly airborne:** Look for involvement of shaded areas and a history of exposure to contact allergens.
B. **Lupus erythematosus, porphyria, polymorphous light eruption, and pellagra** are other diseases associated with photosensitivity. Systemic findings often are present in the absence of photosensitizing compounds.

IV. TREATMENT
A. Identify and avoid the causative agent.
B. Pruritus relief:
1. Use antihistamines such as *hydroxyzine hydrochloride* 10 to 50 mg q4 to 8h prn.
2. Cool compresses, such as cold, wet cloths, applied for 10 to 20 minutes 2 to 3 times a day, are soothing.

C. Topical corticosteroids: for mild or limited involvement.
1. *Hydrocortisone cream* 1%, *hydrocortisone valerate* 0.2%, or *alclometasone dipropionate* 0.05% to the face and neck areas 2 or 3 times daily.
2. *Triamcinolone cream* 0.1% to affected areas on hands, chest, and arms.

D. Systemic corticosteroids: *Prednisone,* 0.5 to 1 mg/kg/day, tapered over 7 to 10 days, is useful for facial involvement or for severe widespread disease.
E. Sun protection: Use a broad-spectrum sunscreen (e.g., UVA Shade containing Parsol 1789) to protect against ultraviolet A *and* B; also wear protective clothing.
F. Referral: Some patients may become persistently light-sensitive and should be referred for consultation.

V. PATIENT EDUCATION
A. Emphasize protection from sunlight, including during daily activities such as going to and from the car.
B. Avoid offending agents and any chemically related compounds.

ANAPHYLAXIS ICD-9 (995.0)

Anaphylaxis as a skin disorder is likely the most urgent condition that the clinician must recognize. Treated appropriately, patient's lives literally are saved. Some patients do not appreciate the seriousness of potential anaphylactic drug reactions and fail to seek prompt medical help.

Anaphylaxis is a systemic type I reaction in which mast cells and/or basophils degranulate in the presence of IgE and the inciting allergen. In the case of radiographic dye, the compound itself may cause a massive release of mediators from mast cells. Other mechanisms include involvement of the complement system or alterations in the arachidonic acid pathway. The most common causes of anaphylaxis are salicylates, nonsteroidal antiinflammatory drugs, penicillins, sulfonamides, ACE inhibitors, blood products, radiographic dye, anesthetics, latex, animal-derived sera, insect stings, and foods, such as nuts and seafood.

The release of multiple mediators causes a massive increase in vascular permeability in the skin and mucous membranes, with subsequent edema in the airways and vascular collapse.

Symptoms include tightness in the throat or chest, hoarseness, stridor, and, if untreated, respiratory failure, with cyanosis, hypotension, arrhythmias, and death.

I. CLASSIC DESCRIPTION
Distribution: Mucous membranes and skin
Primary: Diffuse wheals
Secondary: Erythema, edema

II. DIAGNOSIS
The diagnosis is based on the clinical findings of acute generalized hives and/or angioedema (Fig. 9–4; see also Chapter 17). It is important for clinicians to remember that *systemic manifestations of chest tightness or hypotension may predominate, with few skin findings.*

III. DIFFERENTIAL DIAGNOSIS
Hereditary angioedema: C1 esterase inhibitor deficiency: There is a positive family history of acute, recurrent attacks of angioedema, usually precipitated by minor trauma. Patients have deficient or functionally absent serum C1 esterase inhibitor and decreased C4 levels.

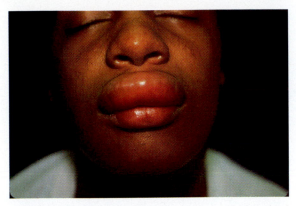

Fig. 9–4
Angioedema of the upper lip, with severe swelling of deeper tissues. (Courtesy Beverly Sanders, MD.)

IV. TREATMENT

A. ABCs: Maintain the airway, ensure adequate breathing, establish and maintain circulation. Assess and treat any cardiac arrhythmias.

B. *Epinephrine:* Use with continuous cardiac monitor.

   1. Administer 0.5 ml 1:1000 subcutaneously, sublingually, or via endotracheal tube or 0.5 mg (5 ml 1:10,000 solution) intravenously.
   2. Repeat q5 to 10 minutes if signs of anaphylaxis are still present.

C. *Aminophylline* 6 mg/kg as a loading dose may be infused IV over 20 to 30 minutes (500 mg in 1000 ml D_5W) to treat bronchospasm, then 0.5 to 0.6 mg/kg/h maintenance dosage.

D. Administer IV fluids to sustain normal blood pressure.

E. Steroids: *Hydrocortisone sodium succinate* 250 mg IV q6h for serious or prolonged reactions.

F. H_1 and H_2 blockers: *Diphenhydramine* 25 to 50 mg IV, IM, or PO q6h, *cimetidine* 400 mg PO bid, *ranitidine* 150 mg PO bid.

G. Observation: All patients should be observed for at least 6 hours.

V. PREVENTION

A. Take a good medical history and accurately document the type and severity of any previous drug reactions.

B. Avoid identified offending drugs and their cross-reacting compounds. In general, avoid mast cell degranulators (e.g., aspirin, opiates, radiocontrast dyes, polymixin B).

C. Consider allergy testing to determine whether the patient has a truly IgE-mediated allergic reaction to penicillin.

D. Hyposensitization:

E. Prescribe an *EpiPen Kit* for sensitive people.

   1. Educate them as to proper storage of the EpiPen Kit (e.g., keep it protected from light and do not refrigerate). The solution should be clear and colorless.
   2. Review symptoms for which use is appropriate (i.e., shortness of breath, throat tightening, dizziness).
   3. Instruct patients about proper injection sites, such as the thigh, and to avoid the buttocks or sites where intravascular injection might be likely.

SUGGESTED READING

Bochner BS, Lichtenstein LM: Anaphylaxis, *N Engl J Med* 324:1785–1790, 1991.

González E, González S: Drug photosensitivity, idiopathic photodermatoses, and sunscreens, *J Am Acad Dermatol* 35:871–85, 1996.

Gould JW, Mercurio MG, Elmets CA: Cutaneous photosensitivity diseases induced by exogenous agents, *J Am Acad Dermatol* 33:551–573, 1995.

Prussick R, Knowles S, Shear NH: Cutaneous drug reactions. In: Callen JP, ed: *Current problems in dermatology,* St Louis, 1994, Mosby.

Roujeau JC, Stern RS: Severe adverse cutaneous reactions to drugs, *N Engl J Med* 331:1272–1285, 1994.

Shear NH: Diagnosing cutaneous adverse reactions to drugs, *Arch Dermatol* 126:94–97, 1990.

CHAPTER 10

Superficial Fungal Infections

Superficial fungal infections comprise a large portion of dermatoses seen by primary care clinicians. Despite their common occurrence, ease of treatment, and relative similarities, such fungal infections are often initially misdiagnosed or mistreated. Because the infections are common, usually fairly innocuous, and often chronic, clinicians may rely too much on initial visual inspection of lesions and fail to confirm a diagnosis with appropriate laboratory specimens. Subsequently the eczematous lesion that "looks like a fungus," or vice versa, may be treated for several weeks with no real improvement. *Therefore the "art" in dermatologic diagnosis and treatment of superficial fungal infections involves a firm understanding of the necessity to confirm initial clinical impressions whenever possible.* Successful treatment requires both knowledge of the underlying disease processes and patience and persistence with treatment alternatives.

Superficial fungal infections involve a complex interaction between a host, an environment, and an organism. A host's genetic predisposition or underlying acquired immune defect may explain disease in some patients, whereas others exposed to the same environment may remain unaffected. T cell-mediated immune responses may limit or cure an infection, but in other cases infections persist or recur. Environmental factors, such as moisture and maceration, influence the infection site and disease course.

Tinea infections are caused by three types of noninvasive fungi known as *dermatophytes: Epidermophyton, Trichophyton,* and *Microsporum.* The word *tinea* itself is derived from the Greek word meaning *moth,* and refers to the clothes moth, which originally was thought to cause the disease. These fungi can be found on humans or other animals and in the soil. Those fungi whose usual hosts are animals tend to cause the most inflammatory response; those occurring in humans (anthrophilic) tend to cause the least amount of host inflammatory response. Tinea infections are named by location: tinea capitis, head; tinea manus, hand; tinea pedis, foot; tinea cruris, groin; tinea corporis, body; and tinea unguium, nail.

Severe inflammatory skin reactions can cause a generalized skin eruption known as an *id reaction* (e.g., a severe tinea pedis infection), which may look quite different from the original skin lesion. Id eruptions, which may break out at distant sites, represent an immunologic reaction to the fungus and the associated severe inflammation.

Tinea versicolor, also known as *pityriasis versicolor,* is a different superficial yeast infection caused by *Pityrosporum orbiculare (Malessezia furfur).* It has a distinctly different appearance from the superficial fungal infections caused by dermatophytes. The common candidal skin infections are caused by *Candida albicans;* manifestations are influenced by location (e.g., mucous membranes, intertriginous areas, nails).

Superficial fungal infections involve the uppermost layers of the skin. Unless a person has a significant immune problem, these organisms do not invade deeper tissues or involve other organ systems. In contrast, deep fungal infections, such as histoplasmosis, frequently present with non–skin findings.

TINEA CAPITIS ICD-9 (110.0)

Tinea capitis is a superficial scalp fungal infection caused by dermatophytes from either the *Trichophyton* or *Microsporum* species. The disease is seen predominantly in children. Tinea capitis may present in a variety of ways, ranging from diffuse generalized scalp scaling to round scaling areas of alopecia (Fig. 10–1). Severe tinea capitis may lead to a *kerion,* an inflamed, exudative, boggy nodule, with marked edema and hair loss (Fig. 10–2). Enlarged cervical lymph nodes frequently accompany the condition.

The clinical presentation is influenced by several factors, including the dermatophyte source (animal sources tend to be more inflammatory) and host response (which can be minimal to severe). Children tend to be exposed to tinea capitis by playmates or infected household pets.

I. CLASSIC DESCRIPTION

Primary: Plaques, papules, pustules, nodules

Secondary: Scale, alopecia, erythema, exudate, edema

The most important point to remember about tinea capitis is that it may have a quite varied presentation, ranging from mild scaling with broken hairs to exudative and inflammatory lesions.

II. DIAGNOSIS

A. Direct microscopic examination of hairs. Obtain by either rubbing a moistened gauze in an area of scaling alopecia or by "plucking" 2 to 3 hairs, and then examine the broken-off hairs with 10% potassium hydroxide (KOH) for hyphae or spores. (See procedure for obtaining a KOH specimen, Chapter 3.)

   1. Look for hyphae or spores either surrounding or involving the hair shaft.
   2. If there is a vigorous inflammatory

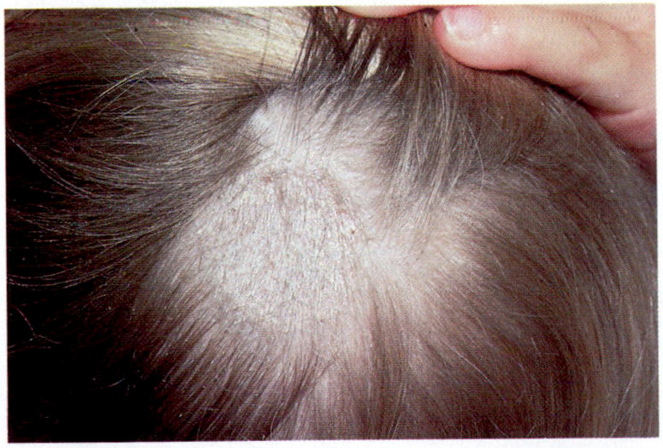

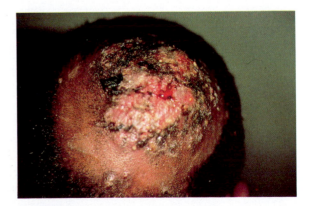

Fig. 10–1. Tinea capitis. Note scaling and alopecia. (Courtesy Department of Dermatology, University of North Carolina at Chapel Hill.)

Fig. 10–2. Tinea capitis with indurated boggy plaque (kerion). (Courtesy Department of Dermatology, Medical College of Georgia.)

response, the KOH test may produce negative results.

B. **Wood's lamp examination:** Bright green fluorescence in hair shafts is indicative of infections caused by *Microsporum canis* and *Microsporum audouinii*. However, *Microsporum* infections are much less common in the United States, with *Trichophyton tonsurans* causing almost 80% of tinea capitis. Therefore Wood's lamp examination is not helpful in the majority of the cases of tinea capitis.

C. **Culture:** (See Chapter 3)
   1. Consider fungal cultures if the KOH test results are negative but a strong suspicion for tinea capitis remains.
      a. Dermatophyte test medium agar contains a color indicator that turns from yellow to pink or red within 2 to 3 weeks.
      b. Incubate infected hairs under dark, slightly aerobic conditions, such as in a cabinet with the lid loosely applied.
   2. Tinea capitis can mimic seborrheic

dermatitis and other conditions; cultures may be useful in defining the differential diagnosis.

III. **DIFFERENTIAL DIAGNOSIS**

A. **Alopecia areata** is discrete, has non-scaling areas of hair loss, and all hairs are lost in the involved area.

B. **Seborrheic dermatitis** is rare in children, yet it may be necessary to do a KOH test or culture to differentiate from tinea capitis.

C. **Cellulitis** or **abscess** may resemble more severe forms of tinea capitis and it is important to address the fungal component in these lesions. It is essential to distinguish tinea capitis from bacterial infections by performing a KOH test or fungal culture. The infections may coexist, particularly in children with kerions.

IV. **TREATMENT**

A. **Systemic therapy is necessary.** Topical therapies, such as *ketoconazole* shampoos, are ineffective.

B. *Griseofulvin* is the drug of choice (see Tables 10–1 and 10–2).

TABLE 10–1.

Treatment of Superficial Fungal Infections

Disease	Preferred Therapy	Alternative Therapy	*Comments
Tinea capitis	Griseofulvin Microsize Children: 15-20 mg/kg/day Adults: 500-1000 mg/day Ultramicrosize Children: 10-15 mg/kg/day Adults: 330-660 mg/day Use for a minimum of 8 wks (2 wks beyond cure) Pills are much less expensive than liquid.	1. Terbinafine 62.5-250 mg/qd x 4 wks 2. Itraconazole 5 mg/kg/qd x 3-6 wks Not FDA approved for tinea capitis or pediatric use in U.S., although regimens are evolving. Consider using if griseofulvin-allergic.	Selenium sulfide 1%-2.5% shampoo for household members reduces shedding of spores in asymptomatic carriers. Treat all combs, brushes, hats, etc.
Tinea corporis Tinea cruris (Majocchi's granuloma)	*Limited disease:* topical agents (See Table 10–3.) *Extensive disease:* Griseofulvin 500 mg qd microsize or Griseofulvin 250-375 mg qd ultramicrosize for 2-4 wks	1. Terbinafine 250 mg qd 2-4 wks 2. Itraconazole 200 mg qd x 1 wk 3. Fluconazole 150 mg/wk up to 4 doses	Alternative therapies are effective and are indicated when disease is recalcitrant or recurrent. Zeasorb AF Powder may be used chronically for drying effect (cruris).

Continued.

TABLE 10–1 (cont.).

Disease	Preferred Therapy	Alternative Therapy	*Comments
Tinea manus and pedis	*Limited disease:* Topical agents (See Table 10-3.) *Extensive disease:* Griseofulvin 500 mg bid microsize x 4-8 wks Griseofulvin 250-375 mg bid x 4-8 wks Terbinafine 250 mg qd x 2-6 wks Itraconazole 200 mg bid x 1 wk	Fluconazole 150 mg/wk up to 4 doses	Terbinafine or itraconazole are appropriate for recalcitrant or recurrent disease. When nails are involved, use the treatment regimen for onychomycosis.
Onychomyosis	*Single nail involvement:* (especially if mold infection) chemical or surgical avulsion + topical therapy (Table 10–3) under occlusion for 1 yr *More than one nail:* Terbinafine 250 mg qd x 6 wks for fingernails; x 12 wks for toenails, or Itraconazole 200 mg bid x 1 wk each mo for 2 mos for fingernails; 3-4 mos for toenails	Fluconazole 300 mg/wk until nails appear clear (3-5 mos for fingernails; 9-12 mos for toenails)	Use topicals chronically to prevent recurrence.
Tinea versicolor	*Limited disease:* Topical agents (See Table 10–3.) See comments. *Extensive disease:* Ketoconazole 200 mg x 2 = 400 mg as one dose, repeat in 1 wk or 200 mg qd *x* 7-10 days	1. Fluconazole 400 mg qd x 1-3 doses. 2. Itraconazole 200 mg qd x 1 wk	Apply selenium sulfide lotion 2.5% to affected areas overnight, repeating monthly in warm weather to prevent recurrence.
Candidiasis: intertriginous	*Limited disease:* Topical agents (See Table 10–3.) *Extensive disease:* Itraconazole 200 mg qd x 1-2 wks	1. Ketoconazole 200 mg qd x 1-2 wks 2. Fluconazole 100-400 mg/qd Regimens not well studied.	Local care with drying is essential. Use cool compresses if maceration is present. More common in obese/diabetic patients.
Oral	Oral nystatin Infants 1 ml each cheek qid Adults 2-3 ml each cheek qid x 10-14 days Fluconazole 200 mg day 1; 100 mg days 2-14 Pediatric: 6 mg/kg day 1; 3 mg/kg days 2-14 Clotrimazole troches: dissolve 1 PO 5 times/day x 2 wks	1. Ketoconazole 200 mg qd x 1-2 wks 2. Itraconazole 100-200 mg/day x 1-3 wks	Regimens for immuno-suppressed patients will vary.
Balanitis	*Limited disease:* Topical agents (See Table 10–3.) *Extensive, recalcitrant, or recurrent disease:* Itraconazole 200 mg qd x 3	Fluconazole 150 mg x 1 dose. May be repeated weekly	Oral treatment is indicated for recalcitrant disease only. Balanitis is more common in diabetics.

*Itraconazole, ketoconazole, and sometimes fluconazole may have significant drug–drug interactions, including: terfenadine, astemizole, oral hypoglycemics, coumarin type of anticoagulants, phenytoin, rifampin, theophylline, cyclosporine, cisapride, triazolam, oral contraceptives, lovastatin, simvastatin, and digoxin. Rare cases of hepatic injury have occurred, therefore laboratory monitoring is indicated in patients with a preexisting history of liver disease or in continuous long-term therapy. Rare cases of hematologic abnormalities have occurred with terbinafine. CBC monitoring is indicated in continuous therapy.

TABLE 10–2.

Oral Agents for Fungi and Yeast

Generic Name	Brand Name	How Supplied	Side Effects*
Fluconazole	Diflucan	50, 100, 150, 200 mg 10 mg/ml; 40 mg/ml	Monitor for liver toxicity if therapy is chronic. Watch for rare cases of lymphopenia, thrombocytopenia, hypokalemia, and skin rashes. Possibly contraindicated with astemizole and terfenadine.
Griseofulvin	Fulvicin P/G ultramicrosize	125, 250 mg	Photosensitivity, headache, GI upset, hypersensitivity reactions; interferes with phenobarbital, warfarin, and other hepatically metabolized drugs. Leukopenia and granulocytopenia occur, rarely, with prolonged use at high dosages. Contraindicated in hepatocellular failure, pregnancy, and porphyria. Avoid alcohol. Monitor CBC and liver function if using meds for more than a few months.
	Fulvicin P/G ultramicrosize	165, 330 mg	
	Grisactin capsules microsize	250, 500 mg	
	Grisactin Ultra Tabs ultramicrosize	250, 330 mg	
	Gris-PEG tablets ultramicrosize	125, 250 mg	
	Grifulvin V suspension microsize	125 mg/5 ml	
	Grifulvin V tablets microsize	250, 500 mg	
Itraconazole	Sporanox	100 mg	Nausea, GI upset, rash, pruritus, hypokalemia, leg edema, rare liver toxicity. Monitor liver function in all patients with a history of preexisting hepatic disease and if therapy is chronic. Contraindicated with astemizole, terfenadine, cisapride, and triazolam.
Ketoconazole	Nizoral	200 mg	Nausea, GI upset, rash, allergic reactions. Contraindicated with astemizole, cisapride, terfendadine, and triazolam. Liver toxicity occurs in 1 in 10,000. Liver function should be monitored pretreatment and during treatment.
Terbinafine	Lamisil	250 mg	Nausea, GI upset, rash, reversible taste disturbances, rare hepatotoxicity and hematologic abnormalities. Lab monitoring indicated if there is a history of preexisting liver disease or if symptoms of liver disease or hematologic abnormalities develop during therapy or if therapy > 1 month.

*Significant drug–drug interactions occur with many of these drugs. H_2 blockers may interfere with absorption of ketoconazole and itraconazole.

V. PATIENT EDUCATION

(See patient education handout in Appendix R.)

A. Compliance with a complete regimen for 2 weeks beyond cure is essential to prevent relapse.

B. Playmates and family members, especially children and pets, should be examined as possible sources of infection.

C. Clean all contaminated objects (e.g., hairbrushes, combs) to help prevent reinfection.

D. Reassure caretakers that it may take up to 1 month to see improvement, especially with kerions.

TINEA CORPORIS ICD-9 (110.5)

Tinea corporis is a dermatophyte infection on the trunk, limbs, or face. Disease onset typically begins as an isolated lesion, with subsequent development of satellite areas. Tinea corporis may be acquired from direct human contact, animal exposure, or, rarely, from the soil, and affects people of all ages.

Majocchi's granuloma, or granulomatous type of tinea corporis, occurs most commonly on the legs of women, with lesions characterized by follicular involvement. The disease often does not present as a typical annular plaque but as nodules or follicular pustules, with significant erythema and exudate.

I. CLASSIC DESCRIPTION
Primary: Papules, plaques
Secondary: Erythema, scale
Lesions typically are annular, with peripheral enlargement, central clearing, and well-demarcated margins (Fig. 10–3).

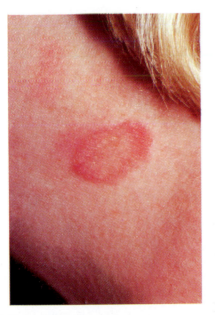

Fig. 10–3
Tinea corporis. Note well-demarcated erythematous plaques with central clearing and peripheral scale.

II. DIAGNOSIS
A. *Perform a direct KOH microscopic examination* of *scale from a leading edge* of a lesion, not from the center, to look for hyphae.
B. *Majocchi's granuloma, or granulomatous type of tinea corporis:* Examine plucked hairs for hyphae. If negative, consider obtaining a 3- to 4-mm punch biopsy specimen and requesting stains for fungi.
C. Prior use of topical corticosteroids may alter the presentation by decreasing the inflammatory response while still allowing for fungal growth. In such cases, classic central clearing with raised edges may not be present.

III. DIFFERENTIAL DIAGNOSIS
A. **Nummular eczema:** Lesions are diffuse and small, and the KOH preparation is negative.
B. **Pityriasis rosea:** Onset is acute, usually with a recent viral illness. Look for multiple small, symmetric papules and plaques that are KOH-negative.
C. **Psoriasis:** Scales are thick and silvery, there is no central clearing, and the KOH is negative.
D. **Granuloma annulare:** No scale is present.
E. **Lyme disease:** Erythema migrans lesions lack scale and are KOH-negative.

IV. TREATMENT
A. **Topical antifungal agents:** (Tables 10–1 and 10–3)
1. First-line therapy. Choose one agent and use as directed.
2. Some of the newer prescription antifungal agents have the advantage of once-a-day dosing and a broader spectrum of activity, but most medications, including nonprescription drugs, also are effective.

TABLE 10–3.

Topical Agents for Fungi and Yeast

Trade Name	Generic Name	Packaging	Dosage
Exelderm*	Sulconazole	Cream: 15, 30, 60 g Solution: 30 ml	qd; bid for t. pedis
Lamisil*†	Terbinafine	Cream: 15, 30 g	qd-bid††
Loprox	Ciclopirox olamine	Cream: 15, 30, 90 g Lotion: 30 ml	bid
Lotrimin	Clotrimazole	Cream: 15, 30, 45, 90 g Lotion: 30, 60 ml Solution: 10, 30 ml	bid
Monistat-Derm	Miconazole	Cream: 15, 30, 90 g	bid
Naftin*†	Naftifine	Cream: 15, 30, 60 g Gel: 20, 40, 60 g	qd
Nizoral	Ketoconazole	Cream: 15, 30, 60 g	qd
Oxistat	Oxiconazole	Cream: 15, 30, 60 g Lotion: 30 ml	qd-bid
Spectazole	Econazole	Cream: 15, 30, 85 g	qd, bid for candidiasis

Over-the-counter Preparations

Desenex	Undecylenic acid*†	Cream: 15 g Ointment: 14, 28 g Powder: 43, 85 g Spray powder: 77 g	bid
	Tolnaftate*†	Spray liquid: 100 g	bid
Desenex AF	Clotrimazole	Cream: 15 g	bid
	Miconazole†	Spray powder: 100 g Spray liquid: 100 g	bid
Fungoid Creme	Miconazole†	Cream: 60 g	bid
Lotrimin AF	Clotrimazole	Cream: 12, 24 g Lotion: 20 ml Solution: 10 ml	bid
	Miconazole†	Spray powder: 100 g Spray liquid: 120 g Powder: 90 g	bid
Micatin	Miconazole†	Cream: 15 g	bid
Mycelex	Clotrimazole	Cream: 15 g Solution: 10 ml	bid
Tinactin	Tolnaftate*†	Cream: 15, 30 g Solution: 10 ml Spray: 120 ml Spray powder: 100, 150 g Powder: 45, 90 g	bid

Prescribe 15 g for bid dosage for 2 to 3 weeks to limited areas, such as hands, feet, or a few isolated plaques. For cost effectiveness, if the infection is chronic or recurrent, prescribe a larger quantity. Emphasize that patients need to use ony a small amount of cream at a time and to rub it in until it disappears.

*Not indicated for use in candidal skin infections.

†These preparations are not effective in treating tinea versicolor.

††Use for 1 week or until significantly clinically improved (7 to 28 days).

3. Avoid chronic use of antifungal/corti-costeroid combination products (e.g., *betamethasone dipropionate* [Lotrisone]), especially for tinea cruris or tinea pedis. These products are sometimes initially helpful to control pruritus or inflammation.
B. **Oral agents** should be considered for extensive or resistant disease.
C. **Majocchi's granuloma:** (Table 10–1)
D. **Immunosuppressed patients** (e.g., AIDS): Such patients often require long-term therapy, as well as more more aggressive therapy (e.g., starting with oral therapies).

V. **PATIENT EDUCATION**
   (See patient education handout in Appendix S.)
   A. Continue topical medication for 7 to 14 days beyond clinical cure to prevent relapse.
   B. Try to identify a source of infection (e.g., animal, playmate).

TINEA CRURIS ICD-9 (110.3)

Tinea cruris is a dermatophyte infection of the groin, most commonly involving the upper thigh–intertriginous inguinal folds and occasionally extending onto the buttocks (Fig. 10–4). Predisposing factors include a warm, humid environment, obesity, and tight clothing. *Tinea cruris often is characterized by pruritus or burning sensations.*

I. CLASSIC DESCRIPTION
Distribution: Groin, sparing the scrotum
Primary: Papules, plaques
Secondary: Erythema, scale
Lesions are sharply marginated, with central clearing.

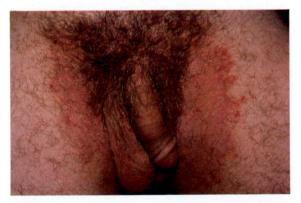

Fig. 10–4
Tinea cruris with well-demarcated erythematous plaques. (Courtesy Department of Dermatology, University of North Carolina at Chapel Hill.)

II. DIAGNOSIS
Perform a direct microscopic examination of scales scraped from the leading edge, cover with 10% KOH, and look for hyphae.

III. DIFFERENTIAL DIAGNOSIS
A. **Candidiasis:** The eruption is beefy red and has poorly defined borders, satellite pustules, and papules; there is often scrotal involvement.
B. **Intertrigo:** An irritant dermatitis, especially in obese patients, where moisture collects between the skinfolds and causes skin irritation. The KOH test is negative.
C. **Erythrasma:** Look for asymmetric velvety patches, fine scales, a negative KOH test, and coral red or pink fluorescence on Wood's lamp examination.
D. **Psoriasis:** Scales are thick, silvery, and adherent, with no central clearing. The KOH test is negative.
E. **Seborrheic dermatitis:** The erythema and scaling are not as well defined, and the scalp, ears, face, and chest are often involved. The KOH test is negative.

IV. TREATMENT
A. **Topical antifungal agents** (Tables 10–1 and 10–3):
   1. Choose one agent and use as directed for 2 to 3 weeks.

2. Some of the newer prescription anti-fungal agents have the advantage of once-a-day dosing and a broader spectrum of activity, but most medications, including the nonprescription drugs, also are effective.
3. Avoid chronic use of antifungal/corticosteroid combination products (*betamethasone dipropionate* [Lotrisone]), especially for tinea cruris or tinea pedis. These products are sometimes initially helpful to control pruritus or inflammation.

B. **Use oral agents in extensive or resistant cases** (Tables 10–1 and 10–2).

C. **Severe inflammatory components:** Use a mild topical steroid, such as *hydrocortisone* 1%, or a moderate topical steroid, such as *triamcinolone* cream 0.1%, for 3 to 7 days, then discontinue to allow healing and to prevent atrophy.

D. **Pruritus relief:** Cetaphil with menthol 0.25%; over-the-counter preparations (e.g., Sarna, Itch X, Prax).

E. **Look for an infection source:** Check feet for tinea pedis as a possible source of infection.

F. **Recurrence:** Usually recurrent in predisposed or immunocompromised people; simple measures may help prevent flare-ups.

V. **PATIENT EDUCATION**
(See patient education handout in Appendix T.)

A. Use topical antifungals (except for terbinafine) for 7 to 14 days beyond clinical cure to prevent relapse.

B. Prolonged topical corticosteroid use, particulary of potent drugs, can produce thinning of the skin and a burning sensation.

C. Educate patients to discontinue use of self-medicating preparations (e.g., alcohol, bleach, neosporin).

D. Avoid hot baths and tight-fitting clothing. Use 100% cotton boxer shorts rather than briefs.

E. Use mild soaps (e.g., White Dove) or a soap substitute (e.g., Cetaphil, Aquanil) if the area is macerated.

F. Antifungal powders (e.g., Zeasorb AF, Desenex) or plain absorbent powders (e.g., Zeasorb) should be used, especially during hot weather. Do not use cornstarch.

G. Keep the area as dry as possible. Use an electric hairdryer on a cool setting to dry the area after showering. Avoid rubbing the area with a towel.

TINEA MANUS ICD-9 (110.2)

Dermatophyte infection of the hand is called *tinea manus. The infection often is unilateral and is virtually always associated with bilateral involvement of the feet.* Tinea manus also may involve the fingernails.

I. **CLASSIC DESCRIPTION** (Fig.10–5)
Primary: Plaque, vesicles
Secondary: Scale, erythema, desquamation
Lesions may show annular or polycylic plaques, especially if they involve the dorsum of the hand. Patients may have only a few isolated vesicles or fine diffuse scaling.

II. **DIAGNOSIS**
Perform a direct microscopic examination of scale or roof of a vesicle with 10% KOH, looking for hyphae. A positive KOH test often is necessary to differentiate this from other disorders with similar features. Check the patient's feet, because with chronic cases the toenails are often involved.

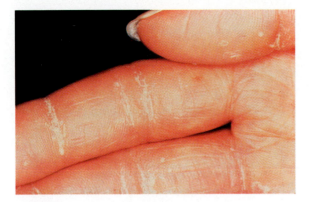

Fig. 10–5
Tinea manus with mild diffuse scaling. (Courtesy Marshall Guill, MD.)

III. DIFFERENTIAL DIAGNOSIS
A. **Eczema:** Eczema usually is bilateral and often has signs elsewhere. The KOH test is negative.
B. **Contact dermatitis:** Acute onset of very pruritic lesions with suspect distribution. Negative KOH test.

C. **Granuloma annulare:** Scale is absent. The KOH test is negative.
D. **Psoriasis:** Pitting nails and signs of psoriasis elsewhere. KOH test is negative.

IV. TREATMENT
A. **Topical antifungal agents** (Tables 10–1, 10–3):
   1. Choose one agent and use as directed for 2 to 4 weeks, except for terbinafine.
   2. Some of the newer prescription antifungal agents have the advantage of once-a-day dosing and a broader spectrum of activity, but most medications, including the nonprescription drugs, also are effective, if the nails are not involved.
B. **Oral agents must be used for fingernail involvement:** (Tables 10–1, 10–2)
C. **Recurrence** is less common with newer agents.

TINEA PEDIS ICD-9 (110.4)

Tinea pedis is a dermatophyte infection involving the feet. Commonly called *athlete's foot,* it's predisposing factors include hot, humid weather and occlusive footwear. Tinea pedis rarely occurs before adolescence.

Secondary eruptions may be present with severe tinea pedis, characterized by papules, vesicles, or bullae at distant sites. Such eruptions represent an immunologic reaction to the fungus and the inflammation. Such lesions, referred to as *dermatophytids,* usually are sterile. The phenomenon, which is not unique to dermatophytes and can occur with any significantly inflamed dermatosis, is referred to as an *id reaction.* The secondary eruption improves with control of the primary infection.

I. CLASSIC DESCRIPTION (Fig. 10–6)
Primary: Plaques, vesicles, bullae
Secondary: Erythema, scale, maceration

Tinea pedis may present with multiple skin variations, ranging from interdigital maceration to fine diffuse scaling to a few isolated vesicles, or as a vigorous vesiculobullous eruption. Interdigital infections often are accompanied by a significant bacterial component.

II. DIAGNOSIS
Although the diagnosis usually is readily accomplished by clinical observation, confirmation is recommended by performing a direct microscopic examination of a scale or the roof of a blister with 10% KOH, to look for hyphae. The toenails are often infected in chronic cases.

III. DIFFERENTIAL DIAGNOSIS
A. **Eczema:** KOH testing is the only reliable way to differentiate these lesions. Look for signs of eczema elsewhere.

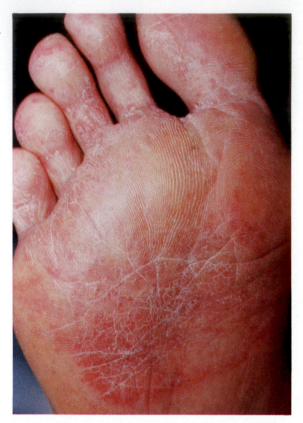

Fig. 10–6
Tinea pedis. Note erythematous, scaling plaques. (Courtesy Department of Dermatology, University of North Carolina at Chapel Hill.)

B. **Contact dermatitis:** The distribution usually is symmetric and located on the dorsum or sole of the foot (e.g., where rubber sneakers contact the foot). The KOH test is negative.

C. **Psoriasis:** Look for signs of psoriasis elsewhere, along with a negative KOH test.

D. **Keratolysis exfoliativa:** Desquamation is often the only finding, and the KOH test is negative.

E. **Toe web infection:** Usually a mixed infection of bacteria, yeast, and/or fungus; look for maceration in the interdigital web spaces. The KOH prep may be negative.

F. **Juvenile plantar dermatosis:** Usually found in prepubertal children. The KOH is negative and there is a history of excessive perspiration, especially wet socks.

IV. TREATMENT

A. **Topical antifungal creams** (Tables 10–1, 10–3):
1. Choose one agent and use as directed for 1 to 4 weeks.
2. Some of the newer prescription antifungal agents have the advantage of once-a-day dosing and a broader spectrum of activity, but most medications, including the nonprescription drugs, also are effective, if the nails are not involved.
3. Long-term therapy often is indicated.

B. **Oral antibiotics:** Use if secondarily infected.

C. **Oral antifungal agents:** (Tables 10–1, 10–2): May be necessary for resistant, recurrent, or extensive cases and always with toenail involvement if attempting to "cure" the toenail component.

D. **Maceration:** If significant, consider Burow's solution soaks for 15 to 20 minutes 2 or 3 times a day, along with elevation of the feet.

E. **Severe inflammation:** Topical and/or oral corticosteroids may be indicated for 5 to 7 days.

V. PATIENT EDUCATION

(See patient education handout in Appendix U.)

A. Use 100% cotton socks to reduce moisture. Nylon socks allow moisture to accumulate.

B. Aerate feet as much as possible; wear sandals or go barefoot.

C. Antifungal powders and creams (e.g., Desenex, Tinactin, Zeasorb AF) may help to control chronic infection and to prevent recurrence.

TINEA VERSICOLOR ICD-9 (111.0)

Tinea versicolor is a common superficial infection caused by a yeast-like organism, *Pityrosporum orbiculare (Malessezia furfur)*. Versicolor refers to the variety and changing shades of colors present in this disease. Tinea versicolor typically involves the upper trunk and extremities but may also involve the face and intertriginous areas, limiting its infection to the outermost layers of the skin (Fig. 10–7). It is most evident in the summer because the organism produces azelaic acid, which inhibits pigment transfer to keratinocytes, thereby making infected skin more demarcated from uninfected, evenly pigmented skin. Predisposing factors include hot, humid weather and use of oils.

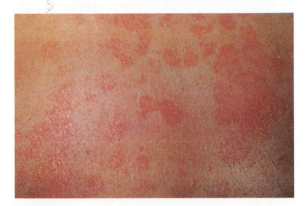

Fig. 10–7
Tinea versicolor. Note individual and coalescing erythematous lesions with a fine brawny scale. (Courtesy Department of Dermatology, University of North Carolina at Chapel Hill.)

I. CLASSIC DESCRIPTION
Primary: Macule, plaque
Secondary: Scale, erythema, hypopigmentation
A fine scale is apparent, especially after scraping.

II. DIAGNOSIS
Perform a direct microscopic examination of scale with 10% KOH to look for hyphae and spores (often described as "spaghetti and meatballs"; see Fig. 3–4).

III. TREATMENT (Tables 10–1, 10–2, 10–3)
A. **Use topical therapies for limited disease.**
B. **Use oral therapies for extensive or recalcitrant infection.** (Note: Griseofulvin is not active against this organism.)
C. **Prevention:** Prophylactic monthly use of selenium sulfide lotion during warm weather is helpful in preventing recurrences.

IV. PATIENT EDUCATION
(See patient education handout in Appendix V.)
A. Educate patients to avoid the use of skin oils.
B. Explain that suntanning will make lesions more evident and that pigmentation irregularities may take several months to resolve after the infection has been eliminated.
C. Emphasize that although infection tends to be recurrent, patients can easily treat themselves, with good response.

CANDIDIASIS ICD-9 (MOUTH 112.0; VULVA/VAGINA 112.1; BALANITIS 112.2; SKIN, NAILS 112.3)

Intertriginous Areas

Intertriginous candidal infections frequently involve large skinfolds, such as those beneath pendulous breasts, overhanging abdominal folds, the groin, rectum, and axillae, or even between the fingerwebs (Fig. 10–8). Hot, humid weather, tight underclothing, and underlying diabetes can make a yeast infection more likely. Fingerweb infections often are seen in patients whose occupations require that they work in a wet environment (e.g., dentists, bakers, dishwashers). The scrotum frequently is involved in male patients.

I. CLASSIC DESCRIPTION

Primary: Plaque, pustules, papules
Secondary: Erythema, scale, maceration, fissures, exudate
Lesions are beefy red, with satellite erythematous papules and/or pustules. A KOH preparation of the scale or exudate will demonstrate pseudohyphae and spores.

II. DIFFERENTIAL DIAGNOSIS

A. Tinea: Lesions have well-defined borders, there are no satellite lesions, and the scrotum is not involved.

B. Intertrigo: The KOH is negative and environmental measures must be used for treatment.

III. TREATMENT

A. Topical antifungal creams (Tables 10–1, 10–3) once or twice a day for limited involvement.

B. Use oral therapies for extensive or recalcitrant infection. (Note: Griseofulvin is not active against this organism.)

C. Environmental measures:
   1. Zeasorb powder is useful to reduce moisture.
   2. If there is maceration, use Burow's soaks for 15 to 20 minutes 3 times a day.

D. Mild topical corticosteroid creams may be used as antiinflammatory agents for 1 to 2 weeks.

IV. PATIENT EDUCATION

A. Discuss the role of moisture control; suggest ways to decrease moisture (e.g., wearing loose undergarments, cool blow-drying of the skin after showers).

B. Tell patients to apply creams sparingly and to rub in creams until they disappear; creams left on "creamy" can cause even more maceration.

C. Avoid use of cornstarch; it may promote growth of Candida organisms.

D. Change diapers frequently or leave off as much as possible.

E. Control underlying diabetes mellitus, if present.

Mucous Membranes

Oral candidiasis, or thrush, is caused by *C. albicans* (Fig. 10–9). Healthy infants are susceptible, especially after administration of antibiotics. Oral candidiasis can develop in adults with diabetes, in elderly patients, after administration of antibiotics or immunosuppressant agents, and in any person with a depressed immune system (e.g., by cancer or AIDS).

I. CLASSIC DESCRIPTION

Look for white, creamy exudates or white, adherent flaky plaques that, when scraped

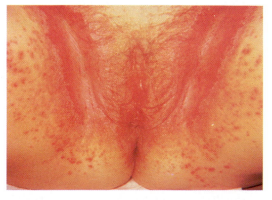

Fig. 10–8
Candidal intertrigo. Note erythematous plaques with multiple satellite papules. (Courtesy Beverly Sanders, MD.)

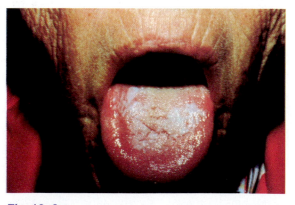

Fig. 10–9
Oral candidiasis. White, creamy exudate is KOH-positive. (Courtesy Beverly Sanders, MD.)

with a tongue blade, appear beefy red and superficially eroded.

II. DIAGNOSIS
A KOH preparation of tongue blade scrapings of the white exudate will demonstrate pseudohyphae and/or spores.

III. TREATMENT (Tables 10–1, 10–2)

Balanitis

Candidal balanitis is an infection of the penis, particularly the glans, with *C. albicans* (Fig. 10–10). It occurs after sexual exposure with an infected partner or in men with diabetes mellitus.

I. CLASSIC DESCRIPTION
Primary: Plaques
Secondary: Erosion, erythema, scale, exudate

II. DIAGNOSIS
A KOH preparation from tongue blade scrapings of the white exudate will demonstrate pseudohyphae and/or spores.

III. DIFFERENTIAL DIAGNOSIS
A. **Erythroplasia of Queyrat:** Velvety erythematous plaques in erythroplasia of Queyrat will be KOH-negative, and biopsy will confirm the diagnosis.
B. **Erythema multiforme:** Erythema multiforme lesions involving the glans are erosive, KOH-negative, and associated with lesions elsewhere.
C. **Fixed drug eruptions:** Fixed drug eruptions involving the glans leave classically hyperpigmented plaques (KOH-negative), which recur on repeated exposure to the same medication.
D. **Contact dermatitis:** Contact dermatitis from topical preparations or poison ivy is characterized by acute onset of pruritic,

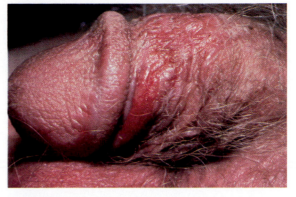

Fig. 10–10
Candidal balanitis. Note beefy red erosion with white exudate. (Courtesy Department of Dermatology, University of North Carolina at Chapel Hill.)

often vesicular, lesions (KOH-negative), which may have marked edema.
E. **Seborrheic dermatitis:** Fine scaling with slight erythema is KOH-negative.

IV. TREATMENT (Tables 10–1, 10–3)
A. **Use topical antifungal creams** once or twice a day for limited involvement.
B. **Use oral therapies for recalcitrant disease.** (Note: Griseofulvin is not active against this organism.)
C. **Laboratory measures:** Consider checking blood glucose level, especially for recurrent or recalcitrant disease.

V. PATIENT EDUCATION
A. Emphasize that the partner also will need treatment if the infection results from sexual exposure.
B. Follow-up in 4 to 6 weeks is necessary to ensure that the disease has resolved (e.g., so as not to miss a smoldering Bowen's cancer).

SUGGESTED READING

Brodell RT, Elewski BE: Clinical pearl: systemic antifungal drugs and drug interactions, *J Am Acad Dermatol* 33:259–260, 1995.

Degreef HJ, DeDoncker PR: Current therapy of dermatophytosis, *J Am Acad Dermatol* 31:S25–S30, 1994.

Drake LA et al: Guidelines of care for superficial mycotic infections of the skin: mucocutaneous candidiasis, *J Am Acad Dermatol* 34:110–115, 1996.

Elewski B, Silverman RA: Clinical pearl: diagnostic procedures for tinea capitis, *J Am Acad Dermatol* 34:498–499, 1996.

Frieden IJ, Howard R: Tinea capitis: epidemiology, diagnosis, treatment, and control, *J Am Acad Dermatol* 31:S42–S46, 1994.

Gupta AK, Sauder DN, Shear NH: Antifungal agents: an overview. I, *J Am Acad Dermatol* 30:677–698, 1994.

Gupta AK, Sauder DN, Shear NH: Antifungal agents: an overview. II, *J Am Acad Dermatol* 30:911–933, 1994.

Hay RJ: Antifungal therapy of yeast infection, *J Am Acad Dermatol* 31:S6–S9, 1994.

Honig PJ et al: Treatment of kerions, *Pediatr Dermatol* 11:69–71, 1994.

CHAPTER 11

Hair and Nails

Hair and nail conditions are frequently encountered dermatologic complaints that cause significant morbidity as a result of their local destructive effects on physical appearance. Hair loss, or alopecia, is classified broadly as either scarring or nonscarring (Table 11–1). Scarring alopecia refers to hair loss with which there is fibrosis and scar tissue replacing, and often permanently destroying, the hair follicle. Nonscarring alopecia refers to hair loss with which there is no permanent destruction of the hair follicle.

All types of hair loss can be psychologically debilitating to patients, especially because of society's association of hair with body image. The loss of hair, particularly if it occurs acutely, may serve as a major emotional stressor.

Therefore psychologic support is essential for all patients with hair loss. Patients that have an opportunity to express their feelings about their condition may have less overall anxiety.

TABLE 11–1.

Classification of Alopecia

Non-scarring	Scarring
Anagen effluvium	Bullous diseases
Androgenic alopecia	Chemical alopecia
Chemical alopecia	Discoid lupus erythematosus
Folliculitis (mild)	Folliculitis (severe)
Inherited disorders of the hair shaft	Lichen planopilaris
Telogen effluvium	Tumors
Traumatic alopecia	
Trichotillomania	

ALOPECIA AREATA ICD-9 (704.01)

Alopecia areata (from the Greek words meaning *fox mange-like areas of disease*) is a type of hair loss, with an estimated incidence of 1 in 1000 in the general population. The disease produces an area of smooth, discrete hair loss (Fig. 11–1). The cause is not known, but an autoimmune factor has been suggested by biopsy findings of involved areas that demonstrate predominantly T cell infiltrates about the hair follicles. Infrequently, other autoimmune diseases, such as vitiligo, thyroiditis, and pernicious anemia, may be associated with alopecia areata. There is a signif-

icant genetic link, with 20% of patients having a positive family history of the disease. Although some patients report severe stress, especially emotional stress, as a precipitating event, many patients have no such history.

Typically, hair loss occurs over a period of a few weeks, with regrowth over several months. The disease recurs in as many as a third of patients. Certain prognostic indicators associated with poor chances of regrowth and/or high likelihood of relapse include atopy, prepubertal state, widespread involvement (alopecia totalis,

111

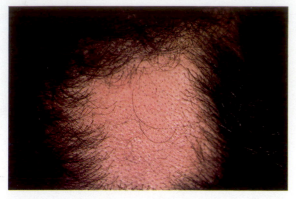

Fig. 11–1
Alopecia areata. Note smooth, discrete area of hair loss.
(Courtesy Department of Dermatology, Medical College of
Georgia.)

i.e., entire scalp hair loss; alopecia universalis,
i.e., scalp, body, and facial hair loss), duration of
more than 5 years, and involvement of the peripheral scalp, or ophiasis. *Ninety percent of discrete patchy hair loss will regrow within 2 years.*

I. CLASSIC DESCRIPTION

Distribution: Most commonly on the scalp,
but may occur on any hair-bearing area
Primary: Alopecia
Secondary: None
Patients usually have smooth, circular, dis-
crete areas of complete hair loss. These
patches may coalesce into bizarre patterns.
Black dots of hairs broken off a few millime-

ters from the scalp ("exclamation point"
hairs; Fig. 11–1, 11–2) are found at expanding edges. Areas of regrowth often are characterized initially by fine, white vellus hairs
(Fig. 11–3). Nail involvement is characterized by fine pitting of the proximal
nailplates.

II. DIAGNOSIS

The diagnosis is made clinically on the
basis of smooth, discrete areas of hair loss.
Exclamation point hairs are present. The
hair root, examined by plucking out the hair,
is narrower and less pigmented than normal. Biopsy specimens usually are not necessary to confirm the diagnosis but, if obtained, should entail a 4- to 6-mm punch
biopsy into the subcutaneous fat from an
expanding area of hair loss.

III. DIFFERENTIAL DIAGNOSIS

A. Tinea capitis: Tinea capitis produces
scaling and possibly inflammation in
areas of hair loss. Alopecia areata produces smooth areas of hair loss, without
any scaling.
B. Secondary syphilis: Areas of hair loss
appear moth-eaten rather than smooth
and discrete, as in alopecia areata.
Serologic testing may be necessary for
differentiation.
C. Discoid lupus erythematosus: Inflammation is present, with plugged, promi-

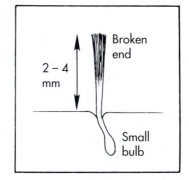

Fig. 11–2
Exclamation point hairs of alopecia areata.

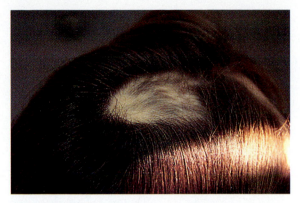

Fig. 11–3
Areas of regrowth in alopecia areata demonstrating fine, light-colored hairs.

nent follicles and scale. Scarring of hair follicles results in permanent hair loss and pigmentary alterations frequently are present.

D. **Androgenetic alopecia:** Onset of hair loss is gradual and with a typical distribution pattern. No exclamation point hairs are found.

E. **Nervous hair pulling (trichotillomania):** There is a bizarre pattern of broken hairs of varying length, as compared with the smooth hair loss of alopecia areata. A biopsy in the area of alopecia will help differentiate the two conditions.

IV. **TREATMENT**

A. **Intralesional corticosteroids:** Treatment of choice for isolated patches of hair loss.
   1. *Triamcinolone* 2.5 to 5.0 mg/ml intradermally on the face for eyebrow or beard involvement and concentrations of 10 to 15 mg/ml on the scalp.
   2. May repeat treatment every 6 to 8 weeks.
   3. Side effects include atrophy, hypopigmentation, and systemic absorption.
   4. Pretreatment with topical anesthetic cream (e.g., lidocaine 2.5% and prilocaine 2.5% EMLA cream, 5 g, 30 g). Apply the cream *generously,* under

occlusion with a tightly fitting shower cap or plastic wrap, 1.5 to 2 hours before treatment.

B. **Potent topical corticosteroids:**
   1. *Betamethasone dipropionate 0.05%* (cream, lotion, ointment) to affected areas and 1 centimeter beyond, twice a day. If a large area is involved, treat the entire scalp.
      a. Use for 3 months, then evaluate treatment.

C. *Anthralin* (Drithocreme 0.5%, 1%; Micanol 1%, 50 g): Often used with recalcitrant psoriasis and is also useful in alopecia areata instead of topical steroids.
   1. Start with 0.5% or 1.0% cream to the affected area and 1 centimeter beyond or to the entire scalp for widespread involvement; leave on for 10 to 20 minutes, then rinse off with cool to lukewarm water. Follow with any shampoo.
   2. An irritant reaction with erythema and scaling occurs. This irritant reaction is desired but should not be allowed to become frankly vesicular.
   3. Warn patients that the preparation will stain hair, scalp, and clothing brown. Wash hands immediately after application with cool to lukewarm water.
   4. Use for 3 months before reevaluating for treatment effectiveness.

D. *Minoxidil* **2% solution:** (OTC)
   1. Use twice daily in combination with *betamethasone dipropionate* in children or adults or with *anthralin* in adults.
   2. This treatment does not induce remission and continued application is required to maintain growth.
   3. Use for 3 months before evaluating effectiveness.
   4. A 5% solution may be more effective.

E. **Oral corticosteroids:** May cause short-term regrowth; however, after treatment is discontinued, any hair regrown as a result of therapy usually will be lost. It is important to weigh the risks of long-term corticosteroid therapy in a disorder such as this, remembering that systemic steroids are not a recommended treatment regimen.

F. Consider screening for underlying autoimmune diseases infrequently associated with alopecia areata, if the history or exam are suggestive (e.g., thyroid disease; more rarely, pernicious anemia).

G. Emotional support:

1. Support is critical because this disease can be devastating for some patients. In children, often it is the parents whose reactions must be addressed for the child to adjust to the hair loss.

2. Wigs or hair pieces may be useful cosmetically and will not adversely influence hair regrowth.

3. The National Alopecia Areata Foundation, a national support group, publishes a newsletter and provides names of local support groups.*

H. Referral is appropriate if the diagnosis is in question or to assist in management.

V. PATIENT EDUCATION

A. Explain in detail that although any of the treatments discussed can induce resumption of normal hair growth, none will cure or alter the course.

B. Encourage the patient to contact the national support group for further information.†

TELOGEN EFFLUVIUM ICD-9 (704.02)

Telogen effluvium is an elegant name for a cosmetically unacceptable disease. Defined as *hair that flows out,* telogen effluvium is the most common cause of diffuse hair loss. The disease involves reversible diffuse loss of mature, terminal hairs, usually secondary to a significant stress (Box 11–1).

Understanding the normal hair cycle (Fig. 11–4) helps explain the characteristics of this disease. At any one time, 80% to 90% of hairs are in the growth, or *anagen,* phase, which typically lasts 2 to 3 years; 1% to 3% will be in the short transition, or *catagen,* stage, which lasts for 2 to 3 weeks; and the remaining 5% to 10% will be in the resting, or *telogen,* phase, which usually lasts 3 to 4 months. The telogen hairs are characterized by a mature root sheath, or "club," at the proximal end (Fig.11–4).

Normal hair loss averages 100 hairs per day. In telogen effluvium, rather than 1% to 5% of hair being lost in a staggered fashion, a stress triggers more hairs into the telogen phase, causing diffuse hair loss that peaks approximately 3 to 4 months after the inciting event. Usually up to 50% of the hair must be lost before it is

BOX 11–1.

Causes of Diffuse Hair Loss

Chronic inflammatory scalp disease
Connective tissue disease
Crash diet
Emotional stress
Hypervitaminosis A
Inherited hair shaft disorder
Iron deficiency anemia
Medications
Nutritional deficiency (zinc/biotin)
Postpartum
Postsurgery
Severe systemic disease (including HIV)
Syphilis
Thyroid disease

cosmetically apparent. Therefore the clinician should not discount complaints of hair loss in someone who still has a full head of hair.

*710 C St. No. 11, San Rafael, CA 94901 or P.O. Box 150760, San Rafael, CA 94915-0760; 415-456-4644; FAX 415-456-4274.

†Alopecia areata internet resource for information: http://weber.u.washington.edu/~dvictor/alopecia.html

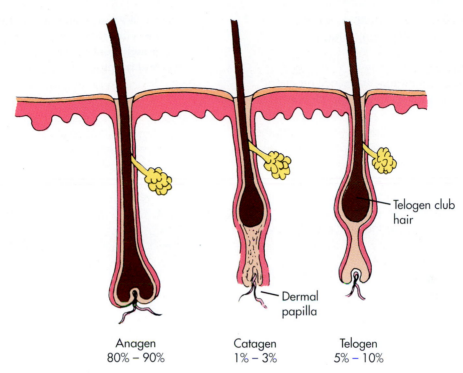

Anagen
80% – 90%

Catagen
1% – 3%

Telogen
5% – 10%

— Telogen club hair

— Dermal papilla

Fig. 11–4
Normal hair cycle and types of hairs.

I. CLASSIC DESCRIPTION

Distribution: Scalp
Primary: Diffuse alopecia
Secondary: None

II. DIAGNOSIS

A. Pull test: Pull gently on 2 to 3 dozen hairs at the same time. Obtaining more than 5 telogen (club) hairs is abnormal.

B. Patients should perform daily counts of hair loss. When the disease peaks, as many as several hundred hairs may be lost each day. The hairs should be mature, telogen hairs (see Fig. 11–5).

C. The patient's history should reveal an inciting event.

III. DIFFERENTIAL DIAGNOSIS

A. **Anagen effluvium** involves loss of growing (anagen) hair. Because the majority of hair is in this phase, acute loss involves 80% to 90% of hair. Disease re-

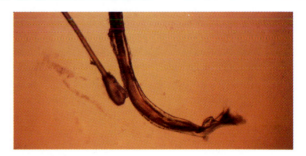

Fig. 11–5
Microscopic examination of telogen *(left)* and anagen *(right)* hairs. (Courtesy Department of Dermatology, University of North Carolina at Chapel Hill.)

sults from alkylating, antimitotic, or cytotoxic agents (e.g., cancer chemotherapy) 10 to 14 days after insult.

B. **Androgenetic alopecia** involves gradual, not acute, loss of hair from the vertex or frontal hairline. In women the disease can be diffuse and difficult to discern clinically from telogen effluvium.

IV. TREATMENT

A. Identify the cause: If no inciting event can be identified, check for other causes of diffuse hair loss, particularly medications (Box 11–2). Consider obtaining the following laboratories: thyroid panel, ferritin, and CBC.

B. Reassure patients that they will not lose all of their hair, that the process is usually reversible, and that regrowth should occur over the next 3 to 4 months.

V. PATIENT EDUCATION

A. Styling options (e.g., permanents) may help existing hair look fuller and will not cause damage.

B. Shampoos such as Progaine (by Upjohn and available in pharmacies) or Vivagen (by Redken and available in hair salons) also will help existing hair look fuller.

C. Regrowth will become evident only after several months.

BOX 11–2.

Some Medications Associated With Hair Loss

Allopurinol	Lithium
Amitriptyline	Lovastatin
Anticoagulants	Methysergide
Antithyroid drugs	Metoprolol
Bromocriptine	Nitrofurantoin
Carbamazepine	Oral contraceptives
Chemotherapeutic agents	Probenecid
Colchicine	Propanolol
Doxepin	Retinoids
Gemfibrozil	Sulfasalazine
Haloperidol	Trimethadione
Indomethacin	Valium
Interferon	Valproic Acid
Levodopa	Vitamin A (excessive)

ANDROGENETIC ALOPECIA ICD-9 (704.00)

Androgenetic alopecia, more simply known as *increasing scalp visibility in a typical distribution,* affects approximately 30% to 40% of adult men and women. Characterized by partial hair loss from the vertex of the scalp, it is typically more diffuse and rarely complete in women, usually in an **M**-shaped pattern in the frontal hair line in men and a more diffuse pattern in women (Fig. 11–6). The incidence increases in women around menopause.

The mechanism of "loss" is due to the shortening of the growth phase (anagen hair cycle), with subsequent production of a shorter, thinner hair shaft, and is often called *follicular miniaturization.* Causes of this miniaturization include genetic influences in which there is a hormonal processing defect at the follicular level.

I. CLASSIC DESCRIPTION

Distribution: Vertex of scalp and frontal hair line; vertex loss is typically more diffuse in women

Primary: Alopecia
Secondary: None

II. DIAGNOSIS

When evaluating females with pattern hair loss, a family history of similar alopecia is especially important. Diffuse vertex thinning in women may provide a problem in diagnosis. Examine the scalp for other signs of hair disease, such as scarring or follicular plugging, that could cause permanent hair loss. Rule out other causes of diffuse hair loss, such as illness, medications, or trauma. Although most women are endocrinologically normal, take a careful history and look for any signs of androgen excess in women, such as menstrual irregularities, acne, hirsutism, or other signs of virilization.

III. DIFFERENTIAL DIAGNOSIS

A. Androgen excess syndrome in women: Inquire about the patient's men-

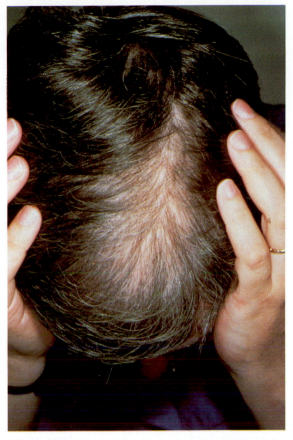

Fig. 11–6
Androgenetic alopecia in a woman. (Courtesy Elise Olsen, MD.)

strual history, any fertility problems, new onset of acne, or signs of hirsutism (often women use techniques to hide hirsutism, so it is important to ask, not just look, for hirsutism).

B. Telogen effluvium: Androgenetic alopecia in women may be so diffuse that it may be difficult to distinguish it from the diffuse hair loss of telogen effluvium. Telogen effluvium is usually associated with an acute event, the results of the hair pull are positive, and a history of a precipitating event or drug is helpful. A biopsy specimen (4 to 6 mm) from an area of alopecia may be helpful to distinguish the condition.

C. Diffuse alopecia areata: This type of alopecia is usually more acute in onset than androgenetic alopecia, does not follow a classic distribution, and is associated with hair loss on other body sites.

IV. TREATMENT

A. Topical *minoxidil* 2% solution, 60 ml (OTC).
   1. A normal, healthy scalp is required to use this medication.
   2. Use 1 ml bid to involved areas on a dry scalp.
   3. Hair shedding usually decreases within 2 months of starting treatment. Hair growth may be seen within 4 to 8 months and stabilizes at 12 to 18 months.
   4. Cosmetically significant hair growth occurs in only 30% to 40% of patients.
   5. The best results are obtained if the baldness pattern is present for less than 5 years, involves a vertex location, and is less than 10 cm in diameter.
   6. Treatment must be continued indefinitely; once discontinued, any hair maintained or regrown as a result of the medication will be lost.
   7. Side effects most common, although infrequent, are contact and irritant dermatitis. Patients with a history of cardiovascular disease should be educated to watch for tachycardia, edema, or weight gain, because systemic absorption can occur if the scalp skin barrier is not intact.
   8. Topical *minoxidil* 5% solution (not FDA approved as of 1/97) may be more effective than the 2% solution.

B. Surgical options, including referral to a dermatologist or plastic surgeon, may be successful in appropriate patients.
   1. Hair transplantation or flaps.
   2. Scalp reduction.

C. Psychologic support:
   1. Support is essential for both men and women, because hair is associated

with total self-image, and hair loss can serve as a major emotional stressor.

2. Allow patients the opportunity to express their feelings about their condition. Monitor closely for associated signs or symptoms of depression or anxiety.

D. Rule out androgen excess syndrome if the history is appropriate in women with male-pattern hair loss. Laboratory tests should include free testosterone, dehydroepiandrosterone sulfate (DHEAS), and prolactin levels. If virilizing tumors have been excluded and there is evidence of excessive production of androgens by the ovaries, patients 20 to 40 years old may be candidates for treatment with birth control pills with a low androgenic potential (e.g., Demulen 1/35). Antiandrogens, such as spironolactone, may be effective in women with elevated adrenal androgens.

V. PATIENT EDUCATION

A. Discourage use of hair treatments and tonics; they are unproved, often expensive, and possibly damaging to remaining hair.

B. Explain that minoxidil solution is to be used for an indefinite time and that it is not usually covered by insurance.

C. Emphasize that minoxidil is a scalp treatment, not a hair treatment, and must be used exactly as prescribed for maximum benefit.

D. Explain that minoxidil solution must be used twice a day for at least 4 months before evaluating the initial response to therapy.

E. Pictures before initiating therapy and 4 months later may be helpful to document for patients any change in appearance.

F. Offer psychologic support.

G. For more information, contact a support group for men.*

TRAUMATIC ALOPECIA ICD-9 (704.9)

Traumatic alopecia (Fig. 11–7) includes alopecia caused by mechanical traction, chemical trauma, and trichotillomania (nervous, self-induced hair pulling). Styling techniques that call for chronic tension on the hair, repeated use of lye-containing chemicals for hair straightening, or hot oils for styling may cause a reversible loss of hair; however, if use of these techniques continues, the hair loss may become permanent. In addition, habits of pulling, twisting, and plucking hairs cause a bizarre distribution of broken off hairs, which is initially reversible but may become permanent if the habits persist.

I. CLASSIC DESCRIPTION

Distribution: Scalp; varies with styling techniques; hair loss most prominent where greatest tension occurs; with trichotillomania, bizarre, asymmetric, and irregular hair loss pattern is characteristic

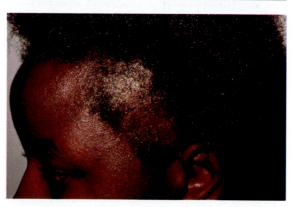

Fig. 11–7
Traumatic alopecia secondary to use of a hot comb. (Courtesy Department of Dermatology, University of North Carolina at Chapel Hill.)

*Bald-Headed Men of America, 901 Arendell St., Morehead City, NC 28557.

Primary: Alopecia; follicular pustules
Secondary: Rare; if present, usually erythema from chronic use of hot oils

II. DIAGNOSIS

Diagnosis is based on the unusual pattern of hair loss. A patient's history should include the exact styling techniques and products used. Occasionally a biopsy specimen is necessary to diagnose trichotillomania if the patient denies any hair-pulling habit. On examination, note that hairs are broken off at varying lengths.

III. DIFFERENTIAL DIAGNOSIS

A. **Alopecia areata:** Hairs are not broken off at various lengths. There should be areas of smooth hair loss in round patches.

B. **Tinea capitis:** Scaling is present.

IV. TREATMENT/PATIENT EDUCATION

A. **Decrease tension on hair roots** by altering styling techniques, avoiding styling practices that require tension on the hair (e.g., rollers, hot combing, braiding hair tightly).

B. **Avoid using harsh chemicals** on the hair, especially those containing lye and hot oils for styling.

C. **Identify any habits or tics** causing trichotillomania. If the patient is recalcitrant to simple education, behavior modification therapy usually is successful. *Fluoxetine hydrochloride* (Prozac) 20 to 40 mg a day in adults or *clomipramine* (Anafranil) 25 to 250 mg/day in adults or a maximum of 3 mg/kg/day in children has alleviated compulsive hair pulling in some patients.

D. **Interdisciplinary approach:** The optimal treatment protocol often involves a team approach with the patient, appropriate medical consultants, and social support from family members.

E. **Follow-up:** Regrowth cannot be evaluated for several months, and if the problem is longstanding, the hair loss may be permanent.

HIRSUTISM ICD-9 (704.1)

Hirsutism is the overgrowth of androgen-dependent terminal hairs in female patients, in a male-pattern distribution. Classically, hirsutism is categorized by cause: idiopathic, familial, drug-induced, and androgen excess (Box 11–3). Most hirsutism is either idiopathic, familial, or associated with polycystic ovary syndrome.

I. CLASSIC DESCRIPTION

Distribution: Male-pattern (beard, chest, upper shoulders, groin)
Primary: Excessive growth of terminal hair
Secondary: None

II. DIAGNOSIS

The diagnosis is based on the presence of terminal male-pattern hair growth in women.

III. DIFFERENTIAL DIAGNOSIS

Hypertrichosis is excessive hair growth in non–androgen-dependent areas.

BOX 11–3.

Common Causes of Hirsutism

Idiopathic
Familial
Drug-induced
  Testosterone, danazol, adrenocorticotropin, phenothiazines, anabolic steroids, acetazolamide
Androgen excess
  Ovarian: polycystic ovary syndrome, ovarian tumors
  Adrenal: Cushing's disease, congenital adrenal hyperplasia, adrenal tumors
  Pituitary: Pituitary tumors

IV. TREATMENT

A. **No treatment** is indicated if a hirsute female patient has a normal menstrual history, a family history of female hirsutism, no findings consistent with an endocrine cause of hirsutism, or the condition is cosmetically acceptable.

B. **Androgen excess syndromes:**

1. The onset of rapidly progressive hirsutism after puberty, associated with hair loss, acne, and deepening voice, should increase clinical suspicion for androgen-excess syndrome.

2. Rule out serious underlying disease, such as Cushing's syndrome or congenital adrenal hyperplasia, when the history and physical examination reveal signs or symptoms to direct this workup. Initial screening tests, especially to rule out tumors, may consist of DHEAS and free testosterone. If there is galactorrhea or significant menstrual abnormalities, obtain a prolactin level and consider obtaining cortisol with dexamethasone suppression test, 17-OH progesterone, sex hormone binding globulin, luteinizing hormone and follicle stimulating hormone (FSH) levels.

3. If there is adrenal source of androgen excess, adrenal suppression is indicated (after a tumor has been ruled out):

    a. *Dexamethasone* 0.25 to 0.75 mg hs or

    b. *Spironolactone* 50 to 200 mg/day and contraceptive counseling.

4. If there is ovarian source of androgen excess, ovarian suppression is indicated:

    a. *Spironolactone* 50 to 200 mg/day and contraceptive counseling.

    b. *Oral contraceptives* that have an estrogen component and a progestin component with low androgenic potential (e.g., Desogen, Ortho-cyclen, Brevicon, Demulen-35).

C. **Idiopathic hirsutism:** If the diagnosis is idiopathic hirsutism and the condition bothers the patient, consider using

spironolactone 50 to 200 mg/day as an androgen antagonist. Such therapy may cause significant reduction in hair growth rate and hair shaft diameter in 20% to 40% of patients after 6 months of therapy. *Flutamide* or *finasteride* may be alternatives in patients with severe disease.

D. **Cosmetic treatments** for removal of excess hair:

1. Temporary:

    a. *Bleaching:* Available in pharmacies OTC, bleaching products are used widely for hair on the upper lip and arms; although painless, it may cause a secondary irritant reaction.

    b. *Shaving:* May cause irritation when hair regrows; does not cause the hair to become thicker.

    c. *Waxing:* Application of wax to relatively long hairs; pain and irritation are limiting factors.

    d. *Depilatory creams:* Usually too irritating for regular use on the face.

    e. *Plucking:* Plucking should be discouraged because it leads to ingrown hairs and folliculitis.

2. Permanent:

    a. *Electrolysis* permanently destroys hair follicles by insertion of a fine needle into them and application of electricity to the matrix. Scarring may occur and multiple sessions are required. Discomfort varies among patients and treatment sites.

    b. *Lasers* are being developed for permanent destruction of follicles. Such treatment is expensive, not widely available, and the long-term effects have not been thoroughly evaluated.

V. **PATIENT EDUCATION**

A. Inform patients that shaving will not increase hair growth or change hair texture.

B. Caution patients to test cream depilatories on a small area before applying them to a large area; severe irritant reactions may occur in some people.

C. If the patient decides to pursue electrolysis, inform her that there is no uniform licensing. Tell patients to determine whether the operator uses sterile techniques.

PARONYCHIA ACUTE: ICD-9 (112.3), CHRONIC: ICD-9 (681.02)

Paronychia is an inflammation involving the lateral and posterior fingernail folds (Fig. 11–8). Predisposing factors include overzealous manicuring, diabetes mellitus, and occupations in which a person's hands are frequently immersed in water.

Paronychia may be either acute or chronic. Acute paronychia usually is caused by *Staphylococcus aureus,* and is characterized by the onset of pain and erythema of the posterior or lateral nail folds, with subsequent development of a superficial abscess. Chronic paronychia is usually secondary to *C. albicans,* and often is due to abnormal separation of the proximal nail fold from the nail plate, allowing for colonization. Acute bacterial paronychia can occur along with chronic fungal paronychia.

I. CLASSIC DESCRIPTION
Distribution: Proximal and lateral nailfolds of fingernails
Primary: Acute: pustules
Secondary: Erythema, edema, maceration, scale

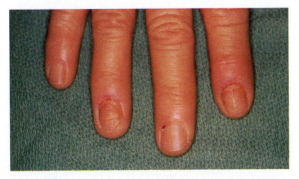

Fig. 11–8
Chronic paronychia with swollen posterior nail folds and nail dystrophy. (Courtesy of Department of Dermatology, University of North Carolina at Chapel Hill.)

II. DIAGNOSIS
The clinical appearance of swollen, tender posterior or lateral nail folds should confirm the diagnosis.

III. DIFFERENTIAL DIAGNOSIS
A. **Subungual onychomycosis:** In onychomycosis the nail plate is friable and the nail folds are not predominantly involved.

B. **Pseudomonal nail infection:** The nail plate has a blue-green tint.

C. **Herpetic whitlow:** Ask the patient about exposure to herpes simplex virus (HSV). Acute onset is associated with vesicles, vesicopustules, severe edema, erythema, or pain. Tzanck staining of vesicles will demonstrate multinucleated giant cells and viral culture will grow HSV.

IV. TREATMENT
A. **Acute paronychia:**
1. Antistaphylococcal agents:
   a. Preferred: *Dicloxacillin* 250 mg tid or *cephalexin* 500 mg tid.
   b. Alternatives: *Erythromycin* 333 mg tid or *azithromycin* 250 mg, 2 on day 1, then 1 daily for 4 more days.
2. Local care: Warm compresses or soaks to the affected digit for 20 minutes 3 times daily.
3. Incise and drain if an abscess is present.

B. **Chronic paronychia:**
1. Apply 3% *thymol* in 95% *ethanol* (must be compounded by pharmacist) to affected areas 3 times daily.
2. In addition, apply *clotrimazole* 1% solution, *ciclopirox* 1% lotion, or

ketoconazole 2% cream to affected areas twice daily.

C. **Resistance:** If lesions remain unresponsive to therapy, perform a KOH test, Gram's stain, and culture with sensitivities to help direct therapy.

D. **Environmental measures:** Have patients keep their hands as dry as possible and use gloves for all wet work.

V. PATIENT EDUCATION

A. Emphasize the importance of patients protecting their hands from moisture (e.g., wearing cotton-lined gloves for wet work).

B. Educate patients to be less aggressive in manicuring.

INGROWN TOENAIL ICD-9 (703.0)

Ingrown toenail is one of the most common conditions of patients seen by primary care physicians and is the source of considerable disability. Clinicians may play a great role in treating the primary lesion and in helping patients prevent future lesions. Ingrown toenails occur when the lateral nail plate pierces the lateral nail fold and enters the dermis (Fig. 11–9). Characteristic signs and symptoms include pain, edema, exudate, and granulation tissue. Predisposing factors include poorly fitting shoes, excessive trimming of the lateral nail plate, and trauma.

I. CLASSIC DESCRIPTION

Distribution: Great toenail, most commonly

Primary: None

Secondary: Erythema, edema, exudate

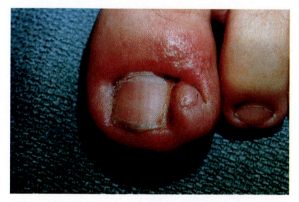

Fig. 11–9
Ingrown toenail. (Courtesy Department of Dermatology, University of North Carolina at Chapel Hill.)

Remember that the lateral nail plate extends into the lateral nailfold.

II. DIAGNOSIS

Diagnosis is based on clinical appearance and rarely is difficult.

III. TREATMENT

A. **Mild to moderate lesion:** Minimal to moderate pain, little erythema, no discharge:

1. Place cotton wedging or dental floss underneath the lateral nail plate to separate the nail plate from the lateral nail fold, thereby relieving pressure (Fig. 11–10).

2. Soak the affected foot in warm water for 20 minutes 3 times a day.

3. Follow up for no improvement, instructing patients on prevention.

B. **Moderate to severe lesion:** Moderate to severe pain, substantial erythema, pustular discharge (Fig. 11–11):

1. Anesthetize with *lidocaine* 1% without epinephrine.

2. Using nail-splitting scissors or hemostat, insert the instrument under the nail plate and remove the involved nail wedge with nail clippers or scissors.

3. Remove any granulation tissue with a curette and/or silver nitrate sticks.

4. Dilute hydrogen peroxide 1:1 with tap water and cleanse the surgical site with cotton swabs 2 or 3 times a day,

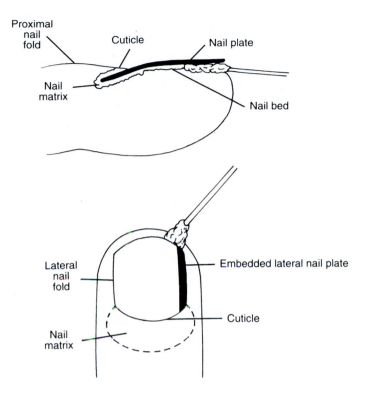

Proximal
nail
fold

Cuticle

Nail plate

Nail
matrix

Nail bed

Lateral
nail
fold

Embedded lateral nail plate

Cuticle

Nail
matrix

Fig. 11–10
Treatment of mild to moderate ingrown toenail by elevation of embedded nail plate.

followed by application of either bacitracin or mupirocin ointment.
5. Treat any secondary infection with
oral antibiotics (e.g., *dicloxacillin*).
6. Follow-up in 3 to 4 days to assess
treatment.
C. **For recurrent ingrown toenail,** consider permanent nail ablation of the lateral nail horn with either phenol or surgical excision. Perform surgical nail
avulsion of involved lateral nail. Then
apply 88% phenol to the lateral nail matrix, with special attention to include the
lateral horns. Repeat 2 to 3 times. Neutralize with water and apply antibacterial
ointment, such as bacitracin, bid until

healed. Surgical ablation is usually best
acheived with electrosurgical techniques, using adapters, which allow
maximum destruction of the matrix. Be
certain to include the lateral nail horns to
prevent regrowth of bothersome nail
spicules.
IV. **PATIENT EDUCATION**
A. Educate patients about proper nail
trimming. The lateral nail plate should
be allowed to grow well beyond the lateral nail fold before trimming
horizontally.
B. Educate patients about the importance
of well-fitting shoes.

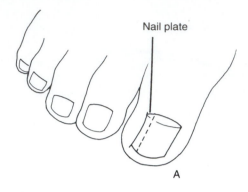

Nail plate

A

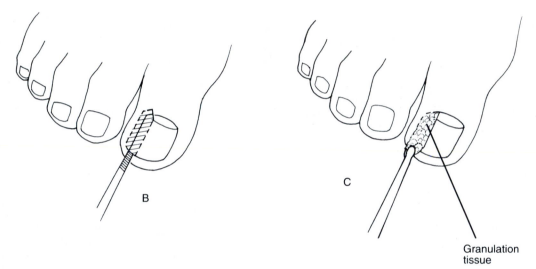

B

C

Granulation
tissue

Fig. 11–11
Treatment of moderate to severe ingrown toenail by surgical removal of embedded nail plate **(A** and **B)** and curettage of granulation tissue **(C).**

ONYCHOMYCOSIS ICD-9 (110.1)

Onychomycosis, or fungal infection of the nail, includes tinea unguium, which is fungal infection of the nail by dermatophytes (90%), nondermatophytic fungi (molds 4%), and yeasts (*Candida, Scytalidium, Trichosporon, Aspergillus, Scopulariopsis,* 6%). Onycholysis is separation of the nail plate distally and laterally from the nail bed. Fungal involvement of the nail causes nail dystrophy, with nail plate thickening, friability,

and crumbling, accounting for the subungual hyperkeratotic scale and debris (Fig. 11–12). Predisposing factors include a positive family history of onychomycosis, abnormal nail anatomy, trauma, and underlying systemic disease (e.g., psoriasis, immunosuppression, poor peripheral circulation).

I. CLASSIC DESCRIPTION
   Distribution: More common on the feet,

especially the great toenails, but may occur on any nail.

II. DIAGNOSIS

The diagnosis is straightforward in a patient with the clinical findings of subungual hyperkeratotic debris, a friable nail, and coexisting tinea pedis. If in doubt, perform a KOH preparation of the subungual debris after trimming back the abnormal nail, using a curette to scrape the most proximal aspect of the infection. Let the KOH test set for at least 10 minutes to aid in viewing. The KOH test is positive in approximately 50% of patients.

III. DIFFERENTIAL DIAGNOSIS

A. **Psoriasis:** Look for psoriatic nail pitting and signs of psoriasis elsewhere on the body. Onychomycosis and psoriasis of the nails may coexist.

B. **Nail dystrophy secondary to eczema:** In eczematous nail changes, the nail plate does not crumble and there is no subungual hyperkeratotic debris. Onychomycosis and eczema of the nails may coexist.

IV. TREATMENT

A. **Oral medications:** (Table 11–2)

B. **Topical therapy:**

1. *Topical therapy alone rarely cures this disease,* but can be used as a supplement to oral therapy to prevent recurrence.

2. Use *sulconazole, econazole, terbinafine, clotrimazole,* or *haloprogin*

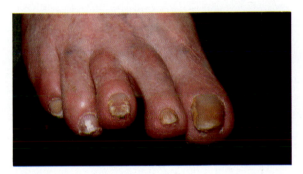

Fig. 11–12
Onychomycosis. Note thickened nails with distal subungual debris. (Courtesy Department of Dermatology, University of North Carolina at Chapel Hill.)

TABLE 11–2.

Oral Treatment for Onychomycosis*

Drug	Dose	Duration	Site
Preferred:			
Terbinafine	250 mg qd	6 wks	Fingernails
	250 mg qd	12 wks	Toenails
Itraconazole	200 mg bid	1 wk each mo for 2-3 mos	Fingernails
	200 mg bid	1 wk each mo for 3-4 mos	Toenails
Alternative:			
Fluconazole	300 mg	2 150 mg tablets once a wk for 3-4 mos	Fingernails
	300 mg	2 150 mg tablets once a wk for 9-12 mos	Toenails

*Itraconazole, ketoconazole, and sometimes fluconazole may have significant drug–drug interactions, See Table 10–2. Laboratory monitoring is indicated in patients with a preexisting history of liver disease or with long-term therapy or signs of hematologic abnormalities with terbinafine, to avoid liver toxicity.

solution twice daily or *naftifine gel* once daily (see Table 10–3). Topical therapy should be started after oral therapy has been completed and continued at least 2 to 3 times a week indefinitely.

3. Some patients with pure toenail involvement may be willing to accept control with topical medications, given the costs of therapy and risks associated with use of oral medications, particularly in patients taking many other medications.

4. Use an antifungal spray in the shoes indefinitely.

C. **Local care:**
   1. Trim back the abnormal nail and scrape away any debris.
   2. Encourage patients to wear protective footwear in common shower areas, pools, and so on.

D. **Consider culturing nail scrapings** on Sabouraud medium with antibiotics to identify the causative organism. Most often, the cause is a dermatophyte that responds to itraconazole, terbinafine, or fluconazole. However some molds and nondermatophyte fungi may be the causative agents. Some of these organisms may not respond to available systemic therapies.

E. **Surgical or chemical nail avulsion** is indicated if there is pronounced nail dystrophy, the infection involves an *isolated* nail, or there is infection caused by a mold that does not respond to oral agents.
   1. Chemical avulsion: 40% urea preparation is available commercially.

a. Apply to the affected nail; instruct the patient to keep the nail dry and covered for 5 to 7 days.
b. Normal skin must be protected with petrolatum; secure paste with a telfa dressing and tape.
c. Scrape away the diseased nail in 5 to 7 days with a curette and begin oral and/or topical therapy.

2. Surgical avulsion:
   a. Anesthesize with lidocaine 1% without epinephrine as a nerve block, followed by local infiltration. Proceed as outlined for ingrown toenail removal.
   b. If more than two or three nails are involved, the prognosis for cure with surgery alone is poor, and avulsion should not be performed.

3. After nail removal, use topical antifungals under occlusion (Bandaid) qhs until a normal nail appears (usually 10 to 12 months).

V. **PATIENT EDUCATION**

A. Educate patients that nails grow slowly and that improvement should be measured over months, not days or weeks. Medications such as *itraconazole* and *terbinafine* will continue to work in the nail bed after the treatment has stopped.

B. Recurrence is seen, even with the newer agents, especially on the toenails. If the patient has no symptoms from the lesions, no treatment might be better than some.

C. Prolonged use of topical antifungal therapy is essential to prevent relapse after completion of oral therapy and avulsion.

SUGGESTED READING

Cohen PR, Scher RK: Topical and surgical treatment of onychomycosis, *J Am Acad Dermatol* 34:S74–S77 1994.

Derksen J et al: Identification of virilizing adrenal tumors in hirsutism in hirsute women, *N Engl J Med* 331:968–973, 1994.

Doncker PD et al: Antifungal pulse therapy for ony-chomycosis, *Arch Dermatol*, 132: 34–41, 1996.

Drake LA et al: Guidelines of care for superfcal my-cotic infections of the skin: onychomycosis, *J Am Acad Dermatol* 34:116–121, 1996.

Fiedler VC: Alopecia areata, *Arch Dermatol* 128:1519–1529, 1992.

Leahy AL et al: Ingrowing toenails: improving treat-ment, *Surgery* 107:566–567, 1990.

Pinner TA, Jones RH, Bandisode MS: Study of efficacy of urea compound versus emollient cream in avul-sive therapy of dystrophic nails, *Cutis* 46:153–157, 1990.

Roberts DT: Oral therapeutic agents in fungal nail dis-ease, *J Am Acad Dermatol* 31:S78–S81, 1994.

Scher RK, Daniel III CR, editors: *Nails: therapy, diag-nosis, surgery,* Philadelphia, 1990, WB Saunders.

Watson RE, Bouknight R, Alguire PC: Hirsutism: eval-uation and management, *J Gen Int Med* 10:282–292, 1995.

CHAPTER 12

Benign Neoplasms

ACROCHORDON (SKIN TAG) ICD-9 (701.9)

Acrochordons, commonly known as *skin tags,* are an outgrowth of normal skin (Fig. 12–1). Twenty-five percent of adults have acrochordons, and there is a familial tendency for these lesions. Acrochordons usually occur in sites of friction and become symptomatic when caught on jewelry or rubbed by clothing. Sometimes they become twisted on their blood supply and turn red or black.

I. CLASSIC DESCRIPTION
Distribution: Axilla, neck, inframammary, inguinal area
Primary: Papules, nodules
Secondary: Hyperpigmentation

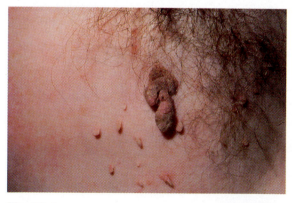

Fig. 12–1
Multiple flesh-colored skin tags. (Courtesy Department of Dermatology, University of North Carolina at Chapel Hill.)

II. DIAGNOSIS
Acrochordons commonly are described as pedunculated lesions on narrow stalks. Diagnosis is based solely on clinical appearance.

III. DIFFERENTIAL DIAGNOSIS
A. **Neurofibromas** usually are larger and firmer than acrochordons.
B. **Pedunculated dermal nevus** sometimes can only be differentiated histologically.
C. **Dermatosis papulosa nigra** is a skin tag variant. Lesions are small, pigmented, pedunculated papules, commonly found on the faces of dark-skinned patients.

IV. TREATMENT
Treatment is indicated if lesions are irritating or a patient desires removal for cosmetic reasons. Local anesthesia with *lidocaine* 1% with *epinephrine,* 0.9% normal saline, or *EMLA* cream may be required in larger lesions. Treatment options include:
A. **Excision** with forceps or fine scissors; larger lesions may require suturing.
B. **Cryosurgery** with liquid nitrogen.
C. **Electrodesiccation.**
D. **Hemostasis:** Lesions often bleed freely. Aluminum chloride, silver nitrate sticks, or electrocautery should be readily available.

V. PATIENT EDUCATION
A. Explain that multiple lesions may develop.

B. Explain that currently there is no way to prevent development of new lesions.

CALLUS/CLAVUS ICD-9 (700)

Calluses and clavi (corns) are among the most frequent skin conditions and may be the source of considerable disability, discomfort, and pain. Many physicians, however, do not feel entirely comfortable examining patients' feet or do not include the foot as part of a routine examination. Considering the degree to which patients' lives are affected by foot problems, the relative ease in diagnosing and treating such conditions, and the great amount of praise that patients bestow on physicians who cure their foot problems, clinicians should strive to master the relatively few conditions that cause the greatest number of problems.

Calluses and corns are two common foot problems that can be readily differentiated and treated. Calluses represent a diffuse thickening of the outermost layer of the skin, the stratum corneum, in response to repeated friction or pressure. Corns represent a similar process, but differ by having a central "core" that is hyperkeratotic and often painful. Corns typically occur at pressure points, secondary to ill-fitting shoes, an underlying bony spur, or abnormal gait.

I. CLASSIC DESCRIPTION
Distribution: Plantar aspect of prominent metatarsals, between toe clefts; dorsal aspect of toe joints
Primary: Papules, plaques
Secondary: Thickening/hyperkeratosis

II. DIAGNOSIS
Clavi (corns) have a central core. The diagnosis is based on clinical appearance (Fig. 12–2).

III. DIFFERENTIAL DIAGNOSIS
Plantar wart: After being pared, warts will have several dark specks that represent punctate capillary thromboses. Warts also disrupt normal skin markings, so that the skin lines are no longer evident. Skin lines are more prominent in callosities.

IV. TREATMENT
A. **Prevention:** Avoid ill-fitting shoes. Consider referring patients for orthotic consultation for fitting innersoles or metatarsal bars.

B. ***Salicylic acid* plasters 40%:** (Available without a prescription).
   1. Debulk the callus or corn by paring skin with a no. 15 scalpel blade.
   2. Cut the plaster to the size of the lesion.
   3. Leave plaster in place for 48 to 72 hours; keep dry.

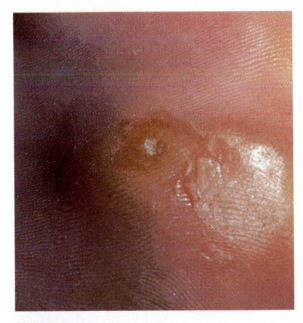

Fig. 12–2
Hyperkeratotic plaques on the sole of the foot, characteristic of clavus and callous. (Courtesy Department of Dermatology, University of North Carolina at Chapel Hill.)

4. Pare down remaining skin; replace plaster patch and let patient resume proper foot care.
5. Follow up if lesions do not resolve.
6. Monitor plaster use carefully in patients with peripheral neuropathies.
C. *Salicylic acid* **10% in petrolatum:** 30 to 45 g (available by prescription and compounded by a pharmacist). Apply at bedtime for maintenance or initially for thinner lesions.
D. **Foot films:** Consider obtaining foot radiographs to evaluate for underlying bony abnormality in lesions that are recalcitrant or recurrent.

V. PATIENT EDUCATION
(See patient education handout in Appendix C.)
A. Educate the patient about the importance of properly fitting shoes.
B. Encourage patients to discuss foot lesions early, before the conditions become chronic.
C. Ask about foot lesions as part of any new patient workup.

CHERRY ANGIOMA ICD-9 (228.01)

Cherry angiomas, also known as *De Morgan's spots,* are mature capillary proliferations and are common in middle-age and elderly patients. Cherry angiomas usually occur as multiple lesions and characteristically bleed profusely with any traumatic rupture.

I. CLASSIC DESCRIPTION (Fig. 12–3)
Distribution: Most commonly on trunk
Primary: Papules
Secondary: Erythema

II. DIAGNOSIS
Cherry angiomas are often dome-shaped and 0.1 to 0.4 cm in diameter. *Lesions always blanch with pressure.*

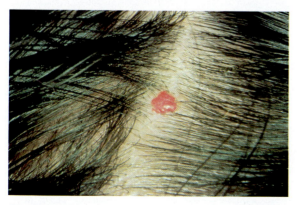

Fig. 12–3
Cherry angioma on scalp. (Courtesy Beverly Sanders, MD.)

III. DIFFERENTIAL DIAGNOSIS
A. **Spitz nevus:** Look for erythematous, isolated, dome-shaped papules or nodules, usually in young children.
B. **Amelanotic melanoma:** Lesions are usually friable and may have recently changed in size or configuration.

IV. TREATMENT
A. **Electrocautery:** Small lesions may be electrocauterized after anesthesia with *lidocaine* 1%. Do not use lidocaine with epinephrine for *small* lesions, because the epinephrine may obscure the lesions.
B. **Shave excision and electrocauterization** of the base may be useful for *larger* lesions.
C. **Pulsed dye vascular laser:** Laser therapy may be useful to remove superficial lesons in isolated cases or for cosmesis, but the high cost rarely warrants this treatment.

V. PATIENT EDUCATION
1. Reassure patients that cherry angiomas are benign.
2. Warn patients that the lesions may bleed profusely if they become traumatized.
3. Explain to patients that many lesions may develop and that there is no known way to prevent new ones.

DERMATOFIBROMA ICD-9 (216.5 TRUNK, .6 UPPER EXTREMITY, .7 LOWER EXTREMITY)

Dermatofibromas are a benign proliferation of fibroblasts that sometimes occur as a result of trauma or insect bites but often are idiopathic. Most patients have isolated lesions, although some have up to 10 at a time. Dermatofibromas are firm, often hyperpigmented nodules, most commonly located on the lower extremities (Fig. 12–4). The lesions usually are asymptomatic but may be pruritic. *Women with dermatofibromas on their legs commonly complain of repeated trauma when shaving their legs and subsequently may seek removal of the lesions.*

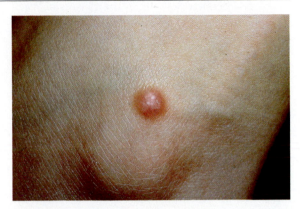

Fig. 12–4
Dermatofibroma on extremity. Note erythematous nodule with rim of hyperpigmentation. (Courtesy Department of Dermatology, University of North Carolina at Chapel Hill.)

I. CLASSIC DESCRIPTION

Distribution: Most common on lower extremities
Primary: Papules, nodules
Secondary: Erythema with rim of hyperpigmentation

II. DIAGNOSIS

Look for discrete, firm lesions, 0.3 to 1.0 cm in diameter, that are nontender and that "buttonhole" or dimple when pinched together, because of the fibrous nature of the lesion. Diagnosis is based on clinical appearance. If the lesion is longstanding, it should have no history of change in appearance.

III. DIFFERENTIAL DIAGNOSIS

A. **Nevus:** Dermatofibromas tend to be firmer than nevi. Nevi do not buttonhole or dimple when pinched.
B. **Basal cell cancer:** Nodular basal cells usually are waxy and have telangiectasias. Biopsy may be necessary to differentiate the two.
C. **Melanoma:** Melanomas are not stable in size, shape, or color. Amelanotic melanomas may initially present as a new pink papule or nodule. A history of any significant change of a lesion should prompt a biopsy.

IV. TREATMENT

A. **Usually, no treatment is required** unless the lesion is symptomatic, has recently changed in size or color, or is bleeding.
B. **When the lesion protrudes above the skin surface and is irritated from repeated trauma, consider partial removal with cryosurgery or shave excision.** Warn patients that the lesion may recur and that the scar may be worse than the initial lesion, especially on the lower extremity. *Excision with suture is indicated for any changing lesion,* because, rarely, dermatofibromas may develop into dermatofibrosarcoma protuberans.

V. PATIENT EDUCATION

A. Explain that removal for cosmetic reasons often results in a scar that looks worse than the initial lesion.
B. Educate patients about the signs and symptoms of abnormal pigmented lesions (e.g., change in size, color, shape, sensation).

EPIDERMAL INCLUSION CYST ICD-9 (706.2)

Epidermal inclusion cysts are discrete nodules that often are referred to erroneously as *seba-* *ceous cysts,* when in fact there is no sebaceous component. The cyst wall consists of normal epidermis that produces keratin. This epidermis may have become lodged in the dermis as a result of trauma or comedone, although often there is no history of an antecedent condition. Lesions may remain stable or progressively enlarge. Spontaneous inflammation and rupture can occur, with significant involvement of surrounding tissue. There is no way to predict which lesions will remain quiescent and which will become larger or inflamed (Fig. 12–5).

Gardner's syndrome is a very rare condition of multiple epidermal inclusion cysts associated with colon cancer. The syndrome is familial and inherited in an autosomal dominant fashion. Cysts are unusual in number and location.

I. CLASSIC DESCRIPTION
Distribution: Face, base of ears, and trunk most commonly
Primary: Cyst, nodule, tumor; often with identifiable central pore
Secondary: None unless inflamed; if inflamed, then erythema, edema, and foul-smelling cheesy exudate

II. DIAGNOSIS
The diagnosis is based on the clinical appearance and palpation of a discrete, freely movable cyst or nodule, often with a central punctum.

III. DIFERENTIAL DIAGNOSIS
A. Pilar cysts occur on the scalp and face

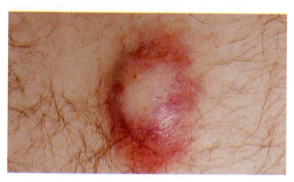

Fig. 12–5
Inflamed epidermal inclusion cyst. (Courtesy Department of Dermatology, University of North Carolina at Chapel Hill.)

and are derived from hair root sheaths. These cysts are benign and can be treated in a similar fashion.

B. Nasal gliomas occur at the nasal root, are often present at birth. These gliomas and other congenital midline facial and scalp lesions may communicate with brain matter and should be evaluated radiographically.

IV. TREATMENT
A. Excise when lesion is not inflamed: The entire cyst wall must be excised or regeneration can occur (see Chapter 3). *When the cyst is acutely inflamed, the cyst wall is very friable and complete excision usually is not possible.* If the cyst is excised while inflamed, recurrence is likely. Wait 4 to 6 weeks after inflammation has resolved before attempting excision.

B. Incise, drain, and pack if inflamed and *fluctuant:*
1. Incise with a no. 11 blade and drain after anesthesia with *lidocaine* 1%.
2. Scrape out the contents with a curette.
3. Place an iodoform gauze wick into the cavity and leave in place for 24 hours.
4. Replace the wick at 24 hours if the cyst is not draining effectively.
5. Treat any secondary infection with oral antibiotics.

C. If inflamed for less than 24 to 48 hours and *not fluctuant:* Consider intralesional *triamcinolone* (Kenalog) 3 mg/ml for the face and 10 mg/ml for the trunk; such therapy may prevent the need for incision and drainage.

V. PATIENT EDUCATION
A. Explain that incision and drainage of acutely inflamed lesions do not prevent recurrence.
B. Explain that despite excision, recurrence of the cyst is still possible, although infrequent.

NEVUS ICD-9 (216- .3 FACE, .4 SCALP AND NECK, .5 TRUNK, .6 UPPER EXTREMITY, .7 LOWER EXTREMITY)

A nevus, or mole, is a benign proliferation of normal skin constituents. Everyone has at least one nevus. *Melanocytic nevus* is a benign proliferation of melanocytes or melanocytic nevus cells that appears in childhood. The number of nevi peaks in early adulthood and decreases thereafter.

Melanocytes present only in the dermal–epidermal junction are referred to as *junctional nevi.* Junctional nevi occur most commonly on the acral surfaces as flat, pigmented macules, but they may occur anywhere. Melanocytes present in the dermal–epidermal junction, as well as the dermis, are referred to as *compound nevi.* Compound nevi are often raised and may even be papillomatous (Fig. 12–6). Melanocytes present in the dermis only are referred to as *dermal nevi.* Dermal nevi typically are flesh-colored (Fig. 12–7).

Congenital nevi are present at birth and have the specific histologic characteristics of nevus cells occurring deep around skin appendages and into the subcutaneous fat. One congenital nevus variant, *giant congenital pigmented hairy nevus,* or bathing trunk nevus, is defined as a

pigmented lesion of melanocytic cells greater than 20 cm in diameter (in adulthood) (Fig. 12–8). Such lesions are important because 3% to 6% may develop into melanomas, most commonly in young children. Because the melanocytes occur deep in the subcutaneous fat and even fascia, excision often is quite disfiguring and may not be feasible. Neural tissue involvement

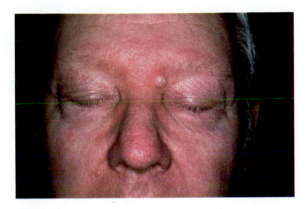

Fig. 12–7
Dermal nevus. Note supraorbital, flesh-colored nodule. (Courtesy Department of Dermatology, Medical College of Georgia.)

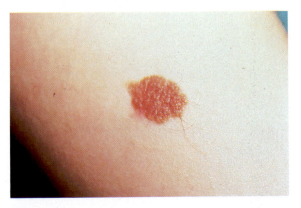

Fig. 12–6
Compound nevus. Note hyperpigmentation and papillomatous surface. (Courtesy Department of Dermatology, University of North Carolina at Chapel Hill.)

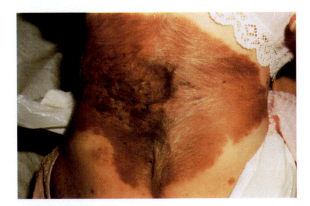

Fig. 12–8
Giant congenital hairy nevus. (Courtesy Department of Dermatology, University of North Carolina at Chapel Hill.)

is not uncommon with extensive lesions of the axial trunk, and melanomas may also develop there.

Dysplastic, or *atypical, nevi* are pigmented lesions with irregular borders, which occur in a variety of colors, ranging from red-pink to brown to tan or, less often, black (Fig. 12–9). Such nevi typically are flat, with raised, palpable components, and are larger than usual nevi (about 1.0 cm; typical nevi are less than 0.6 cm). The severity of disease ranges from atypical isolated lesions, with a low risk of melanoma, to *atypical nevus syndrome,* in which patients may have more than 75 to 100 nevi, a strong family history of melanoma, and an extremely high risk of developing melanoma.

Halo, or *Sutton's, nevi* are pigmented nevi with a surrounding white halo caused by the presence of lymphocytes (Fig. 12–10). The cause of these lesions is unknown, but the lymphocytes are reactive against melanocytes. Such lesions are common in adolescents. Occurrence in adults should prompt concern about a melanoma in the lesion or elsewhere on the body.

I. CLASSIC DESCRIPTION
Distribution: Anywhere, especially trunk
Primary: Macules, papules, plaques

Secondary: Hyperpigmentation

II. DIAGNOSIS
Diagnosis is based on clinical appearance. Dysplasia or atypia will be confirmed on histopathologic examination.

III. DIFFERENTIAL DIAGNOSIS
A. Seborrheic keratosis lesions appear to be "stuck on," are scaly, and, on close inspection with a hand lens, will reveal horn cysts.

B. Melanoma usually is larger than 0.6 cm in diameter. Look for irregular borders, asymmetry, variable pigmentation, or pruritus. A history of change in a longstanding pigmented lesion or development of a new pigmented lesion with the aforementioned features are sensitive indicators of atypia.

IV. TREATMENT
A. Suspicious or unusual nevi:
1. If there is any suspicion that the lesion might be malignant, elliptical excision is indicated.
2. Excise with a no. 15 blade.
3. Include the entire pigmented lesion for complete architectural evaluation.
4. A deep shave excision may be an acceptable alternative to elliptical exci-

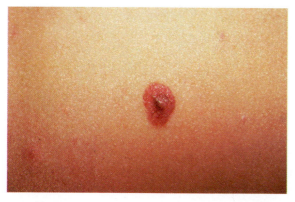

Fig. 12–9
Dysplastic nevus. Note red-brown discoloration and raised central papular component ("fried egg" appearance). (Courtesy Department of Dermatology, University of North Carolina at Chapel Hill.)

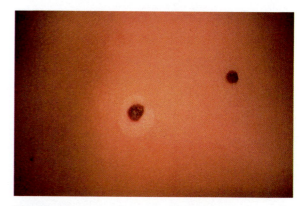

Fig. 12–10
Halo nevus. (Courtesy Department of Dermatology, University of North Carolina at Chapel Hill.)

sion only for lesions that are less suspicious.

B. Halo nevi:
1. When discovered in children, halo nevi do not require treatment.
2. Halo nevi in adults may be a sign of melanoma in that lesion or elsewhere. A thorough skin examination and removal of the lesion are indicated.

C. Pathologic consultation:
1. It is important to give the pathologist all available information about any suspect pigmented lesion. Include the patient's age, the location and size of the lesion, any significant characteristics of the lesion (e.g., variable pigmentation, irregular borders, long-standing lesion with history of recent change), and the presence or absence of personal or family history of melanoma.
2. Reliable histologic examination of pigmented lesions requires certain expertise and experience. Inquire how experienced your pathologic consultant is in reading pigmented lesions. If there is any doubt about a specimen's interpretation, consider a second opinion from a dermatopathologist.

D. Referral: Patients suspected of having atypical nevus syndrome or who have a giant congenital pigmented hairy nevus should be referred to a dermatologist.

V. PATIENT EDUCATION

A. Educate patients about the signs and symptoms of melanoma. (See patient education handout in Appendix K.)

B. Teach patients to carefully and properly examine their skin 5 minutes each month. With the help of a spouse or friend or with a mirror, patients should look over the entire body and note any suspect moles. Instruct patients to note the size, shape, and color of moles. If moles change in size or appearance, patients should bring them to the attention of their physician.

C. Patient education handouts that have color pictures of abnormal moles are available from The Skin Cancer Foundation.* A good Web site for patients: http://www.derm-infonet.com/Moles.html

PYOGENIC GRANULOMA ICD-9 (686.1)

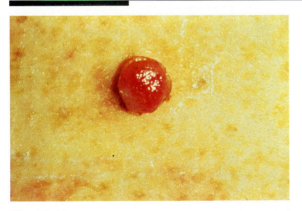

Fig. 12–11
Pyogenic granuloma. Note friable red nodule. (Courtesy Beverly Sanders, MD.)

Pyogenic granuloma, also known as *granuloma telangiectaticum,* is not an infection caused by bacteria, as the name suggests, but is associated with capillary proliferation (Fig. 12–11). Pyogenic granulomas often occur after a history of antecedent trauma but, in some cases, no prior trauma is evident. Pyogenic granulomas also occur more frequently during pregnancy, especially on the gingiva. Lesions usually are solitary and develop over the course of several weeks.

I. CLASSIC DESCRIPTION

Distribution: Head, neck, extremities, gingiva in pregnancy

*The Skin Cancer Foundation, 245 Fifth Ave., Suite 1403, New York, NY 10016, 212-725-5176 or 1-800-SKIN-490.

Primary: Papule, nodule
Secondary: Erythema, maceration, exudate
Lesions are dome-shaped, often macerated, and bleed easily.

II. DIAGNOSIS
The diagnosis is based on the clinical history of an erythematous papule that bleeds easily and has developed over a few days to weeks.

III. DIFFERENTIAL DIAGNOSIS
Amelanotic melanoma: Melanoma usually does not develop rapidly, but if there is any doubt, histologic confirmation is recommended.

IV. TREATMENT
A. Excision:
1. Anesthetize with *lidocaine* 1%.
2. Perform a shave excision and/or curettage.
3. Cauterize the base.

B. Recurrence: If the original lesion or multiple satellite lesions recur after treatment, reexcision or consultation is indicated.

SEBACEOUS HYPERPLASIA ICD-9 (706.9)

Sebaceous hyperplasia is a common skin condition involving hypertrophy of sebaceous glands. Lesions occur particularly on the central face of adults. Patients usually are concerned about the lesions either because of fear of skin cancer or because of cosmesis.

I. CLASSIC DESCRIPTION
Distribution: Face
Primary: Papule
Secondary: Yellow, telangiectasia

II. DIAGNOSIS
The diagnosis is clinical and based on the appearance of an isolated, yellow papule on the face of an adult (Fig. 12–12) and no history of recent change.

III. DIFFERENTIAL DIAGNOSIS
A. Basal cell carcinoma: Basal cell carcinomas usually have a history of recent change in size and tend not to be yellow.
B. Sebaceous carcinoma: A rare lesion; the yellow papule has a history of recent change in size or shape.

IV. TREATMENT
A. No treatment unless worried about cancer or condition is cosmetically bothersome.
B. Electrocautery:
1. Anesthetize with *lidocaine* 1%.
2. Cauterize, using low energy levels to prevent scarring.
3. Use a small curette or gauze to remove charred tissue.

C. Shave excision: Useful for isolated, large lesions or to rule out malignancy.
D. *Trichloroacetic acid 35%:* Useful to superficially "peel" the lesions, although more than one application may be necessary. Hypopigmentation may occur.
E. Diffuse lesions: Consider referral for carbon dioxide laser or dermabrasion.

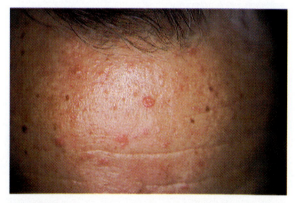

Fig. 12–12
Sebaceous hyperplasia on the face of an adult. Note the isolated yellow papules.

SEBORRHEIC KERATOSIS ICD-9 (702.11 IRRITATED, 702.19 NONIRRITATED)

Seborrheic keratoses are extremely common epidermal tumors, occurring usually in people older than 50 years but also seen in young adults. Seborrheic keratoses represent a benign proliferation of immature keratinocytes. Such skin changes can occur as an isolated lesion or hundreds may be present in the same person. The tendency for seborrheic keratoses may be inherited in an autosomal dominant fashion or associated with the healing phase of inflammatory skin diseases.

I. CLASSIC DESCRIPTION

Distribution: Trunk, face, upper extremities most commonly
Primary: Papules, plaques
Secondary: Hyperpigmentation, scale

II. DIAGNOSIS

The diagnosis is based on the clinical appearance of "stuck on," warty, well-circumscribed, often scaly hyperpigmented lesions (Fig. 12–13). Close inspection with a hand lens often will demonstrate the presence of horn cysts or dark keratin plugs. Lesions should be able to almost be picked off with a no. 15 blade. If lesions are atypical, biopsy may be necessary to confirm the diagnosis.

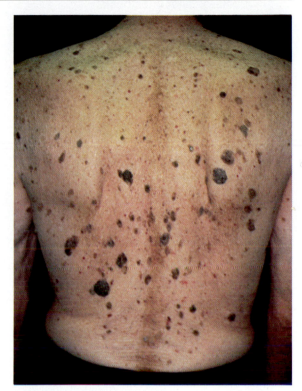

Fig. 12–13
Multiple truncal seborrheic keratoses. (Courtesy Department of Dermatology, Medical College of Georgia.)

III. DIFFERENTIAL DIAGNOSIS

A. **Nevus** does not have a stuck-on or warty appearance, and there is an absence of scale.
B. **Melanoma** usually does not have a stuck-on warty appearance. Look for blurring of borders, asymmetry, and history of a changing mole.
C. **Pigmented basal cell carcinomas** should have a history of a slowly changing lesion, along with a waxy appearance. Look for dilated blood vessels and any ulceration.

IV. TREATMENT

A. **No treatment is indicated for most lesions.** Remove lesions that are symptomatic or those causing cosmetic problems. Any of the treatments below is acceptable.
B. **Liquid nitrogen therapy:**
1. Thicker lesions may not respond as well.
2. Hypopigmentation often occurs with healing.
C. **Liquid nitrogen therapy with curettage:**
1. Helps with anesthesia and easy removal.
2. Useful for thinner lesions.
3. Curette while the freeze ball is present.
D. **Snip or shave excision** after anesthesia with *lidocaine* 1%.

E. **Use electrocautery** alone or followed by curettage after anesthesia.

F. **Excisional biopsy** with a no. 15 scalpel blade into the subcutaneous fat is indicated to rule out a melanoma or biopsy a pigmented basal cell carcinoma in any suspect lesion.

V. PATIENT EDUCATION

A. Educate patients about the signs and symptoms of melanoma. (See patient education handout in Appendix K.)

B. Explain postinflammatory changes seen after lesion removal with liquid nitrogen, shave excision, or electrocautery.

C. Tell patients that there is no effective way to prevent development of new lesions.

SOLAR LENTIGO ICD-9 (709.0)

Solar lentigo, most commonly known as *liver spots* or *old age spots*, is a proliferation of normal melanocytes secondary to chronic solar damage (Fig. 12–14). These lesions occur most commonly in those with fair complexion and a history of chronic sun exposure.

I. CLASSIC DESCRIPTION

Distribution: Face, dorsa of hands, shoulders, back
Primary: Macules
Secondary: Hyperpigmentation
Hyperpigmentation may vary from light to dark brown but is uniform within an individual lesion.

II. DIAGNOSIS

Diagnosis is based on clinical appearance:

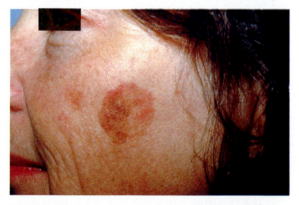

Fig. 12–14
Large hyperpigmented macule of solar lentigo. Watch carefully for variation in pigment or texture. (Courtesy Department of Dermatology, University of North Carolina at Chapel Hill.)

flat, oval, evenly pigmented macules in areas of chronic sun exposure.

III. DIFFERENTIAL DIAGNOSIS

A. **Seborrheic keratosis:** Early on, these lesions may be difficult to differentiate. Scale and palpable components are features of seborrheic keratoses.

B. **Lentigo maligna:** Lesions have variable pigmentation and irregular borders.

C. **Lentigo maligna melanoma:** This cancerous lesion has an irregular border, variable pigmentation, and may have a raised papule or nodule within the plaque. The history is of gradual change, usually over years.

IV. TREATMENT

A. **No treatment is needed** unless the patient desires removal for cosmetic reasons.

B. **Use liquid nitrogen** for 10 seconds or less if treatment is needed. Melanocytes are very sensitive to liquid nitrogen and are destroyed easily with small amounts and short exposure times. Lesions may heal with hypopigmentation.

C. **Use *tretinoin* (Retin A):** 0.025%, 0.05%, 0.1% cream (20, 45g) or (Renova): .05% cream (40, 60g) qhs for at least 4 to 6 months to lighten areas or prevent new lesions. Causes photosensitivity.

D. **Biopsy** any area that has changed color or developed a papular or nodular component.

V. PATIENT EDUCATION

A. Explain to patients that these lesions arise from chronic, cumulative sun damage.

B. Educate patients on the proper use of sunscreens and sunprotection.

(See patient education handouts in Appendix O.)

C. Explain to patients that many lesions may develop and that there is no known way to "undo" sun damage.

VENOUS LAKE ICD-9 (215.0)

Venous lakes are lesions of dilated capillaries on the face, lips (Fig. 12–15), and ears of elderly patients. Venous lakes bleed easily following minor trauma.

I. CLASSIC DESCRIPTION

Distribution: Vermillion border of the lip, ear, face

Primary: Papules

Secondary: Lesions are blue and easily compressible.

II. DIAGNOSIS

Diagnosis is based on the lesion disappearing when compressed with a glass slide.

III. DIFFERENTIAL DIAGNOSIS

A. **Blue nevus** will not disappear with compression. Such nevi do not usually appear on the face, ears, or lips.

B. **Nodular melanoma** will not disappear with compression and remains a firm nodule.

IV. TREATMENT

A. If the lesion causes a bleeding prob-

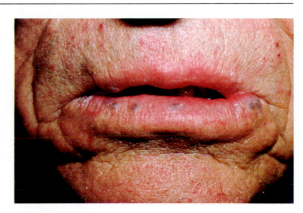

Fig. 12–15
Venous lake. Note multiple compressible venous dilations of the lower lip. (Courtesy Department of Dermatology, University of North Carolina at Chapel Hill.)

lem or is unsightly, electrocauterize after anesthesia with *lidocaine* 1%.

B. **Pulsed dye vascular laser** may remove lesions without causing a scar.

SUGGESTED READING

Drake LA et al: Guidelines of care for nevi. I. (Nevocellular nevi and seborrheic keratoses), *J Am Acad Dermatol* 26:629–631, 1992.

Drake LA et al: Guidelines of care for nevi. II. (Non-melanocytic nevi hemartomas, neoplasms, and potentially malignant lesions), *J Am Acad Dermatol* 32:104–108, 1992.

Goldberg DJ: Benign pigmented lesions of the skin, *Dermatol Surg* 19:376–379, 1993.

Kang S, Barnhill RL, Mihm MC: Melanoma risk in individuals with clinically atypical nevi, *Arch Dermatol* 130:999–1001, 1994.

Marghoob AA et al: Risk of cutaneous malignant melanoma in patients with "classic" atypical mole syndrome, *Arch Dermatol* 130:993–998, 1994.

Marghoob AA et al: Large congenital melanocytic nevi and the risk of development of malignant melanoma, *Arch Dermatol* 132:170–175, 1996.

Stern RS, Boudreaux C, Arndt KA: Diagnostic accuracy and appropriateness of care for seborrheic keratoses: a pilot approach to quality assurance for cutaneous surgery, *JAMA* 265:74–77, 1991.

CHAPTER 13

Premalignant and Malignant Neoplasms

ACTINIC KERATOSIS/CHEILITIS ICD-9 (702.0/692.72)

Actinic keratoses are common premalignant lesions resulting from chronic, cumulative sun exposure and occurring most commonly in fair-skinned people (Fig. 13–1). Some actinic keratoses may progress to squamous cell carcinomas. Squamous cell carcinomas arising from actinic keratoses tend to be very indolent and not highly invasive unless they occur on the lip (cheilitis).

I. CLASSIC DESCRIPTION
Distribution: Sun-exposed skin, including face, dorsa of hands, scalp in men
Primary: Papules, plaques

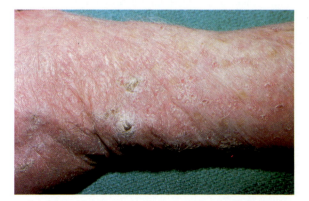

Fig. 13–1
Actinic keratosis. Note rough scaling papules and plaques on sun-damaged skin. (Courtesy Department of Dermatology, University of North Carolina at Chapel Hill.)

Secondary: Erythema, scale, occasionally hyperpigmentation

II. DIAGNOSIS
Patients often describe actinic keratoses as having a sticking or stinging sensation. Diagnosis is based on clinical appearance. *Some lesions are identified better by palpation*, and are usually recognized by their sandpapery texture.

III. DIFFERENTIAL DIAGNOSIS
A. **Squamous cell carcinoma:** If the papule or plaque is indurated, shave or punch biopsy is indicated to rule out carcinoma.
B. **Seborrheic keratosis:** Seborrheic keratoses are pigmented and have a "stuck on" appearance. Actinic keratoses may be pigmented but do not appear stuck on.
C. **Nummular eczema:** Look for coin-shaped, erythematous, pruritic, scaling lesions on the trunk and proximal extremities. Lesions resolve with emollients and topical corticosteroids.

IV. TREATMENT
A. **Cryosurgery with liquid nitrogen:**
  1. Because actinic keratoses are superficial, lesions should be frozen for only 10 to 20 seconds for one or two freeze–thaw cycles.
  2. Judge freeze–thaw cycles based on the site and thickness of the lesion.

Depending on how the liquid nitrogen is applied, the freeze balls are roughly 1 and ½ times as wide as they are deep.
3. Side effects: Patients should be informed before therapy of the possibility of hypopigmentation or erythema after healing. If the freeze is too deep, scarring may result.
B. *5-Fluorouracil (5-FU):*
Solution: 1% (30 ml), 2%, 5% (10 ml).
Cream: 1% (30 g), 5% (25 g).
1. Apply once or twice daily for 3 to 8 weeks. Use 1% to 2% preparations on the face for shorter periods and 5% preparations on the extremities for longer treatment times.
2. 5-FU is especially useful when treating multiple lesions.
3. Patient selection is essential, because there will be striking erythematous reactions and, often, crusting in response to the medication, alarming many patients. Warn patients that the severe erythematous reaction is a sign that the medication is working.
4. 5-FU causes extreme photosensitivity and should be used with strict instructions regarding sun protection (e.g., clothing, hats, gloves, sunscreen, sun avoidance). 5-FU often is best used in winter.
5. Obtain a biopsy specimen of any indurated, ulcerated, or bleeding lesions before using 5-FU or for any lesions that fail to resolve despite therapy.
6. Use caution when the lesions involve the face; there may be reepithelialization of normal skin over a carcinoma, hiding a cancerous lesion until it has progressed.
C. *Masoprocol* **cream** 10% (Actinex, 30 g):
1. Apply bid for 30 days.
2. Masoprocol cream is useful for treating multiple lesions and, unlike 5-FU cream, does not induce photosensitivity.

3. As with 5-FU, patient selection is essential, because there will be striking erythematous reactions and, often, crusting in response to the medication, alarming many patients. Warn patients that the severe erythematous reaction is a sign that the medication is working.
4. Up to 10% of patients may develp a true allergic contact dermatitis reaction to the drug, over and above the expected irritant dermatitis. Although redness and crusting are expected, if swelling, pruritus, or vesicles develop, the medication should be discontinued.
5. Obtain a biopsy specimen of any indurated, ulcerated, bleeding, or recurrent lesions.

V. PATIENT EDUCATION
A. Patient education brochures about 5-FU that provide pictures of typical reactions are useful.*
B. Explain that although lesions result from chronic and cumulative sun exposure, using sun protection now and in the future may decrease the development of subsequent lesions.
C. Explain that most patients will develop new lesions and explain the signs and symptoms of precancers and cancers. (See patient education handout in Appendix N.)
D. Educate patients about prevention of continued sun damage through use of protective clothing (e.g., hats, gloves, long sleeves) and sunscreens. (See patient education handout in Appendix O.)
E. Explain about the postinflammatory changes of erythema and hypopigmentation after treatment.

*Available from Allergan, Inc. (Fluoroplex), 714-752-4500 and Roche Dermatologic Division (Efudex) 1-800-526-6367.

F. Discuss in detail the use of topical medications, including sun avoidance, and patient expectation of severe, erythematous skin reactions during the course of therapy.

KERATOACANTHOMA ICD-9 (701.1)

Keratoacanthomas are tumors of epithelial origin that typically appear with the sudden onset of a solitary, rapidly growing dome-shaped nodule with a central keratotic core (Fig. 13–2). First described by Sir Jonathen Hutchinson in 1889, keratoacanthomas were so named because they resembled "crateriform ulcers of the face." Keratoacanthomas usually are seen in male patients, most commonly age 50 to 70, and are distributed over sun-exposed areas. Lesions may be associated with tar exposure; an increased incidence is seen in immunosuppressed patients. Controversy exists as to whether this lesion is better thought of as a carcinoma or a benign tumor. Although keratoacanthomas are not invasive, they can become quite large and involute and cause severe scarring. If the scarring occurs on structures such as the ears or nose, disfigurement results. Rarely, eruptive keratoacanthomas with multiple lesions are seen, sometimes associated with multiple other carcinomas (Muir-Torre syndrome).

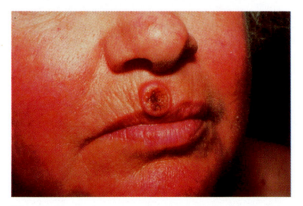

Fig. 13–2
Keratoacanthoma is a rapidly growing tumor with a central crater. (Courtesy Department of Dermatology, University of North Carolina at Chapel Hill.)

Some researchers have found evidence of human papillomavirus in lesions; however, confirmation of the virus as an etiologic agent remains to be seen. Chronic sun exposure and chronic immunosuppression are predisposing factors.

I. CLASSIC DESCRIPTION
Distribution: Sun-exposed areas, including cheeks, nose, ears, dorsa of hands, forearms
Primary: Papules, nodules, tumor
Secondary: Erythema, crust
Lesions are classically described as having a central keratotic, dome-shaped core.

II. DIAGNOSIS
A history of a rapidly growing lesion, as described above, should alert the clinician to the diagnosis. *Excisional biopsy is essential for diagnosis and to differentiate keratoacanthoma from squamous cell carcinoma.* Be sure to biopsy into the subcutaneous fat. A superficial shave biopsy will not provide adequate architecture to rule out an invasive squamous cell carcinoma.

III. DIFFERENTIAL DIAGNOSIS
Squamous cell carcinoma: Biopsy often is the only way to differentiate these lesions. Squamous cell carcinomas are slower growing and typically do not have a central keratotic plug.

IV. TREATMENT
A. Surgical ellipse excision through the dermis may be performed with a no. 15 scalpel blade, allowing for healing with secondary intention or by primary closure.
B. Curettage with electrodessication is adequate therapy for this lesion and is

especially useful in concave areas and on the extremities, where primary closure is difficult.

C. **Observation: These are rapidly growing lesions and therapy should not be delayed.** Although spontaneous regression may occur over several months, lesions may heal with significant scarring and disfigurement, especially those located on the central face.

D. **Referral:** Consider referral to a dermatologic surgeon, especially for multiple lesions. Oral retinoids (*isotretinoin, etretinate*) or intralesional chemotherapy may be options in such cases.

V. **PATIENT EDUCATION**
Educate patients about the role of chronic sun exposure and especially about preventing future sun exposure to help prevent development of new lesions.

MELANOMA ICD-9 (172.3 HEAD, EAR; 172.4 SCALP, NECK; 172.5 TRUNK, GROIN; 172.6 UPPER EXTREMITY; 172.7 LOWER EXTREMITY; 232 IN-SITU LESIONS BY SITE)

Melanoma, which literally means *black tumor,* is the malignant proliferation of pigment cells called *melanocytes.* Malignant melanoma deserves all of the attention given it, because of its potentially fatal nature, rapidly increasing incidence, and excellent prognosis if treated early. Malignant melanoma also is unique in that it is a visible tumor, unlike many other potentially fatal malignancies. *The importance of early diagnosis cannot be overstated.*

Malignant melanoma represents 3% of all cancers, with 38,000 new cases in the United States annually. Representing 1% to 2% of all cancer-related deaths, the increase in melanoma mortality rates is second only to lung cancer. One of every 75 whites born in the United States in the year 2000 will develop melanoma. In 1994 alone, more than 6,700 deaths occurred as a result of the disease. Although the causes of melanoma are not fully understood, excessive sunbathing, sunburns, and deterioration of the earth's ozone layer almost certainly play important roles in the increasing number of melanomas seen by clinicians. Educational efforts remain the mainstay of treatment; the public must be made aware of the warning signs (e.g., changing moles) and encouraged to seek treatment much earlier in the disease process.

Melanoma is classified by gross and microscopic characteristics correlated with the clinical history of the particular lesion. Melanomas are classified as *superficial spreading, nodular, lentigo maligna melanoma, acral lentiginous, amelanotic,* or *unclassified* (Table 13–1).

Superficial spreading melanoma is the most frequently reported melanoma and affects adults of all ages. Predisposing factors include a history of blistering sunburns in childhood, a history of atypical and congenital nevi, and a family history of atypical nevi or melanoma. The most common sites of occurrence are the upper back, face, lower legs, and trunk; the arms and lower legs are more common sites in women and the trunk is a more common site in men. Superficial spreading melanoma occurs as either a change in a preexisting mole or as a new mole (Fig. 13–3). Features include asymmetry, irregular borders, variable pigmentation, enlarging diameter, change in sensation (e.g., pruritus), and development of a nodular component. Typically, there is a horizontal growth phase, which lasts from months to years while the lesion is very superficial, followed by development of a nodular component, signaling invasive disease.

Lentigo maligna melanoma occurs in sun-exposed areas in elderly patients, most commonly on the face, head, and neck of fair-skinned whites. Predisposing factors include a history of chronic sun exposure. Lentigo maligna melanoma typically has a prolonged horizontal

TABLE 13–1.

Types of Melanoma and Distinguishing Features

	Superficial Spreading	Nodular	Lentigo Maligna	Acral Lentiginous
Percent	75	15	5	<5
Risk factors	White race, blistering childhood sunburn, personal or family history of melanoma or atypical nevus syndrome	Low index of suspicion	White race, sunburn	Low index of suspicion
Distribution	Face, trunk, back, legs	Anywhere	Face, sun-exposed areas	Palms, soles, terminal phalanges
Age (yr) (commonly)	40–60	50–70	60–80	40–60
Growth characteristics	Horizontal, slow (6 mo–2 yrs)	Rapidly invasive	Prolonged horizontal growth (often years)	Very invasive, metastasizes early (within months)

growth phase, when the lesion appears as a slowly expanding, irregularly pigmented macule that lasts for several years. Invasive disease is heralded by the development of raised areas, which often reach several centimeters in diameter (Fig. 13–4).

Nodular melanoma develops *de novo* as a blue or blue-black nodule or elevated plaque (Fig. 13–5). It typically has a rapid vertical growth phase, with invasion occurring early in the disease.

Acral lentiginous melanoma is less common. It does occur in whites but is found more often in blacks and Asians. Architecturally it may resemble lentigo maligna melanoma but can have a more aggressive course, with invasive disease occurring sooner and more fulminantly. Acral lentiginous melanoma is seen most frequently on hands, feet, and mucous membranes (Fig. 13–6).

Amelanotic melanoma is a nonpigmented tumor of melanocytes that commonly occurs as a pink nodule. The increased morbidity seen with this lesion is secondary to clinician and patient failure to recognize it as an abnormal growth.

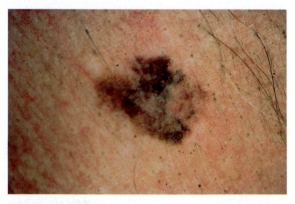

Fig. 13–3
Superficial spreading melanoma. Note asymmetry, irregular borders, and variation in color. (Courtesy Department of Dermatology, Medical College of Georgia.)

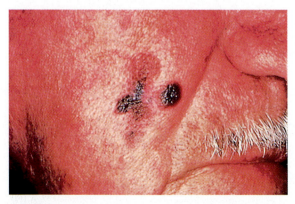

Fig. 13–4
Lentigo maligna melanoma, characterized by raised areas, asymmetry, and pigmentary variations. (Courtesy John Cook, MD.)

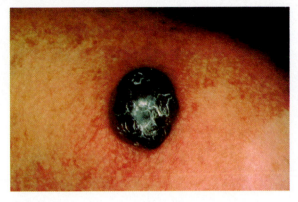

Fig. 13–5
Nodular melanoma with rapidly growing black nodule. (Courtesy Department of Dermatology, Medical College of Georgia.)

Precursor risk factors for malignant melanoma include lentigo maligna, dysplastic nevi, and giant congenital nevi (greater than 20 cm in diameter in adulthood). Malignancy can occur in long-standing lesions of solar lentigo after many years of slow growth, in a preexisting nevus, in a new nevus, or even as a rapidly growing nodule, as in nodular melanoma.

The prognosis is based on the thickness of the primary tumor, measured histologically from the top of the granular layer to the deepest melanoma cell (Breslow's measurement; Table 13–2 and Fig. 13–7). Histologic grading by melanoma location in the dermis is known as *Clark's levels* (Box 13–1 and Fig. 13–7).

I. CLASSIC DESCRIPTION
Primary: Macule, papule, plaque, nodule, tumor
Secondary: Hyperpigmentation, including

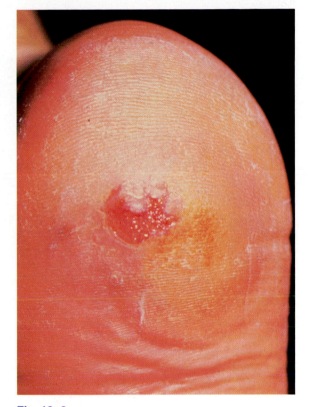

Fig. 13–6
Acral lentiginous melanoma presenting as a nonhealing foot ulcer. (Courtesy Marshall Guill, MD.)

black, brown, blue-gray, red, tan, white, purple-gray; later, ulceration
Look for asymmetry, irregular borders, variation in color, or a nodular component.

II. DIAGNOSIS
Diagnosis is based on excisional biopsy and characteristic histologic findings. However, any patient with a history of change in

TABLE 13–2.
Five-Year Survival Based on Tumor Thickness (Breslow's Measurement)

Tumor Thickness (mm)	5-Year Survival (%)
<0.75	98–99
0.76–1.50	94
1.51–2.25	83
2.26–3.00	72–77
>3.00	<50

BOX 13–1.
Clark's Levels

I	Confined to epidermis in "in situ" disease; not considered invasive
II	Melanoma cells into papillary dermis
III	Melanoma cells filling papillary dermis
IV	Melanoma cells in reticular dermis
V	Melanoma cells in subcutaneous fat

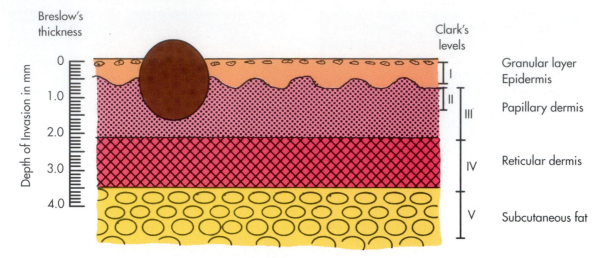

Fig. 13–7
Melanoma classification by Breslow's measurements and Clark's levels.

a long-standing pigmented lesion or a new lesion with suspect features should alert the clinician to the possible diagnosis of melanoma. A mnemonic that can be used to remember suspect features is:

    A = asymmetry
    B = borders irregular and blurred
    C = color change or variable pigmentation
    D = diameter greater than 6 mm
    E = elevation of previously flat lesion

III. DIFFERENTIAL DIAGNOSIS

  A. Nevus: A nevus is a benign pigmented lesion that typically is symmetric, has regular borders, is less than 6 mm in diameter, and has even or stable pigmentation throughout the life of the lesion (e.g., a congenital nevus may be brown and black, so variability in pigmentation is not necessarily ominous of itself; however, the history of recent change in pigmentation is cause for concern). A biopsy may be necessary to differentiate the diseases.

  B. Recurrent nevus: A previously treated nevus that recurs in a scar site often looks bizarre. Biopsy may be necessary to confirm the benign nature of the le-

sion. It is essential to notify the pathologist of any history of previous treatment, so that the lesion is not labeled erroneously as a melanoma.

  C. Seborrheic keratosis: Seborrheic keratosis has a stuck-on appearance, a scaly surface, well-demarcated borders, and horn cysts in the epidermis on gross examination. Any atypical pigmented lesion suspected of being a melanoma or for which the clinician is unsure of the diagnosis should be excised, biopsied, or referred.

  D. Pigmented actinic keratosis: This lesion has a rough, sandpapery feel and is not indurated.

  E. Pigmented basal cell carcinoma: This lesion often has a waxy appearance and is associated with telangiectasia. Biopsy is indicated for differentiation.

  F. Hemangioma/angiokeratoma: A hemangioma is a compressible blood vessel tumor that should blanch with compression. Amelanotic melanoma may resemble a hemangioma. Hemangiomas may thrombose and turn black. Biopsy often is indicated for differentiation.

G. **Subungual hematoma:** In subungual hematoma, often there is a history of trauma, and the lesion grows as the nail grows. Diffusion of pigment into the cuticle area is more consistent with a melanoma.

IV. TREATMENT

A. **Elliptical excision:**
   1. Remove all visible pigment, even into the superficial subcutaneous fat.
   2. Wider excisions are necessary with a confirmed melanoma, with margins ranging from 1 to 3 cm, depending on the depth of the lesion.
   3. If the lesion is thinner than 1 mm by Breslow's measurement, a 1-cm margin is adequate (0.5-cm margins may be adequate for some in situ lesions).

B. **Referral to a dermatologist** or a plastic surgeon is indicated for consultation and management, particularly if the lesion cannot easily be excised.

C. **Long-term follow up:**
   1. Patients with malignant melanoma should be examined every 3 months for 2 years, because 3% will develop a second melanoma within 3 years.
   2. Include annual chest x-ray examination and liver profiles for at least 3 to 5 years for invasive lesions.
   3. Give special attention to the site of surgery for recurrence of new pigmented lesions or adenopathy.

D. **Extensive patient education** (see discussion of patient education).

E. **Examine family members:** Examine and educate family members about the signs and symptoms of malignant melanoma.

F. **Spontaneous resolution** of advanced metastatic cases has occurred rarely, but the frequency of occurence or reasons for such regression are unknown.

V. PATIENT EDUCATION

A. Educate about the signs and symptoms of suspect pigmented lesions: ABCDEs (*a*symmetry; irregular *b*orders; *c*hange or variation in pigmentation; increase in *di*ameter, especially greater than 6 mm [size of a pencil eraser]; *e*levation, change in sensation).
   (See patient education handout in Appendix K.)

B. Discuss sun protection and sunscreens, emphasizing that patients must never sunburn. Use protective clothing (e.g., hats, long sleeves), and avoid the sun between 10:00 AM and 4:00 PM.

C. Emphasize the importance of the patient performing a total body skin examination on a regular basis. The examination should include the use of mirrors to adequately examine the back.

D. Explain that other family members are at risk for melanoma and that any suspect pigmented lesions must be evaluated.

E. For further information about melanoma, including clinical trials, patients may contact the American Melanoma Foundation or use either of two excellent Web sites.*

MYCOSIS FUNGOIDES/CUTANEOUS T CELL LYMPHOMA ICD-9 (202.1)

Mycosis fungoides initially was described by Jean Louis Alibert, a French physician, in the eighteenth century. He described tumorous skin lesions that resembled mushrooms evolving from an eczematous rash, thus the name mycosis fungoides.

Mycosis fungoides is a neoplasm of T helper cells and now is referred to as cutaneous T *cell*

*American Melanoma Foundation, UCSD Cancer Center, 9500 Gilmer Dr. 0658, La Jolla CA 92093-0658; 619-534-3840, FAX 619-534-7628. Web sites: (1) http://www.sonic.net/~jpat/getwell.html (2) http://cancer.med.upenn.edu/disease/melanoma/

lymphoma. Initially this lymphoma involves only the skin; subsequently it can disseminate, involving the viscera, especially lymph nodes. Although the tumor is rare, it is the most common cutaneous lymphoma in adults, usually becoming apparent during the fifth or sixth decade of life.

Typically the patient has a therapeutically resistant dermatitis that has evolved over years into cutaneous T cell lymphoma (Fig. 13–8). Rarely, the disease presents with fulminant tumors and nodules. Some patients may have lesions that have evolved into a generalized exfoliative erythroderma, associated with a leukemic component and lymphadenopathy, known as *Sézary syndrome*. Such systemic involvement also is characterized by poor temperature regulation, fever, chills, weight loss, malaise, and often intractable pruritus.

The prognosis is variable, ranging from death within a year to chronic disease lasting for decades, with the patient often dying of an unrelated illness. The median survival after diagnosis is 7 to 8 years. Advanced age, black race, previous malignancy, and presence of Sézary syndrome are associated with decreased survival.

I. CLASSIC DESCRIPTION

Distribution: Unexposed sites initially; nodules have predilection for face and intertriginous areas

Primary: Early: Macules, patches; some present as areas of atrophy, with surface wrinkling and telangiectasia

Later: Indurated plaques, then nodules, tumors, and generalized exfoliation

Secondary: Erythema, scale; plaques, nodules, and tumors may be dusky red or violescent or ulcerate. Nail dystrophy and alopecia may develop, along with peripheral adenopathy.

Early patches are well-demarcated and often bizarre in configuration (e.g., arciform, annular).

II. DIAGNOSIS

Diagnosis is made by biopsy and light microscopic examination. Collections of atypical lymphocytes (Pautrier's microabscesses) are seen in the epidermis. Early in the disease process, histopathologic diagnosis is difficult and may require multiple biopsies. Therefore, *when ruling out the disease, at least three or four sites should be biopsied*. Choose the most evolved and indurated lesions for biopsy (e.g., a plaque over a patch, a nodule over a plaque). Immunophenotyping and molecular biologic testing (T-cell receptor gene rearrangement analysis) are helpful but not always definitive in confirming the diagnosis. Clinicians should remain suspicious of refractory, long-standing eczema.

III. DIFFERENTIAL DIAGNOSIS

A. **Chronic eczematous dermatitis,** including atopic dermatitis: Early in the course of cutaneous T cell lymphoma the clinical appearance can be identical to that found in chronic eczematous eruptions; however, cutaneous T cell lymphoma is refractory to standard therapy. Repeat biopsies over several years may be necessary before a definitive diagnosis is made.

B. **Skin metastases** from other tumors usually do not evolve from eczematous eruptions. Such metastases have a more fulminant onset, and biopsy will confirm the diagnosis.

C. **Erythroderma** can occur from many

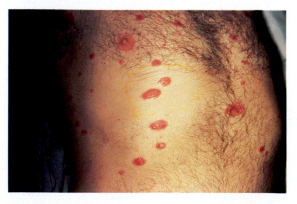

Fig. 13–8
Cutaneous T cell lymphoma with multiple infiltrative papules, plaques, and early tumors. (Courtesy Marshall Guill, MD.)

other underlying skin diseases (e.g., psoriasis, seborrhea, drug eruption). Again, cutaneous Tcell lymphoma is refractory to therapy, and biopsy usually will differentiate these conditions.

IV. TREATMENT

A. Referral to a dermatologist is indicated for confirmation of diagnosis and treatment.

B. Initial treatment often consists of topical therapy because aggressive systemic therapies have not altered the course of the disease and only increase morbidity (except in Sézary syndrome or fulminant disease). The patch, or plaque, stage usually is treated first with topical corticosteroids, then with topical nitrogen mustard, and then with various therapies (e.g., psoralens with ultraviolet A light therapy [PUVA], electron beam therapy, radiation therapy of tumors, or, more recently, extracorporeal photophoresis or immunotherapy).

C. Evaluation for systemic involvement: If adenopathy is present, biopsy the lesions and examine the peripheral smear for Sézary cells.

D. Treat any underlying secondary infection.

E. Control pruritus with antihistamines and emollients.

F. For detailed treatment approaches, contact: http://cancer.med.upenn.edu/disease/t-cell/

PAGET'S DISEASE OF BREAST ICD-9 (174.0)

Paget's disease, named after the nineteenth-century British surgeon Sir James Paget, is an eczematous process secondary to epidermal invasion of the nipple and areola by malignant cells from an underlying intraductal breast carcinoma (Fig. 13–9). Paget's disease is seen most commonly in women between the ages of 50 and 60 and rarely in men. Extramammary Paget's disease is rare. It resembles Paget's disease in appearance but occurs in the axillae and anogenital region. The greatest significance is its association with underlying carcinoma, especially adenocarcinoma of the gastrointestinal tract.

I. CLASSIC DESCRIPTION
Distribution: Nipple, areola; unilateral
Primary: Plaque
Secondary: Erythema, scale, exudate, erosion
Other signs of underlying breast cancer may be present, such as retracted nipple, induration, or even a palpable mass.

II. DIAGNOSIS
The diagnosis is suspected in a patient with a chronic scaling plaque that occurs on one nipple and that has remained unresponsive to topical therapy. Diagnosis is confirmed by biopsy, which may demonstrate the underlying carcinoma.

III. DIFFERENTIAL DIAGNOSIS
A. Chronic eczematous dermatitis: Eczema usually is bilateral and responds to mild corticosteroids. Paget's disease is very rarely bilateral. Follow-up is essential.

B. Bowen's disease of the nipple, while

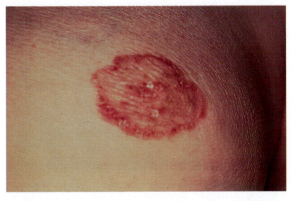

Fig. 13–9
Paget's disease of the left areola, destroying the nipple. (Courtesy Department of Dermatology, University of North Carolina at Chapel Hill.)

rare, is also unilateral. Biopsy is required for differentiation.

C. **Superficial basal cell carcinoma** of the nipple is unilateral and rare. Biopsy is required for differentiation from Paget's disease.

IV. TREATMENT

A. **Biopsy is essential** if there is no response to empirical treatment or if the clinician has any suspicion of underlying breast cancer. In addition, if there is concern about patient compliance for follow-up, initial biopsy is warranted.

B. **Rule out breast carcinoma:** If biopsy confirms the diagnosis of Paget's disease, mammography and evaluation for underlying breast carcinoma are essential.

C. **Empiric treatment is acceptable if there are no signs of breast carcinoma:** In such cases, try treating empirically for eczematous dermatitis, with a mild topical corticosteroid (e.g., Westcort or Des-Owen cream twice a day for 3 weeks).

D. **Follow-up is essential.**

V. PATIENT EDUCATION

Educate patients about the possibility of underlying breast carcinoma and the importance of follow-up after any empirical therapy of nipple eczema.

BASAL CELL CARCINOMA ICD-9 (173.3 HEAD, EAR; 173.4 SCALP, NECK; 173.5 TRUNK, GROIN; 173.6 UPPER EXTREMITY; 173.7 LOWER EXTREMITY)

Basal cell carcinoma is a malignancy of the basal cells of the epidermis. It is the most common human malignancy, with approximately 750,000 new cases in the United States each year. This skin cancer occurs more commonly in men, almost exclusively in whites, and most frequently between the ages of 40 and 80. Eighty-five percent occur on the head and neck, with the nose being the most common site. Predisposing factors include chronic ultraviolet sunlight exposure, arsenic, ionizing radiation, and a rare inherited syndrome, basal cell nevus syndrome, an autosomal dominant disease characterized by development of myriad basal cell carcinomas and xeroderma pigmentosum.

Basal cell carcinomas are classified by histologic appearance. Classification is significant, because certain types of tumors have more aggressive growth traits than others, and treatment should be based on the type of basal cell cancer. In addition to histologic classification, the location and size of the lesions influence treatment (see below).

Nodular basal cell carcinoma is the most frequent type, occurring as a translucent, waxy papule with a rolled, pearly border, telangiectasia, and often central ulceration (Fig. 13–10).

Superficial spreading basal cell carcinomas occur as irregularly shaped erythematous, scaling plaques with telangiectasia and often a thready, well-defined border (Fig. 13–11). Superficial spreading basal cell carcinomas occur most commonly on the trunk.

Morpheaform, or **sclerosing,** basal cell carcinomas resemble scar tissue or morphea, occurring as a thick, firm plaque with atrophy, hypopigmentation, erythema, and prominent telangiectasia (Fig. 13–12). Morpheaform basal cell carcinomas have an irregular growth pattern such that the margins are difficult to discern both clinically and grossly, without histologic confirmation.

Pigmented basal cell carcinomas may have any of the above characteristics, along with hyperpigmentation.

I. CLASSIC DESCRIPTION

Distribution: Sun-exposed areas, most commonly the head and neck

Primary: Papule, plaque, nodule, tumor, telangiectasia

Secondary: Erythema, scale, erosion, ulcer

II. DIAGNOSIS

The diagnosis of basal cell cancer is confirmed by histologic examination of tissue

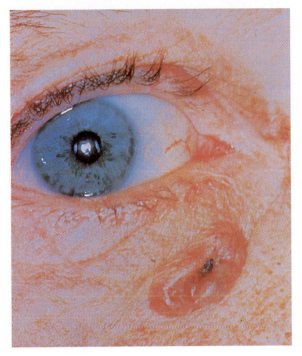

Fig. 13–10A
Basal cell carcinoma, nodular type. Note waxy nodule with prominent telangiectasias. (Courtesy Robert Clark III, MD, PhD.)

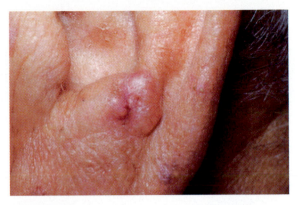

Fig. 13–10B
Basal cell carcinoma, nodular type. Waxy nodule with telangiectasia.

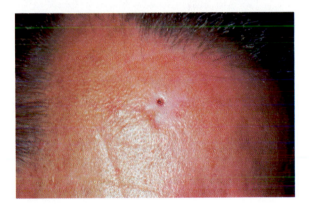

Fig. 13–12
Basal cell carcinoma with biopsy site; morpheaform type, resembling a scar. (Courtesy Department of Dermatology, University of North Carolina at Chapel Hill.)

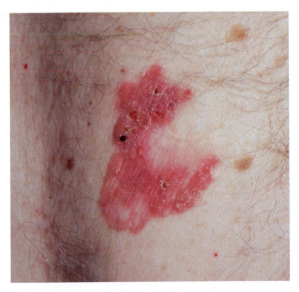

Fig. 13–11
Basal cell carcinoma, superficial type, with slowly expanding erythematous plaque. (Courtesy Department of Dermatology, University of North Carolina at Chapel Hill.)

from a clinically suspect lesion. The history should reveal a persistent lesion that has increased in size gradually over several months to years. A shave biopsy or a 2- to 4-mm punch biopsy usually provides sufficient tissue for diagnosis, although excisional biopsy is acceptable for small lesions. Diagram the area from which the biopsy specimen was taken, because healing of small lesions may make the site difficult to discern if futher treatment is necessary.

III. DIFFERENTIAL DIAGNOSIS

A. **Dermal nevus** is a firm, flesh-colored papule that has not gradually enlarged. Occasionally, dermal nevi may have telangiectasia, and biopsy may be necessary to differentiate them from a basal cell carcinoma.

B. **Squamous cell carcinoma** may look very similar to either a nodular basal cell carcinoma that has ulcerated or a superficial basal cell carcinoma. Squamous cell carcinomas typically lack waxy, thready borders and prominent telangiectasias. Biopsy will confirm the diagnosis.

C. **Keratoacanthomas** have a classic history of rapid growth, whereas basal cell carcinomas typically have a slow growth phase, over months to years. The clinical appearance of keratoacanthomas includes a central keratotic plug, which usually is not present in basal cell carcinomas.

D. **Scarring** may be explained by a history of trauma. Scars usually are stable lesions that do not increase in size. Sometimes minor trauma to an area will bring a long-standing underlying morpheaform basal cell carcinoma to the attention of the patient.

E. **Morphea** may be difficult to discern from morpheaform basal cell carcinoma. Look for characteristics of basal cell carcinoma (e.g., location in sun-exposed areas, prominent telangiectasia, and rolled borders).

F. **Melanomas** should be considered in the differential diagnosis of pigmented basal cell carcinomas. Biopsy is often the only definitive way to differentiate these two lesions.

G. **Eczema** is a consideration when a localized, erythematous, scaling plaque is present, especially on the trunk. A lesion that is well-defined but irregularly shaped and has a thready border and telangiectasia is indicative of a basal cell carcinoma.

IV. TREATMENT

A. **Biopsy any suspect lesions:**
   1. Include an adequate tissue sample to allow for pathologic confirmation of the diagnosis.
   2. Carefully record the biopsy site, because healing may make identification of lesions difficult, especially in patients in whom multiple areas have been treated.
   3. If the diagnosis is not in doubt, definitive therapy is acceptable, simultaneous with biopsy.
   4. *Even if healing of the biopsy site seems to indicate "cure" of the lesion, definitive therapy for a basal cell cancer still is indicated; rates of recurrences as high as 30% have been reported with the wait-and-see approach.*

B. **Definitive therapy:** Histologic type, location, and size of the basal cell carcinoma will guide surgical treatment of the lesion (Table 13–3). For most basal cell carcinomas, treat with either excision with appropriate margins or with curettage and electrodesiccation.

C. **Radiation therapy:** Indicated in patients, often elderly or severely debilitated, who are unable to undergo surgery. Multiple visits are required.

D. **Investigational:** Current research includes using intralesional interferon and photodynamic therapy (photosensitizing agent and laser).

E. **Follow-up:**
   1. Follow-up is essential, not only for primary recurrences but also because in 40% to 50% of patients a second basal cell carcinoma will develop within 3 to 5 years.
   2. Examine the scar site and sun-exposed skin, including the trunk, for changes (e.g., elevation, induration,

TABLE 13–3.

Treatment of Basal Cell Carcinomas

Lesion	Preferred*	Alternative	Comments
Nodular basal cell	Excision with 3-4 mm margins	Curettage and desiccation	A 5-6 mm punch biopsy may be adequate for a small (2 mm) lesion.
Superficial spreading	Curettage and electrodesiccation†	Excision with 3-4 mm margins	Potential for hypertrophic scar formation
Morpheaform	Referral for Mohs' microsurgery for excision with margin control	—	Tumor margins often extend well beyond gross examination.
Basal cell of the nose, posterior ear, and eye	Excision with margin control	Referral for Mohs' microsurgery for excision with margin control. Curettage and electro-desiccation may be acceptable for small, defined lesions	These lesions are the most likely to recur. Recurrence near the eye, ear, and nose may be very destructive.
Recurrent lesions	Referral for Mohs' microsurgery for excision with margin control for areas involving key structures (i.e., face, fingers)	Excision with margin control for areas where vital structures are uninvolved	Biopsy any suspicious recurrent lesion.

*Lesions larger than 2 cm in diameter are best excised.
†Curettage and electrodesiccation often offers a better cosmetic result over concave surfaces and for superficial spreading basal cell carcinomas.

ulceration) every 6 months for 1 year and yearly thereafter.

3. Any lesion suspicious for recurrence should be biopsied. If the biopsy is positive, refer for Mohs' or other margin-controlled surgery.

V. PATIENT EDUCATION

(See patient education handouts in Appendixes N and O.)

A. Explain the direct relationship of basal cell carcinomas and cumulative sun exposure.

B. Discuss sun-protection measures (e.g., wearing hats and long sleeves, avoiding midday sun, and using lotions with a sun-protection factor of 15 or higher).

C. Teach skin self-examination with attention to any new lesions that do not resolve within 6 to 8 weeks.

D. Educate patients to watch for changes in scar sites (e.g., elevation, ulceration, induration).

E. Emphasize the importance of follow-up, because new lesions will develop in 40% to 50% of patients.

F. Before performing surgery, document explanations about possibilities of scar, recurrence, need for further surgery, and damage to possible underlying structures, such as nerves.

G. A good patient Web site is maintained by the American Academy of Dermatology: http://www.derm-infonet.com/SkinCa.html

SQUAMOUS CELL CARCINOMA ICD-9 (173.3 HEAD, EAR; 173.4 SCALP, NECK; 173.5 TRUNK, GROIN; 173.6 UPPER EXTREMITY; 173.7 LOWER EXTREMITY; 232 IN SITU BY SITE)

Squamous cell carcinoma is the second most frequent skin carcinoma, and, similar to basal cell carcinoma, its incidence is increasing greatly. Squamous cell carcinomas occur most commonly in white men older than 55 and in sun-exposed areas. The carcinomas are tumors of malignant keratinocytes, whose main function is the production of keratin.

Predisposing factors to the development of squamous cell carcinomas include ultraviolet radiation, old burn scars, sites of chronic inflammation, PUVA therapy, radiation therapy, arsenic, pitch, tar, immunosuppression, smoking (lip lesions), and a rare genetic disease, xeroderma pigmentosum. Squamous cell carcinomas can develop from a precursor lesion, an actinic keratosis, or *de novo*. Carcinomas that develop from an actinic keratosis are not aggressive and have little or no tendency to metastasize. Lesions involving old burn scars or sites of chronic inflammation and those located on the lower lip or other mucous membranes have the greatest tendency to metastasize, with some reports as high as 30%.

I. CLASSIC DESCRIPTION
Distribution: Sun-exposed areas; legs more commonly involved in female patients

Primary: Papule, plaque, nodule, tumor
Secondary: Erythema, scale, erosion, crust, ulcer (Figs. 13–13 and 13–14) Adenopathy may be present in larger lesions, especially those involving the lower lip, other mucous membranes, old burn scars, and sites of radiation or chronic inflammation.

II. DIAGNOSIS
The diagnosis is confirmed by histologic examination of tissue from a clinically suspect lesion. The history should reveal a persistent lesion that gradually has increased in size over months to years. A shave biopsy or a 2- to 4-mm punch biopsy usually provides sufficient tissue for diagnosis. *Diagram the area from which the biopsy specimen is taken, because healing of small lesions may make the site difficult to discern if further treatment is necessary.*

III. DIFFERENTIAL DIAGNOSIS
A. Eczema will respond to topical corticosteroids. Signs of induration or elevation on manipulation of the skin are more indicative of squamous cell carcinoma.
B. Basal cell carcinoma: Squamous cell carcinomas may look very similar to ei-

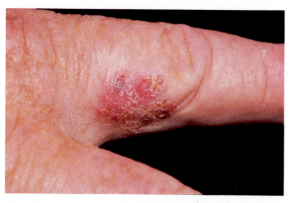

Fig. 13–13
Squamous cell carcinoma of the finger, with erythematous and scaling plaque. (Courtesy Department of Dermatology, Medical College of Georgia.)

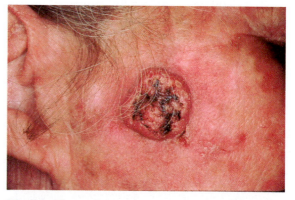

Fig. 13–14
Squamous cell carcinoma with extensive ulceration on sun-damaged skin. (Courtesy Department of Dermatology, Medical College of Georgia.)

ther a nodular basal cell that has ulcerated or a superficial basal cell carcinoma. Squamous cell carcinomas lack the waxy, thready border and prominent telangiectasias typical of basal cell carcinomas. Biopsy will confirm the diagnosis.

C. **Keratoacanthomas** have a classic history of rapid growth, whereas squamous cell carcinomas typically have a slow growth phase, over months to years, and the clinical appearance of keratoacanthomas includes a central keratotic plug. Keratoacanthomas actually may be a less aggressive form of squamous cell carcinoma. A full-thickness biopsy specimen, including all layers of the skin, will be necessary to differentiate invasive squamous cell carcinoma from a keratoacanthoma.

D. **Actinic keratosis:** Actinic keratoses are precursor lesions for squamous cell carcinomas but are not typically indurated; however, if lesions are inflamed or hypertrophied, biopsy may be needed for differentiation.

IV. TREATMENT

A. **Biopsy:**
1. Include adequate tissue sample to allow for pathologic confirmation of the diagnosis. A biopsy is recommended before definitive therapy in most cases.
2. Carefully record the biopsy site, because healing may make identification of lesions difficult, especially in patients in whom multiple areas have been treated.
3. Even if healing of the biopsy site seems to indicate "cure" of the lesion, definitive therapy is indicated.

B. **Squamous cell carcinomas arising from actinic keratoses, identified as in situ, or very superficial, on biopsy:**
1. Curettage and electrodessication.
2. Topical *5-FU* is a treatment option on the extremities for in situ lesions. Use

twice daily for 4 weeks, with close follow-up for in situ lesions.

C. **Excision: All other squamous cell carcinomas should be excised.**
1. Excisional surgery involves either excision with primary closure or saucerization with healing by secondary intention or later with a second procedure.
2. Any technique should be done such that all of the tumor is removed with a 5 mm margin.
3. Attention to underlying vital structures is essential.
4. Refer for microscopically controlled surgery (e.g., Mohs') when excision with margin control is indicated for lesions involving structures where histologic findings reveal a poorly differentiated tumor, the lesion is large or long-standing, margins are not well-defined, and in sites where deeper extension may occur (e.g., nasolabial folds, nose, eyes, posterior auricular areas). The Mohs' technique involves intraoperative evaluation of horizontally oriented tissue sections for optimal evaluation of margins and tissue preservation.

D. **Rule out metastatic involvement.** Check for adenopathy in lesions that are advanced, those that involve the lower lip or other mucous membranes, and those in sites of radiation therapy, old burn scars, or chronic inflammation.

E. **Radiation therapy** is indicated in rare circumstances, such as when surgery is not an option.

F. **Experimental therapies** include *isotretinoin,* especially in patients with multiple skin tumors (e.g., patients with xeroderma pigmentosum).

G. **Follow-up:**
1. Follow-up is essential for recurrences and to monitor for development of new lesions.

2. Examine the scar site and sun-exposed skin, including the trunk, every 6 months for 1 year and yearly thereafter.
3. Any lesion suspicious for recurrence should be biopsied. If positive, refer for Mohs' or other margin-controlled surgery.

V. PATIENT EDUCATION

(See patient education handouts in Appendixes N and O.)

A. Emphasize the direct relationship of squamous cell carcinomas and cumulative sun exposure.
B. Educate about sun protection measures (e.g., wearing a hat and long sleeves, avoiding midday sun, using lotions with a sun-protection factor of 15 or higher).
C. Teach skin self-examination; stress attention to any new lesions that do not resolve within 6 to 8 weeks.
D. Educate about the signs to watch for in scar site changes (e.g., elevation, ulceration, induration).
E. Explain chances of developing new lesions and the importance of follow-up examinations.
F. Before performing surgery, document explanation of the possibilities of scar, recurrence of disease, the need for further surgery, and possible involvement of underlying structures, such as nerves.
G. A good patient Web site is maintained by the American Academy of Dermatology: http://www.derm-infonet.com/SkinCa.html

SUGGESTED READING

Bernstein SC, Li KK, Brodland DG: The many faces of squamous cell carcinoma, *Dermatol Surg* 22:243–254, 1996.

Ceballos PI, Ruiz-Meldonado R, Mihm MC: Melanoma in children, *N Engl J Med* 332:656–662, 1995.

Cohen LM: Lentigo maligna and lentigo maligna melanoma, *J Am Acad Dermatol* 33:923–936, 1995.

Drake LA et al: Guidelines of care for basal cell carcinoma, *J Am Acad Dermatol* 26:117–120, 1992.

Drake LA et al: Guidelines of care for cutaneous squamous cell carcinoma, *J Am Acad Dermatol* 28:628–631, 1993.

Drake LA et al: Guidelines of care for melanoma, *J Am Acad Dermatol* 28:638–641, 1993.

Drake LA et al: Guidelines of care for actinic keratoses, *J Am Acad Dermatol* 32:95–98, 1995.

Drake LA et al: Guidelines of care for Mohs' micrographic surgery, *J Am Acad Dermatol* 33:271–278, 1995.

Gloster HM, Brodland DG: The epidemiology of skin cancer, *Dermatol Surg* 22:217–226, 1996.

Johnson TJ et al: Current therapy for cutaneous melanoma, *J Am Acad Dermatol* 32:689–707, 1995.

Kuflik AS, Schwartz RA: Actinic keratosis and squamous cell carcinoma *Am Fam Physician* 49:817–820, 1994.

Malignant melanoma in CA-A, *Can J Clinicians* 46:4, 1996.

Olsen EA et al: A double-blind, vehicle-controlled study evaluating masoprocol cream in the treatment of actinic keratoses on the head and neck, *J Am Acad Dermatol* 24:738–743, 1991.

Onuigbo WI: Paget's 1874 article on the breast: modern misconceptions, *Int J Dermatol* 24:537–538, 1985.

Preston DS, Stern RS: Nonmelanoma cancers of the skin, *N Engl J Med* 327:1649–1662, 1992.

Schwartz RA: Keratoacanthoma, *J Am Acad Dermatol* 30:1–19, 1994.

Schwartz RA: Premalignant keratinocytic neoplasms, *J Am Acad Dermatol* 35:223–242, 1996.

Willemze R: New concepts in the classification of cutaneous lymphomas, *Arch Dermatol* 131:1077–1080, 1995.

CHAPTER 14

Papulosquamous Diseases

ECZEMA ICD-9 (692.9)

Eczema is the broad term used to describe an array of inflammatory skin disorders. The term *dermatitis* often is used interchangeably with *eczema*. To confuse matters, the descriptive term *eczematous dermatitis* has been used when describing red, scaly, inflamed skin.

Eczema, or dermatitis, can be categorized by several classification schemes, including cause (contact, stasis), location (hand and foot eczema), degree of involvement (exfoliative dermatitis), or a generalized condition (atopic dermatitis). The inflammation can be *acute* and severe, with significant edema, vesicles, and bullae; *subacute,* with scaling plaques; or *chronic,* with thickened, accentuated skin markings known as *lichenification.* Such chronic inflammation also is characterized by scales and pigmentary alterations. Regardless of the cause or stage, *the common, similar feature in an eczematous skin disorder is inflamed skin.*

Atopic Dermatitis ICD-9 (691.8)

Atopic dermatitis is a very pruritic skin disorder involving cutaneous hypersensitivity. The disease is probably caused by combinations of immunologic dysregulation, epidermal barrier dysfunction, and increased genetic susceptibility. Atopic dermatitis often is associated with *atopy* (derived from the Greek word meaning *out of place*), and atopic individuals may have allergic rhinitis, asthma, elevated levels of immunoglobulin E (IgE), and a chronic, dry, pruritic, erythematous, scaling skin eruption occurring in classic areas (Fig. 14–1).

Atopic dermatitis usually begins in early infancy (after 6 weeks of age), childhood, or adolescence. The disease course is variable, although most often the symptoms lessen progressively with increasing age and complete resolution is not infrequent. In some patients, however, atopic dermatitis may be chronic and persist into adulthood or disappear for many years, then suddenly reappear.

Associated skin problems include keratosis pilaris, generalized xerosis, and scaly, hypopigmented plaques (pityriasis alba) on the face and extremities. Atopic dermatitis also is associated with decreased cellular immunity, especially to the herpes simplex and wart viruses. The skin often becomes colonized with increased counts of *Staphylococcus aureus*. In addition, atopic skin is more sensitive to several substances, wool and lanolin in particular. Rarely, there may be eye involvement, with cataracts and corneal abrasions in patients with severe disease.

I. CLASSIC DESCRIPTION (Figs. 14–1 and 14–2)

Distribution: Extensor surfaces and face in infants, flexural areas in children and adults
Primary: Plaques, papules
Secondary: Erythema, scale, excoriation,

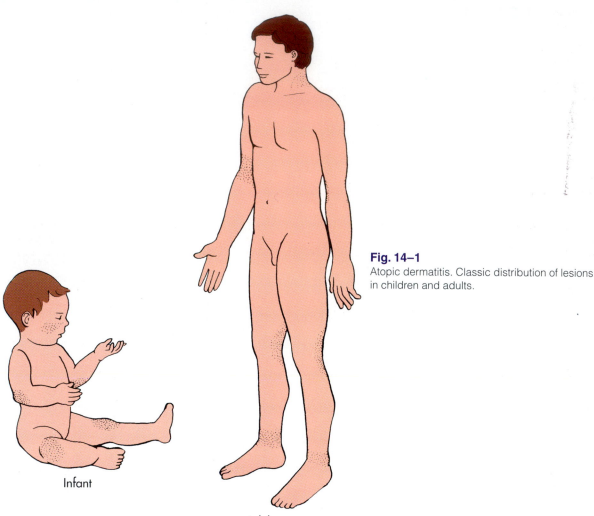

Fig. 14–1
Atopic dermatitis. Classic distribution of lesions in children and adults.

Infant

Adult

fissures, crust, and lichenification in chronic lesions

Follicular reactions are common in dark-skinned individuals. *Dennie-Morgan folds* are prominent lower eyelid folds often seen with atopy but also seen in other diseases.

II. DIAGNOSIS

The diagnosis of atopic dermatitis is based on a personal and/or family history of atopy, in the presence of a chronic, recurrent, pruritic skin eruption in classic locations.

Several features may assist in distinguishing atopic dermatitis from similar-appearing inflammatory skin conditions:

- Flexural involvement
- Pruritus
- Dry skin
- Personal history of asthma or allergic rhinitis
- Family history of atopic dermatitis
- Early age of onset (less than 2 years)

III. DIFFERENTIAL DIAGNOSIS

A. Seborrheic dermatitis: Seborrheic dermatitis in infants has a predilection for the scalp; atopic dermatitis has a predilection for the face and extensor surfaces.

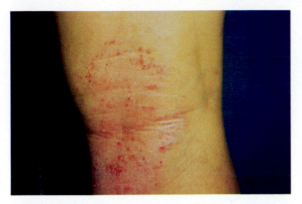

Fig. 14–2
Atopic dermatitis. Note erythematous plaque with excoriation in the posterior popliteal fossa. (Courtesy Beverly Sanders, MD.)

B. **Wiskott-Aldrich syndrome:** An X-linked recessive inherited syndrome, this rare disorder is found in conjunction with atopic dermatitis, thrombocytopenia, and recurrent, severe bacterial infections.

C. **Hyper-IgE syndrome:** This very rare disorder is characterized by increased levels of IgE, T-cell deficiencies, recurrent respiratory tract infections, staphylococcal abscesses, candidiasis, and skin lesions identical to those of atopic dermatitis.

D. **Psoriasis:** The scales of psoriasis are thicker, involvement is extensor rather than flexural, and nails may be affected.

E. **Scabies:** Although the pruritus is severe, scabies distribution, acute onset, and involvement of other household members are distinguishing factors.

F. **Allergic contact dermatitis:** If baseline atopic dermatitis suddenly worsens, look for secondary contact dermatitis, especially to a new soap, lotion, or prescription cream. Patch testing may be helpful.

G. **Cutaneous T-cell lymphoma:** Be suspicious of recalcitrant eczema in adults that remains unresponsive to topical corticosteroids. Biopsy of 3 to 4 indurated lesions may assist in differentiation.

BOX 14–1.
Treatment of Atopic Dermatitis

Mild cleansers for bathing
Daily emollients
Mild laundry detergents
Topical corticosteroids
Oral or topical antibiotics
Oral antihistamines
Cool compresses
Psychologic support for patient and family

IV. TREATMENT (Box 14–1)

A. **General skin care:**

1. *Cleansers:* Use mild cleansers for bathing (e.g., unscented White Dove, unscented Neutrogena, Aveeno) or a soap substitute (e.g., Aquanil, Cetaphil). Avoid hot water.

2. *Lubrication:* Lubricate the body daily, immediately after bathing, when the skin has been "patted" dry. Use unfragranced, lanolin-free moisturizers (e.g., Snow Drift shortening by Martha White, Lubriderm, Nutraderm, Eucerin Plus, or Moisturel). Use creams (e.g., Eucerin) for extremely dry skin.

3. *Avoid potentially offending substances:* Avoid wool, lanolin, and cosmetic agents with fragrances, including bubble bath for children.

4. *Keep children's nails trimmed* and consider covering their hands with socks at night so that rubbing, rather than scratching, occurs.

5. *Use fragrance-free laundry detergents:* (Ivory Snow Flakes, Cheer-Free, etc.)

6. *Use 100% cotton clothing,* because it is less irritating.

7. *Humidifying* the indoor environment may be helpful.

B. **Topical corticosteroids:**

1. Use a topical corticosteroid of the lowest potency that will control the disease. Be aware that systemic

absorption of topical corticosteroids, particularly in young children and infants with extensive areas of application, can cause growth retardation and hypothalamic-pituitary-adrenal gland axis suppression.

2. *Mild disease: Hydrocortisone* 1% to 2.5% or *desonide* 0.05% cream (or ointment for very dry skin).

3. *Moderate disease:* For thicker or unresponsive areas:
   a. Use *triamcinolone* 0.1% cream or ointment 2 or 3 times daily, less often with improvement, or *mometasone furoate* 0.1% cream or ointment daily, less often with improvement. Avoid using on the face and groin.
   b. When the disease is under control, resume using hydrocortisone or desonide cream.

4. *Severe disease:* For disease that remains unresponsive to above:
   a. Use *fluticasone propionate* (Cutivate) cream or ointment, *fluocinonide* (Lidex) or *flucinolone acetonide* (Synalar) qd to bid.
   b. For isolated lichenified lesions in older children or adults, consider using *betamethasone dipropionate* 0.05% cream or ointment bid for 2 to 3 weeks.
   c. Caution patients against prolonged use of these medications because of risk for atrophy; systemic absorption, causing hypothalamic-pituitary-adrenal gland axis suppression; and tachyphylaxis. Avoid use in face and groin.

5. Prescribe sufficient quantity for adequate application:
   - 15 g for an isolated lesion
   - 120 to 240 g for extensive involvement

6. Allow for ample refills because of the chronic and recurrent nature of the disease.

C. **Oral corticosteroids:** Although systemic steroids provide rapid relief in many cases, their use often leads to steroid dependence or rebound when discontinued. Use of systemic steroids should be limited to severe, acute flares in older children and adults (e.g., *prednisone* 0.5 to 1 mg/kg/day for a *maximum* of 7 to 10 days).

D. **Antibiotics:**
   1. Because atopic skin often is colonized with increased numbers of *S. aureus,* consider a course of antibiotic therapy for recalcitrant cases or those with secondary infection (in addition to topical corticosteroids), even if the skin does not appear overtly infected. Treat with oral antibiotics effective against *S. aureus* (e.g., *cephalexin, dicloxacillin, erythromycin*).
   2. Topical *mupirocin* (Bactroban 15, 30 g) ointment 3 times daily for 10 days is useful for limited involvement (in addition to topical corticosteroids). Use in place of oral antibiotics in these cases.
   3. Culture exudative lesions for bacterial antibiotic sensitivities in patients in whom multiple antibiotic regimens are required to control the disease.

E. **Antiviral agents:**
   1. Treat herpes infections aggressively, because patients with atopy are predisposed to more severe and disseminated infections, especially with primary exposure.
   2. Antiviral therapy:
      a. *Herpes simplex: Valacyclovir* 500 mg PO bid for 5 to 7 days for adults or *acyclovir* 200 mg/5 ml, 20 mg/kg/day in four divided doses for children.
      b. *Varicella (chickenpox) infections: Valacyclovir* 500 mg 2 PO or *famciclovir* 500 mg tid × 7 days for adults or *acyclovir* 200 mg/5 ml 20 mg/kg

4 times a day for 5 days in children (do not exceed 800 mg/dose).

3. Varicella vaccine: Encourage immunization of all children with atopic dermatitis, because varicella tends to be more severe in patients with atopic disease. The use of topical steroids is not a contraindication to varicella immunization.

F. **Psychologic support:** Atopic dermatitis can be very debilitating, particularly for children and their families.

1. Encourage parents to discuss any anxiety, apprehension, or feelings of aggression about having a child with atopic dermatitis.
2. Explain that atopic infants are not fragile, and that frequent affectionate touching will not hurt the child but will in fact help to alleviate anxiety for both the child and the parent.
3. Increased anxiety in an affected child or stress in an adult may manifest itself through increased scratching, which worsens the disease.
4. Stress-management techniques, such as muscle relaxation, meditation, imaging, or biofeedback, may be appropriate treatment modalities, particularly for disease flares precipitated by stress.

G. **Pruritus control:**

1. Oral antihistamines:
   a. *Hydroxyzine hydrochloride* 10 mg/5 ml elixir or 10-, 25-mg tablets. Sedating antihistamines are especially useful at bedtime.
      (1.) *Children less than 6 years:* Up to 50 mg/day in divided doses; more than 6 years: 50 to 100 mg/day in divided doses.
      (2.) *Adults:* 10 to 50 mg PO q6h prn.
   b. *Terfenadine* 60 mg PO bid, *astemizole* 10 mg qd, *loratidine* 10 mg qd, or *cetrizine* 10 mg qd on an empty stomach sometimes are useful as

nonsedating antihistamines for daytime use in adults. *Loratidine,* 10 mg qd (10 mg/10 cc) or *cetrizine* 5-10 mg qd (5 mg/5 ml) may be used in children less than 6 years old.

   c. *Doxepin* 10 to 50 mg qhs may be useful for pruritus control if sleep disturbances are not relieved by above. Watch for anticholinergic and other side effects.

2. Topical antihistamines:
   a. Pramoxine HCL, Prax, or Itch-X (OTC): May be useful for pruritus relief, in addition to topical steroids.
   b. *Doxepin* HCl cream 5% (30 g): Indicated for short-term (less than 8 days) management of pruritus in adults. Patients may apply qid prn, in addition to topical steroids. The medication may cause drowsiness and a rare contact dermatitis.
3. Topical compresses: Wet washcloths kept in the freezer and applied to affected, exudative skin may be quite soothing. Lukewarm baths with oatmeal (Aveeno) can also soothe acute pruritus.

H. **Allergy skin testing has not proved especially helpful** in treating most cases of atopic dermatitis. Avoiding particular animals, grasses, or foods (e.g., eggs, wheat, fish, soy, peanuts, cow milk) that seem to cause worsening of the skin disorder on exposure may be more helpful than extensive testing or elimination diets in the home.

I. **Alternative therapies:** Recent reports of Chinese herbal therapy being helpful may herald new approaches; however, the formulas are not yet standardized and the risks are not defined.

J. **Follow-up:** See patients initially monthly, then every 3 months for a year, offering emotional support and practical tips for dealing with potential physical and psychologic sequelae.

K. Referral: If the disease at any stage is unresponsive to routine therapies as outlined, refer the patient to a dermatologist. Other treatments may include topical tar preparations, ultraviolet B light therapy, PUVA light therapy, *azathioprine,* and *cyclosporine.*

V. PATIENT EDUCATION

(See patient education handout in Appendixes B and H.)

A. Educate patients that the disease is chronic and often recurrent.

B. Emphasize the need to maintain daily therapy with mild cleansers and lubricating lotions.

C. Explain the need to avoid wool products, creams with lanolin, and OTC products, especially those containing fragrance.

D. Write detailed instructions for using corticosteroid creams and explain that if there is not an adequate response, antibiotics may be needed.

E. Explain how and why patients should not be exposed to herpes simplex virus (e.g., don't let grandma with a cold sore kiss a baby with atopic dermatitis).

F. Consider advising patients to avoid occupations in which the work involves contact with irritating chemicals.

G. Advise patients that need additional support or desire further information to contact the National Eczema Association for Science and Education.*

Contact Dermatitis ICD-9 692.9

Contact dermatitis is any pruritic, reactionary skin disorder that results when a particular substance comes in contact with the skin. Contact dermatitis most commonly occurs in teenagers and young adults and is the second most common cause of occupational disability, with at

*National Eczema Association for Science and Education, 1221 S.W. Yamhill, #303, Portland, OR 97205; 1-800-818-SKIN, 503-228-4430.

A useful Web site: http://www.hkma.com.hk/std/eczema.htm

least 5 million physician visits yearly. Contact dermatitis often is subdivided into allergic contact dermatitis and irritant contact dermatitis. Clinically, both forms may occur in combination.

Allergic contact dermatitis occurs when an allergen or related compound causes a delayed type of hypersensitivity reaction on reexposure. This dermatitis usually appears as an acute, vesicular dermatitis within a few hours to 72 hours after contact. The course peaks within 7 to 10 days and resolves within 21 days if there is no repeat exposure. The most common reaction is *Rhus dermatitis,* which includes allergic reactions to poison ivy and poison oak. Table 14–1 lists other common allergens. A predisposing factor to developing allergic contact dermatitis includes any condition in which the skin integrity has been altered, such as stasis dermatitis.

Latex allergies are another kind of allergic contact dermatitis that has become an important cause of occupational morbidity over the past few years. Latex allergy must be differentiated from irritant contact dermatitis secondary to frequent handwashing or the powder on the gloves. With wheal development, rather than dermatitis, upon exposure, *anaphylaxis* (e.g., nasal stuffiness, wheezing, and shortness of breath) is possible.

Primary irritant dermatitis occurs secondary to any nonallergic skin irritation resulting from exposure to an offending agent, either with initial or repeated exposures. A common example includes frequent handwashing in harsh de-

TABLE 14–1.

Common Causes of Contact Dermatitis

Cause	Source
Fragrance	Perfumes, colognes, lotions
Nickel	Jewelry, clothing
Dichromate	Cement, leather
Paraphenylenediamine	Hair dye, clothing
Rubber chemicals	Clothing, shoes
Neomycin	Topical antibiotic ointments
Benzocaine	Topical anesthetic creams
Parabens	Sunscreens, lotions

tergents. Unless contact with the offending substance is discontinued, irritant contact dermatitis can be a chronic problem similar to allergic contact dermatitis. Other common irritants include lye, nitric acid, turpentine, gasoline, paint remover, soaps, solvents, laundry bleaches, and metal cleansers.

I. CLASSIC DESCRIPTION (Figs. 14–3 and 14–4)

Distribution: Site of contact
Primary: Vesicles, bullae, papules, plaques, wheals
Secondary: Erythema, edema, exudate, excoriation, fissures; chronic lesions may show lichenification and hyperpigmentation

Look for sharply demarcated lesions (e.g., linear lesions, where a leaf rubbed across the skin, indicate poison ivy; in glove dermatitis, the lesion stops abruptly above the wrist).

II. DIAGNOSIS

Diagnosis is based on a history of exposure to an allergen or a related compound, pruritic lesions, and a distribution pattern suggestive of contact dermatitis (Table 14–2). The history should center around exposure to common allergens. Be sure to inquire about any occupational, recreational, or household exposure. A good deal of detective work may be necessary to identify the inciting agent(s). See Table 4–1 for an outline of causes of occupational dermatitis.

III. DIFFERENTIAL DIAGNOSIS

A. Nummular eczema is characterized by discrete coin-shaped, erythematous, scaling plaques that are pruritic, similar to contact dermatitis, but there is no history of allergen exposure and the lesions are round, not of other configurations.

B. Atopic eczema is usually more chronic, occurs in a flexural distribution, and may be associated with atopy.

C. Hand eczema has no identifiable allergens, although this condition is often differentiated from allergic contact dermatitis only by patch testing. Contact dermatitis may precipitate flare-up of underlying hand eczema.

D. Dermatitis herpetiformis is usually localized to the elbows, knees, buttocks, and posterior scalp, has severe pruritus, and has less prominent cutaneous findings.

E. Scabies usually begins in the finger-webs and on the wrists, spreading to the

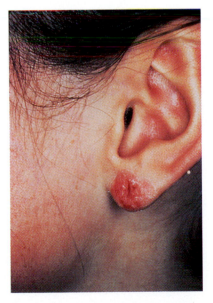

Fig. 14–3
Allergic contact dermatitis secondary to earrings. (Courtesy Department of Dermatology, Medical College of Georgia.)

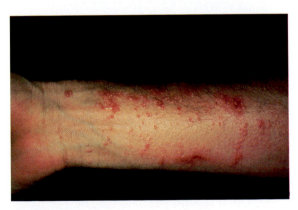

Fig. 14–4
Allergic contact dermatitis secondary to poison ivy.

TABLE 14–2.

Causes of Contact Dermatitis by Region

Eyelids:	Nail polish
	Facial cosmetics
	Hair cosmetics
	Ophthalmic medications
	Airborne contactants
Facial:	Facial cosmetics
	Nail cosmetics
	Airborne contactants
	Sunscreens
Scalp:	Hair products
Forehead:	Hair pomades
External ear:	Nickel (jewelry)
Earlobes:	Eyeglass frames
	Hearing aides
	Medications (neomycin, sulfonamides)
Neck:	Nickel (jewelry)
Chest:	Nickel (jewelry)
	Perfume
Beltline:	Underwear: rubber or chlorine-bleach
Umbilicus:	Metallic buttons
Trunk:	Perfume, detergents, deodorants
Axillae:	Clothing dye or finishes
Forearms:	Irritants that may splash above protective gloves
Thighs:	Nickel-containing objects (coins, keys)
	Hosiery
Vulva:	Feminine hygiene products
	Medications
	Chemical contraceptives
	Latex condoms
	Dyes and resins in clothing
	Bubble baths
Penis:	Poison ivy
	Medications
	Contraceptive chemicals
	Latex condoms
	Hygiene products used by partner
Rectum:	Medications (antibiotics, oil-containing laxatives)
	Perfumed or colored toilet tissue
	Certain foods (spices)
Lower legs:	Medications, especially in stasis dermatitis
	Clothing dyes, resins
	Detergents
	Insecticides

axillae, waist, groin, knees, and feet. Other family members may be symptomatic.

BOX 14–2.

Treatment of Contact Dermatitis

Identify inciting agents
Control pruritus with cool compresses, lotions, oral antihistamines
Use topical steroids for limited involvement
Use oral steroids for involvement of face, generalized body, or for uncontrollable pruritus
Psychologic support for potential extensive morbidity

IV. TREATMENT (Box 14–2)

A. Identify exposure and remove inciting agent(s) from patients. This often is difficult, especially in chronic cases.

B. Pruritus control: Use alone or in combination:

1. Oral antihistamines:
   a. *Hydroxyzine hydrochloride* 10 mg/5 ml elixir, 10-, 25-mg tablets. Sedating antihistamines are especially useful at bedtime.
      (1.) *Children less than 6 years:* Up to 50 mg/day in divided doses; more than 6 years: 50 to 100 mg/day in divided doses.
      (2.) *Adults:* 10 to 50 mg PO q6h prn.
   b. *Terfenadine* 60 mg PO bid, *astemizole* 10 mg qd, *loratidine* 10 mg qd, or *cetrizine* 10 mg qd sometimes are useful as nonsedating antihistamines for daytime use in adults.
   c. *Doxepin,* 10 to 50 mg qhs, may be useful for pruritus control if sleep disturbances are not relieved by the treatment suggested above. Watch for anticholinergic and other side effects.
2. Topical lotions that contain menthol, phenol, or pramoxine are useful to temporarily soothe itching and are not sensitizing, unlike benzocaine and diphenhydramine. Over-the-counter drugs include Sarna lotion, Itch X gel and Prax lotion; Cetaphil with menthol 0.25% and phenol 0.25% is available by prescription.

3. Topical compresses: Wet washcloths kept in the freezer and applied to affected, exudative skin for 20 minutes 3 times daily may be quite soothing. Avoid heat around lesions.

C. **Topical corticosteroids are useful if the involvement is limited** or if oral corticosteroids are contraindicated. Potent topical corticosteroids are necessary to blunt the allergic contact dermatitis reaction. Use agents for no more than 3 weeks and avoid using potent agents on the face, groin, or axillae.

1. Children: *Triamcinolone* 0.1% cream tid or *fluocinonide* 0.05% cream, gel, or lotion qd to tid.
2. Adults: *Betamethasone dipropionate* 0.05% cream, gel, or lotion; *diflorasone diacetate* 0.05% cream; or *clobetasol propionate* 0.05% cream or gel bid.
3. Face, groin, and axillary involvement: *Hydrocortisone* 2.5% cream or ointment.
4. Potent topical corticosteroid preparations are very expensive (at $30 to $40 for a 15-g tube). If the cost is prohibitive to the patient, prescribe *triamcinolone* 0.1% cream or ointment, but results may not be so dramatic.

D. **Oral corticosteroids are very useful for generalized allergic contact dermatitis, dermatitis involving the face or groin, or cases in which the pruritus cannot be controlled with local measures.**

1. *Prednisone:* 0.5 to 1 mg/kg, tapered over 2 to 3 weeks. One regimen might include 50 mg/day for 2 days, 45 mg/day for 2 days, 40 mg/day for 2 days, etc.
2. *Avoid dose packs,* because the dosage usually is inadequate and the treatment course far too short, resulting in a frustrated patient and clinician.

3. Oral steroids are inappropriate for irritant contact dermatitis or for use as chronic therapy.

E. **Treat any secondary bacterial infection.**

F. **Patient education strategies are vital to cure the disease.** (See below.)

G. **Referral:** Patients with chronic disease unresponsive to therapy or who do not respond after an adequate trial of therapy should be referred to a dermatologist.

V. **PATIENT EDUCATION**
(See patient education handout in Appendixes D and E.)

A. Educate patients on the need to identify and avoid inciting agents.

B. Instruct patients about the use of protective clothing, such as 100% cotton gloves, or protective barrier creams, such as Stokogard or Ivy Block to prevent contact of the skin with poison ivy if repeated exposure to an offending agent is expected.

C. Repeatedly explain that allergic contact dermatitis usually lasts 2 to 3 weeks, and that the purpose of treatment is to try to blunt the allergic reaction. Patients should expect to get a few new lesions even though they are receiving effective therapy.

D. Thoroughly explain to patients that they will not spread the rash on themselves or to other family members or friends by touching or scratching lesions.

E. Educate patients to discontinue any therapies that may be harmful or likely to cause secondary contact dermatitis. For instance, instruct patients to avoid self-medications, such as topical Benadryl or topical benzocaine, because such medications may cause an additional allergic or irritant reaction.

F. Instruct patients on the proper use and potential side effects of potent topical and oral steroids.

G. Provide patients with resource information.*

Exfoliative Dermatitis/Erythroderma
ICD-9 (695.89, or by etiology)

Exfoliative dermatitis, also known as *erythroderma,* is a rare, total skin erythema, followed by desquamation. The disease can have an acute or gradual onset, and about three fourths of cases are caused by either an underlying skin disease (Box 14–3), drug (Box 14–4), or malignancy. Exfoliative dermatitis secondary to an underlying skin disease usually lacks the typical skin features of the underlying disorder.

Typical signs and symptoms include malaise, fever, chills, and generalized adenopathy. The disorder is systemic, and the increased body stress is manifested by temperature dysregulation, transepidermal water loss, enteropathy, increased metabolic rate, and tremendous protein loss. Associated laboratory abnormalities include anemia, hypoalbuminemia, and, sometimes, eosinophilia. Sepsis, pneumonia, and heart failure are not uncommon, and prognosis depends on the underlying cause. Men are affected twice as often as women, usually after age 40.

I. CLASSIC DESCRIPTION (Fig. 14–5)
Distribution: Generalized, sparing mucous membranes
Primary: Papules, plaques
Secondary: Diffuse monomorphous erythema, scale/desquamation, edema, alopecia, and nail dystrophy

Lymphadenopathy (60%) and hepatomegaly (20% to 35%) may also be present.

II. DIAGNOSIS
Diagnosis is based on the clinical presence of diffuse, monomorphous erythema with scaling. Obtain two or three 4-mm punch biopsy specimens from early representative lesions to rule out an underlying skin disorder, especially cutaneous T-cell lymphoma. Obtain a complete blood cell count, liver and renal profile, serum protein electrophoresis, and chest radiograph examination. Consider bone marrow biopsy to rule out leukemia and lymphoma. Consider lymph node biopsy if adenopathy is present and the underlying cause is not identified.

III. DIFFERENTIAL DIAGNOSIS
A. Staphylococcal scalded skin syndrome: Diffuse erythema often is tender and occurs most commonly in infants. A source for underlying staphylococcal infection usually is present.
B. Toxic epidermal necrolysis: The onset is acute; bullae may be present, along with severe pain; and frozen section will reveal deeper involvement of the dermis.

IV. TREATMENT
A. Discontinue any suspect drugs.
B. Watch for systemic signs and symptoms: Observe and treat for any signs of dehydration, cardiac stress (high-output cardiac failure), malnutrition (hypoalbuminemia), and infection.

BOX 14–3.
Underlying Skin Disorders That Cause Exfoliative Dermatitis/Erythroderma

Atopic dermatitis	Pityriasis rubra pilaris
Contact dermatitis	Psoriasis
Cutaneous T cell lymphoma	Scabies
Lichen planus	Seborrheic dermatitis
Pemphigus foliaceus	

BOX 14–4.
Drugs That Can Cause Exfoliative Dermatitis:

Allopurinol	Hydantoins (phenytoin)
Barbiturates	Isoniazid
Captopril	Penicillin
Carbamazepine	Phenothiazine
Chloroquine	Sulfonamides
Gold	

---

*An internet resource for information is:
http://www.mc.vanderbilt.edu/vumcdept/derm/contact/

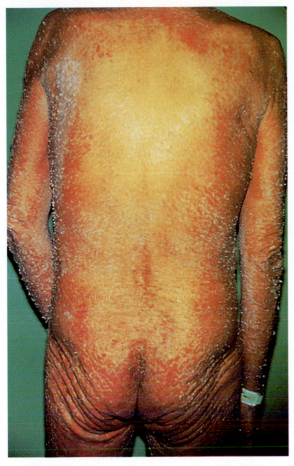

Fig. 14–5
Generalized exfoliative dermatitis with diffuse monomorphous erythematous scaling. (Courtesy Department of Dermatology, University of North Carolina at Chapel Hill.)

C. **General skin care** includes lukewarm baths and bland emollients qid (e.g., Aquaphor ointment, Eucerin cream, or Snow Drift shortening by Martha White).

D. **Topical corticosteroids:** *Triamcinolone acetonide* 0.1% cream or ointment 2 to 4 times a day. If folliculitis develops with ointment use, switch to cream. Prescribe sufficient quantity (1-lb jars) and be aware that systemic absorption will occur because of extensive involvement.

E. **Systemic steroids:** Consider systemic steroids for erythroderma that is caused by severe contact dermatitis, atopic dermatitis, or medications. Oral corticosteroids are contraindicated if psoriasis is the underlying skin disorder, because they can exacerbate the condition and cause rebound on withdrawal.

F. **Pruritus control:** Oral antihistamines (e.g., *hydroxyzine hydrochloride* 10 to 50 mg PO q4 to 8 hours). If no response, add another class of antihistamine (e.g., *cyproheptadine* 4 mg q8h).

G. **Referral or consultation:** Referral or consultation with a dermatologist is indicated to assist in diagnosis and management, particularly when the cause is unclear or the course is chronic.

Hand and Foot Eczema ICD-9 (692.9)

Hand and foot eczema are chronic, often pruritic, inflammatory skin disorders that can range from acute vesicular lesions to painful fissures or chronic scaling plaques. Hand eczema occurs more often in people who frequently have their hands immersed in water (e.g., housewives, cooks, nurses, bartenders). Acute vesicular hand dermatitis that is characterized by deep-seated vesicles occurring in a cyclical pattern is known as *pompholyx,* or *dyshidrotic,* eczema.

Underlying atopic dermatitis can predispose to these conditions. Contact dermatitis also may play a role in either initiating flare-ups in a predisposed person or in prolonging resolution of a flare-up. Sweat abnormalities have no relation to the disorder.

I. **CLASSIC DESCRIPTION** (Fig. 14–6)
Distribution: Palms, including sides of fingers, soles; usually symmetric
Primary: Vesicles, papules, plaques
Secondary: Erythema, scale, fissures, exudate, lichenification, erosions

Nail dystrophy can occur if the eczema involves the nail matrix.

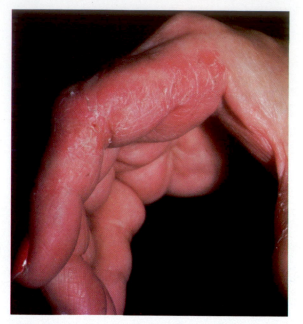

Fig. 14–6
Inflamed hand eczema.

II. DIAGNOSIS

Diagnosis is based on a history of recurrent eruptions, localized to either the palms or soles, when other causes of dermatitis, such as contact dermatitis or dermatophyte, have been excluded.

III. DIFFERENTIAL DIAGNOSIS

A. **Contact dermatitis:** Irritant or allergic contact may initiate or cause persistence of underlying hand or foot eczema, but contact dermatitis usually is linked with an exposure history (e.g., use of detergents on hands, hobbies, occupational, etc.). Contact dermatitis on the feet usually is not diffuse but is limited to weight-bearing aspects and dorsa of feet and is the result of rubber or leather tanning.

B. **Dermatophyte infections (tinea manus or tinea pedis):** Dermatophyte infections are rare in preadolescent children. When the hands and feet are involved, the pattern may be asymmetric, often in the distribution of one hand and two feet. Exceptions, such as an id reaction, occur when both hands are involved. Potassium hydroxide testing must be done on the involved areas to rule out a dermatophyte infection before diagnosing hand or foot eczema.

C. **Atopic dermatitis:** Atopic dermatitis can be localized to the hands and feet, and atopic individuals are more likely to develop eczema on exposure to precipitating agents (e.g., an atopic beautician or health care worker who develops eczema after frequent handwashing). A personal or family history of atopy and a history of typical atopic dermatitis lesions elsewhere should be present.

D. **Psoriasis:** Psoriasis can occur on the hands and feet as well-demarcated plaques with thicker, silvery scales. Look for the pustules of pustular psoriasis, psoriatic lesions elsewhere on the body (e.g., elbows, knees, scalp), and the typical nail changes of pitting or distal onycholysis.

IV. TREATMENT

A. **General skin care** (Box 14–5)
1. Use only mild cleansers or soap substitutes.
2. Use lanolin-free and fragrance-free emollients frequently.
3. Avoid constant skin wetting and wear protective cotton-lined gloves.

BOX 14–5.
General Skin Care Guidelines

Mild cleansers (e.g., White Dove or Eucerin cleansing lotion)
Soap substitutes (e.g., Cetaphil, Aquanil) for sensitive skin
Emollients as frequently as possible that are lanolin-free and fragrance-free (e.g., Neutrogena Norwegian Hand Formula, Aquaphor, Eucerin, Lubriderm, or Moisturel cream)
Moisturizers after bathing
Protective barriers (e.g., gloves)
Prescription creams or ointments *only* as directed

B. Topical corticosteroids:
1. Start with a medium-potency steroid (e.g., *triamcinolone* 0.1%, *desoximetasone* [Topicort] 0.25% cream) 2 or 3 times daily; instruct the patient to taper the medication gradually as improvement occurs (e.g., daily, then every other day, then as necessary).
2. For maintenance, try a lower-strength steroid (e.g., *desonide* 0.05% [Tridesilon], *hydrocortisone butyrate* 0.1% [Locoid], *hydrocortisone valerate* 0.2% [Westcort]).
3. For more severe or resistant cases, consider a 2-week course of *betamethasone dipropionate* 0.05% ointment or cream or other class I or II topical steroids twice daily, then return to using a medium- or low-potency corticosteroid for long-term use.
4. Ointments are stronger than creams; however, some patients will not use ointments because they are "greasy."

C. Oral antibiotics: Treat any secondary infections with an antibiotic effective against both *S. aureus* and *Streptococcus pyogenes.*

D. Avoid over-the-counter medications: Some OTC agents, such as Caladryl and Neosporin, may be sensitizing, contributing to a contact dermatitis on top of the eczema.

E. Referral: If the lesions remain unresponsive or there is strong suspicion for contact dermatitis underlying the chronic hand eczema, refer the patient to a dermatologist for possible patch testing and consideration of alternative therapies (e.g., light treatment).

V. PATIENT EDUCATION
(See patient education handout in Appendix G.)
A. Educate patients about the chronic and recurrent nature of the disease.

B. Try to identify and avoid any precipitating substances and OTC preparations that may contain fragrance or other irritating substances.
C. Educate patients about appropriate preventive measures (e.g., use of protective gloves).
D. Write instructions for the appropriate use of topical corticosteroids, especially high-potency drugs, explaining carefully the risk for systemic absorption, atrophy, and other side effects.

Stasis Dermatitis ICD-9 454.1

Stasis dermatitis is a chronic eczematous process resulting from suboptimal lower extremity circulation and chronic venous insufficiency. Clinically, early stasis dermatitis is characterized by hyperpigmentation, caused by leakage of blood into the dermis and its subsequent breakdown into hemosiderin. Predisposing conditions include varicose veins, thrombophlebitis, cardiac failure, hypoalbuminemia, or surgery or trauma to the limb. It more commonly occurs in people older than age 50 and in women more often than men. Chronic ulceration can occur and is associated with substantial morbidity.

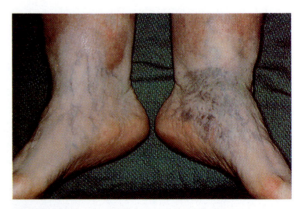

Fig. 14–7
Moderate stasis dermatitis with hyperpigmentation and bilateral venous insufficiency. (Courtesy Department of Dermatology, University of North Carolina at Chapel Hill.)

I. CLASSIC DESCRIPTION (Fig. 14–7)

Distribution: Medial aspect of ankles; lower extremities from ankle to midcalf

Primary: Plaques, vesicles; bullae, if severe edema is present

Secondary: Hyperpigmentation, scale, erythema, edema, ulcers, exudate

II. DIAGNOSIS

The diagnosis is clinical, based on the presence of hyperpigmentation, location of skin findings, and the history of a predisposing condition.

III. DIFFERENTIAL DIAGNOSIS

A. **Contact dermatitis:** With contact dermatitis there is no history of edema or predisposing factors. However, *contact dermatitis can easily occur with stasis dermatitis* because some common topical agents, such as *neomycin* (found in Neosporin) or *benzocaine,* may not be tolerated in the area of stasis, even if the medication is tolerated elsewhere on the body.

B. **Ulcers:** Consider other causes of chronic ulcers (Box 14–6). Arterial ulcers usually involve the pretibial area or the toes. Neuropathic ulcers often are found on weight-bearing areas of the toes or heel.

IV. TREATMENT (Generalized stasis dermatitis)

A. **Localized measures to control edema:**
   1. Elevate the affected extremity above the level of the heart when sitting down and at bedtime.
   2. Use pressure-graded support hose (at least medium [20 mm Hg] or strong [30 mm Hg]). Stockings should extend at least to midthigh.
   3. Encourage lower extremity muscle use, such as walking or flexing, and elevating the involved extremity when reclining.
   4. General skin care: See Box 14–5.

B. **Topical corticosteroids:** Use low-dose topical steroids (e.g., *hydrocortisone* 1%) once or twice daily. For very inflamed lesions, use a medium-strength steroid (e.g., *triamcinolone* 0.1% cream) once or twice daily. Monitor for signs of atrophy.

C. **Oral antibiotics are useful to treat any secondary infection.**

D. **Avoid sensitizing or tissue-toxic agents** (e.g., povidone, alcohol).

E. **For stasis dermatitis with small to moderate ulcer formation:** Consider one or more of the following.
   1. *Duoderm patches for isolated small ulcers:*
      a. Clean and debride the ulcer with dilute hydrogen peroxide (4 parts water to 1 part water) or normal saline.
      b. Cut patch to size of ulcer, leaving 1¼ inches beyond the ulcer margin.
      c. Hypoallergenic paper tape may be used to secure the edges if necessary.
      d. Leave on for 3 to 7 days at a time, replacing sooner if exudate leaks from dressing.
      e. It is normal for the ulcer base to have a thick yellow base from the dressing.
      f. May be used in conjunction with Duoderm or other compression bandages, after establishing the presence of adequate arterial blood flow.

BOX 14–6.

Causes of Leg Ulcers

Venous insufficiency (90%)	Vasculitis
Carcinoma	Syphilis
Leukemia	Metabolic diseases
Cryoglobulinemia	Sickle cell disease
Infections: bacterial, fungal, parasitic	Peripheral neuropathy
Panniculitis	Arterial insufficiency
Bites	Trauma
Pyoderma gangrenosum	Sarcoidosis
	Necrobiosis lipoidica

g. Avoid potentially sensitizing topical antibiotics, (e.g., *bacitracin, genatmicin, neomycin*). If a topical antibiotic is desired, use topical *Silvadene, erythromycin,* or *mupirocin.*

2. Unna boot application for ulcers with associated leg edema:
   a. Change no more frequently than once or twice a week.
   b. Wrap to just below the knee.
   c. Continue dressings for 2 weeks after ulcer heals, to help the new delicate skin become established.
   d. Debride the ulcer with each dressing change.
3. Compression stockings: Indefinite use of graduated compression stockings of 30 to 40 mm Hg may be useful.
4. Consider biopsy to rule out carcinoma and other unusual causes or an x-ray examination to rule out osteomyelitis if the ulcer fails to show some improvement with the above therapies after several weeks.

V. PATIENT EDUCATION

A. Educate the patient about the importance of elevating the involved extremity, writing specific instructions on duration and technique.
B. Educate patients on general skin care measures, including using a mild soap (e.g., White Dove), using bland emollients (e.g., Lubriderm), avoiding trauma, and using pressure-graded stockings on a regular basis.
C. Educate about avoiding OTC preparations.
D. Educate on proper topical steroid use; *instruct patients to avoid applying corticosteroid creams in ulcers.*

Xerotic Eczema ICD-9 (706.8)

Xerotic eczema, or xerosis, is a common inflammatory disorder characterized by severe skin dryness and pruritus. The dryness is thought to be related to decreases of surface skin lipids in affected people, although the exact cause is unknown. Xerotic eczema most commonly occurs in older adults. Predisposing factors include atopic dermatitis, low humidity, and renal disease. Underlying hypothyroidism, protein and essential fatty acid deficiency, hypervitaminosis A, and certain drugs can cause the same clinical symptoms. **Nummular eczema** refers to xerotic lesions that are coin-shaped and quite pruritic.

I. CLASSIC DESCRIPTION (Fig. 14–8)
Distribution: Generalized or localized, especially on the legs, arms, or hands
Primary: Plaques
Secondary: Scale, erythema, fissures; occasionally lichenification, excoriation, and crust

II. DIAGNOSIS
Diagnosis is based on the clinical presentation of diffuse or localized areas of dry, scaling, pruritic skin lesions.

III. DIFFERENTIAL DIAGNOSIS
A. **Scabies:** Scabies lesions have a characteristic distribution (see Fig. 6–1), and other family members often are affected. Excoriations can be severe in scabies. Do a scabies scrape to demonstrate mites in suspect lesions.

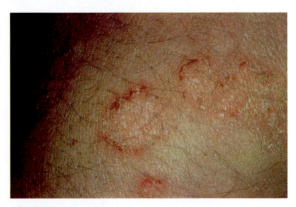

Fig. 14–8
Xerotic eczema. Note excoriated, coin-shaped, or nummular, erythematous plaques. (Courtesy Beverly Sanders, MD.)

B. Pruritus: If the pruritus is present on a daily basis for more than a few weeks, despite adequate management, investigate other causes (e.g., underlying systemic disease, such as thyroid disease, lymphomas or hematologic malignancies, hepatitis, renal disease, diabetes, medications; see Chapter 23).

IV. TREATMENT

A. General skin care: See Box 14–5.

1. Have patients use mild cleansers or soap substitutes for bathing.
2. Encourage daily lubrication after bathing, with unfragranced, lanolin-free moisturizers. Alpha-hydroxy acid-containing moisturizers may be even more effective. (OTC: [Lactic acid: Lacticare, Lachydrin, Lubriderm Moisture Plus, Aquaglycolic lotion]; Rx: [Lachydrin 12%, 225, 400 g] qd after a shower or bath) Transient stinging is expected with lotions containing alpha-hydroxy acids.

3. Avoid wool and hot baths.
4. Consider humidification for low-humidity environments, especially in winter.

B. Topical corticosteroids:

1. Low-potency topical corticosteroids: *hydrocortisone* 1% cream (or ointments if the skin is very dry) or *desonide* 0.05% lotion (2, 4 oz).
2. For thicker, lichenified areas or for those unresponsive to *hydrocortisone* 1% cream, use *triamcinolone* 0.1% cream or ointment 2 or 3 times daily; taper with improvement. When the disease is under control, return to using *hydrocortisone* cream.
3. Prescribe sufficient quantity for adequate application (e.g., 240 g for diffuse truncal involvement).
4. Avoid using oral corticosteroids.

V. PATIENT EDUCATION:

(See patient education handout in Appendixes G and H.)

KERATOSIS PILARIS ICD-9 (757.39)

Keratosis pilaris is a very common and chronic disorder of the *hair follicle*. Patients usually seek medical care either because the disorder is cosmetically unattractive or because of symptoms such as itching. The disease is characterized by follicular plugging with keratin debris and is *usually found on the extensor surfaces of the proximal upper and lower extremities, buttocks, and trunk* (Fig. 14–9). Lesions often are asymptomatic, but this varies among individuals. Tight clothes may aggravate the condition. Patients with atopic dermatitis and ichthyosis more frequently have the disease.

If the lesions are pruritic or painful, the disease is known as **inflammatory keratosis pilaris.** These patients will have erythematous papules and pustules in the characteristic distribution.

I. CLASSIC DESCRIPTION

Primary: Papules, pustules
Secondary: Erythema, scale

II. DIAGNOSIS

The diagnosis is clinical, based on the morphology and distribution of lesions. A hair piercing the center of a papule or pustule confirms a follicular location.

III. DIFFERENTIAL DIAGNOSIS

A. Acne vulgaris: Distribution of acne is on the face, chest, upper back, and shoulders.

B. Miliaria pustulosa: Miliaria, or prickly heat, involves the sweat glands and not the hair follicle; thus a hair will not be seen piercing the pustule. Onset of miliaria is acute.

C. Drug eruption: The onset of drug erup-

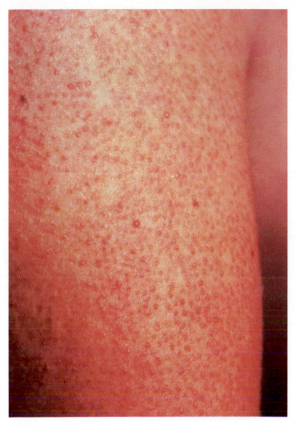

Fig. 14–9
Keratosis pilaris. Note prominent, mildly inflamed follicles on the upper arm. (Courtesy John Cook, MD.)

tions usually is acute and eruptive, whereas keratosis pilaris tends to be chronic. The history of onset often correlates with recent drug ingestion for drug eruptions.

IV. TREATMENT
  A. **Keratolytic agents:** (Table 14-3)
    1. Choose either the urea, glycolic, or lactic acid preparations, to be used alone twice daily or alternate (e.g., urea lotion in the morning, lactic acid lotion at night).
    2. These agents remove keratin debris, keeping follicles "unplugged." Some agents may cause transient stinging.

TABLE 14–3.
Keratolytic Agents as Treatment for Keratosis Pilaris

	Product	Dosages
OTC	Urea 10% lotion	6, 8 oz
	Urea 10% cream	2.5 oz
	Urea 20% cream	3 oz, 1 lb
	Glycolic 10% acid lotion	4 oz
	Lactic acid 5% lotion	4, 8 oz
Px	Lactic 12% acid lotion	225, 400 g
	Tretinoin 0.05% cream	45 g
	Tretinoin 0.1% cream	45 g

OTC: Available over the counter
Px: Available by prescription

    3. If tretinoin is used, apply it at bedtime; it may cause irritation and photosensitivity.
  B. **Inflammatory keratosis pilaris:**
    1. Treat with long-term antibiotic therapy, as in acne vulgaris, in conjunction with the keratolytic agents mentioned above.
    2. Use *tetracycline* or *erythromycin* 500 mg PO twice daily or *doxycycline* 100 mg daily, for 2 months. Taper monthly to daily, every other day, and so on, to the lowest dose that will control new lesions.

V. PATIENT EDUCATION
  A. Educate patients that the treatment goal is control, not cure, of the disorder.
  B. Teach patients that long-term therapy is necessary to prevent new lesions as long as the skin has a tendency for plugged follicles.
  C. Explain that it will take at least 6 to 8 weeks before the patient should judge the effectiveness of treatment.
  D. Give guidelines on general skin care for using mild cleansers and keratolytic agents (e.g., 10% or 20% urea or 5% or 12% lactic acid).

LICHEN PLANUS ICD-9 (697.0)

Lichen planus is a disorder of unknown cause, most commonly affecting middle-age adults. The disease is characterized by polygonal violaceous papules and plaques; its course may be short or chronic, although most cases remit within 1 year. Buccal mucosal or genital involvement can be severe and debilitating in some patients, as a result of painfulness of the lesions. Lesions usually heal with significant postinflammatory hyperpigmentation.

I. CLASSIC DESCRIPTION (Fig. 14–10)
Distribution: Mouth, genitals, volar wrists, ankies; may be generalized; symmetric
Primary: Papules, plaques
Secondary: Erythema, violescent appearance, scale, erosions, rarely ulcers; postinflammatory hyperpigmentation may be marked
Wickham's striae are characteristic white lacelike patterns on the surface of the papules and plaques. Mucous membrane involvement may consist solely of these lacelike lesions (Fig. 14–11). When nails are involved, the disease spectrum varies from minor dystrophy to total nail loss.

II. DIAGNOSIS
Diagnosis usually is based on the lesion's clinical appearance in a characteristic location. With buccal involvement, look for Wickham's striae in the individual lesions to help confirm the diagnosis. Rule out drug-related lichenoid eruptions so that an offending agent can be withdrawn if this diagnosis is likely. If a biopsy is necessary to confirm the diagnosis, perform a deep shave or punch biopsy of the most-developed lesion.

III. DIFFERENTIAL DIAGNOSIS
A. **Lichenoid drug eruptions** historically should correlate with drug intake, most commonly gold, antimalarials, quinidine, captopril, thiazide, methyldopa, and penicillamine.
B. **Chronic graft-versus-host disease** can produce a "lichenoid" eruption similar to lichen planus.
C. **Secondary syphilis** involves the palms and soles. The white lacelike patterns on buccal mucosa or genitals is absent. Serologic studies will differentiate the two.

IV. TREATMENT
A. **Medium- to high-potency topical corticosteroids:**

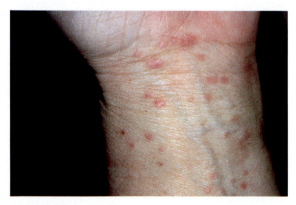

Fig. 14–10
Lichen planus. Note discrete polygonal scaling erythematous papules on the wrist. (Courtesy Department of Dermatology, Medical College of Georgia.)

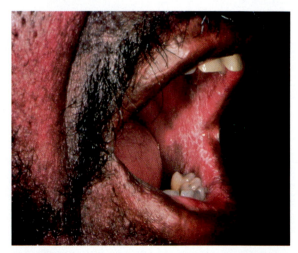

Fig. 14–11
Oral lichen planus with white lacelike lesions on the buccal mucosa. (Courtesy Department of Dermatology, Medical College of Georgia.)

1. *Mouth lesions: Flucinonide* 0.05 ointment or gel 2 or 3 times daily.
2. *Body lesions: Betamethasone dipropionate* 0.05%, *diflorasone diacetate* 0.05%, or other class I cream or ointment 2 times daily. Caution patients about steroid atrophy.
3. *Genital lesions: Desonide* cream 0.05% bid initially, although higher-potency creams may be necessary.
4. *Hypertrophic lesions:* Intralesional injections, such as *triamcinolone* 5 to 10 mg/ml, injecting 0.5 to 1 ml per 2-cm lesion are helpful for pruritus relief. Use cautiously in dark-skinned patients because of risk of hypopigmentation.

B. **Lichenoid drug eruptions:** If drug eruptions are a strong possibility, identify the suspected agent and discontinue its use.

C. **Oral antihistamines** (e.g., *hydroxyzine hydrochloride* 10 to 50 mg 4 times a day, as necessary) may be helpful in controlling pruritus.

D. **Rule out candidal infections:** Such infections may coexist with lichen planus eruptions in oral and genital locations.

E. **Referral** is indicated if there is no response to the above treatments.

V. **PATIENT EDUCATION**

A. Explain to patients that although the disease can be chronic, most cases resolve, often spontaneously.

B. Educate patients to avoid particular drugs that are identified as inciting.

LICHEN SCLEROSUS ICD-9 (701.0)

Lichen sclerosus is a chronic disorder of unknown cause that *affects prepubertal children and older adults.* The disorder is seen more commonly in female patients. Lesions may be asymptomatic but often are quite uncomfortable, especially when they occur in the groin area. Many patients complain of a burning, rather than an itching, sensation. Because the skin tears easily in this disease, erosions or fissures may be seen. Dyspareunia or anal or genital bleeding may occur. In male patients, penile inflammation can lead to urethral strictures or phimosis, requiring circumcision. Spontaneous remission occurs at menarche in two thirds of prepubertal girls. Controversy exists as to whether there is an increased incidence of squamous cell carcinoma in affected genitalia.

I. **CLASSIC DESCRIPTION** (Fig. 14–12)
Distribution: Genitalia, neck, axillae, flexural area of extremities
Primary: Macules, papules, plaques; rarely, bullae
Secondary: Atrophy, ivory-white lesions, hemorrhage into lesions, erosions, fissures

Erythema in genital areas may be the only initial sign. Thinned, atrophic skin is likened to wrinkled tissue paper. A "keyhole" distribution pattern is described in vulval and perineal involvement. Follicular plugs, called dells, are seen in some lesions.

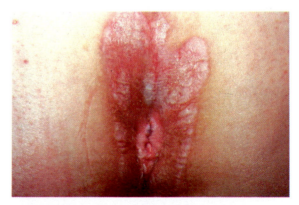

Fig. 14–12
Lichen sclerosus. Perianal area is thinned and chalk white (keyhole distribution). (Courtesy Department of Dermatology, University of North Carolina at Chapel Hill.)

II. DIAGNOSIS

Diagnosis is based on the clinical appearance of ivory-white atrophic lesions in the characteristic locations. Close inspection may reveal the presence of follicular plugs. Early lesions, especially of the vulva, may have only mild erythema despite an extensive burning sensation. Punch or deep shave biopsy of the most developed areas will confirm the diagnosis of lichen sclerosus. Use of EMLA cream (prilocaine and lidocaine mixture) applied 2 hours before the local anesthetic injection will ease the pain associated with the injection and subsequent biopsy.

III. DIFFERENTIAL DIAGNOSIS

A. **Morphea:** The ivory-white plaques of morphea may be difficult to distinguish but look for the characteristic distribution and follicular plugs associated with lichen sclerosus.

B. **Lichen planus:** Look for Wickham's striae, as seen in lichen planus, especially the lacelike network on the mucosa. Look for follicular plugs in lichen sclerosus.

IV. TREATMENT

A. **Topical corticosteroids:**
1. Start with *hydrocortisone* 1% cream or *desonide* 0.05% ointment or cream bid (15, 30 g) in groin areas.
2. Advance to medium-potency steroids, such as *triamcinolone* 0.1% cream, for more severe disease, but monitor closely for thinning in areas that already are atrophic. (*Aristocort A* 0.1% ointment may be indicated to avoid any irritation from vehicles of generic steroid preparations.)
3. For severe, symptomatic disease, consider *clobetasol propionate* 0.05% ointment bid (15 g), with close monitoring of patients every 4 weeks for signs of skin atrophy.

B. **Testosterone 2% cream** may be useful only if disease is resistant to topical steroids.
1. Apply to affected areas twice daily.
2. No commercially prepared creams are available. Instead, mix 5 ml testosterone propionate in 25 g white petrolatum.
3. Judge response after using for 6 to 12 weeks.

C. **Biopsy any nonhealing areas.** A biopsy should also be made of the raised white plaques of leukoplakia in the genital region to rule out squamous cell carcinoma.

D. **Secondary infection:** Watch for and treat any secondary candidal or bacterial infections, particularly when there are disease flares in the genital region.

E. **Pruritus Relief:** *hydroxyzine hydrochloride,* 10 to 50 mg qid may be helpful in controlling pruritus.

F. **Follow-up:** With genital involvement, follow up every 6 months.

G. **Referral:** Consider referral for advanced or recalcitrant disease, for a trial of *tretinoin* cream or oral retinoids or to monitor for signs of skin atrophy when strong topical steroids are used in the genital area. Circumcision may be indicated if dysuria, urethral strictures, or painful erections persist after an adequate trial of *clobetasol.*

V. PATIENT EDUCATION

A. Educate parents of prepubertal patients that lichen sclerosus is sometimes confused with sexual abuse, and although the two conditions may coexist, there is no causal association.

B. Inform patients that pruritus and pain control, not cure, may be the realistic therapeutic goals.

PITYRIASIS ROSEA ICD-9 (696.3)

Pityriasis rosea is a common, eruptive dermatitis that primarily affects people age 10 to 35. The cause is unknown but is speculated to be viral, because many patients have a history of upper respiratory tract symptoms preceding the skin lesions. The characteristic eruption begins with a *herald patch* 1 to 2 weeks before onset of the truncal eruption. Herald patches can be several centimeters in diameter and mimic tinea corporis. Symptoms vary among patients and range from no symptoms to severe pruritus. Most patients seek medical care either because of the pruritus or because of concern about a long-standing rash. The course is usually 2 to 10 weeks, and the disease remits spontaneously.

I. CLASSIC DESCRIPTION (Fig. 14–13)
Distribution: Trunk, upper extremities; inverse variety may occur with primary involvement of flexural areas
Primary: Papules, plaques
Secondary: Scale, erythema; hyperpigmentation in dark-skinned patients
Scales tend to be centrally located. Plaques are oriented along skin cleavage lines, with

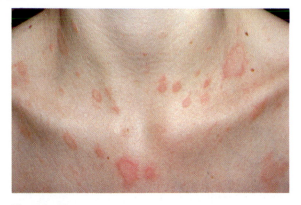

Fig. 14–13
Pityriasis rosea. Note left supraclavicular herald patch and diffuse scaling papules and plaques in a Christmas tree distribution. (Courtesy Department of Dermatology, University of North Carolina at Chapel Hill.)

distribution often described as similar to a Christmas tree pattern.

II. DIAGNOSIS
Diagnosis is based on the clinical history, the presence of a herald patch (although not always present), a characteristic distribution, and the appearance of central scale. A test to rule out syphilis is indicated in most patients, regardless of age or social status. A KOH preparation should be prepared from the herald patch and/or other scaling lesions to rule out fungal infection.

III. DIFFERENTIAL DIAGNOSIS
A. Secondary syphilis: Involvement of the palms, soles, and mucous membranes is more typical of syphilis. Serologic tests easily differentiate the conditions.
B. Guttate psoriasis: Like pityriasis rosea, there often is a history of a preceding upper respiratory tract infection, but psoriasis does not have a herald patch and the scale is thicker.
C. Drug eruptions: The history should suggest an etiologic agent. A herald patch is absent and lesion distribution differs. Look for scales in pityriasis rosea.
D. Eczema: Eczema typically does not have a Christmas tree distribution or a herald patch, and onset usually is not so eruptive as in pityriasis rosea.
E. Tinea corporis: A herald patch must be scraped and tested with KOH for the presence of hyphae. Testing any remaining lesions for the presence of dermatophytes also will distinguish the lesions.
F. Tinea versicolor: Tinea versicolor is a yeast infection, and the KOH-prep test will reveal pseudohyphae and spores.

IV. TREATMENT
A. Pruritus control: Select any agent listed below, in isolation or combination, depending on severity of pruritus.

1. *Topical antipruritic agents* as necessary (e.g., Prax, Pramegel, or Sarna lotion [OTC] or Cetaphil with menthol 0.5% [prescription]).
2. *Topical corticosteroids* (e.g., *triamcinolone* 0.1% cream) to affected areas 2 to 3 times daily. Instruct patients to avoid using on the face, groin, and axillae.
3. *Oral antihistamines:*
   Hydroxyzine hydrochloride 10 mg/5 ml elixir, 10-, 25-mg tablets. Sedating antihistamines are especially useful at bedtime.
   Children less than 6 years: Up to 50 mg/day in divided doses; more than 6 years: 50 to 100 mg/day in divided doses.
   Adults: 10 to 50 mg PO q6h prn.
B. **Referral:** Consider referring the patient to a dermatologist for ultraviolet B light therapy daily for 5 days if the pruritus is severe and unresponsive to the above measures. If available, exposure to natural sunlight will often lessen pruritus. Caution patients to avoid sunburns.
C. **Rule out secondary syphilis.**
D. **Follow-up is not usually needed** unless the symptoms of pruritus do not resolve or if the eruption remains after 2 to 3 months.

V. **PATIENT EDUCATION**
A. Explain to patients that the eruption may last 2 to 3 months.
B. Educate patients that new lesions may continue to develop during treatment but that the lesions will spontaneously resolve.
C. Reassure patients that once the rash occurs they will not infect others.
D. Educate patients that brief periods of natural sunlight (e.g., 30 minutes of midday exposure) may help symptoms of pruritus.

PSORIASIS ICD-9 (696.1)

Psoriasis, which literally means *an itching condition,* is a chronic, recurrent, hyperproliferative inflammatory disorder of unknown cause. Because of the chronicity and unpredictability of the disease and the associated severe symptoms, psoriasis is often very disruptive to patients' lives, contributing significant physical and psychologic burdens.

Psoriasis is common, affecting 2 to 3 million people in the United States at any one time. The disease initially appears most commonly in people younger than age 20 but can occur at any age, even after age 60. Males and females are affected equally. Approximately 30% of patients have a family history of psoriasis.

Psoriasis is characterized by erythematous plaques with thick, adherent, silvery scales (Fig. 14–14). The spectrum of clinical involvement is diffuse, ranging from limited to generalized involvement, which may flare up at any time in life. This unpredictability is a contributing factor in difficulty for many patients in living with this disease.

Several cellular events are key to understanding the clinical course of the disease, including increased growth and differentiation of keratinocytes and the accumulation and activation of T cells and other inflammatory cells within a lesion.

The onset of psoriasis commonly occurs as a *guttate* form, characterized by small, scattered, teardrop-shaped papules and plaques, after a streptococcal infection as a child or young adult; chronic, larger plaques occur later in life. A *pustular* variant may occur, with predominant involvement of the hands and/or feet, including nails.

Psoriatic lesions have a predilection for sites of trauma, a process known as *Koebner's phenomenon.* Emotional or physical stress also is

A

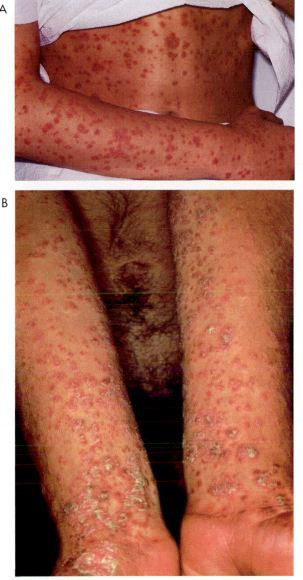

B

Fig. 14–14 A, B
Guttate type of psoriasis, with multiple diffuse erythematous papules and plaques. (**B,** courtesy Marshall Guill, MD.)

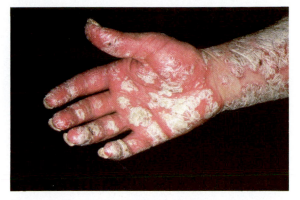

Fig. 14–15
Plaque type of psoriasis. Note thick, silvery scale of well-developed lesions. (Courtesy Department of Dermatology, Medical College of Georgia.)

riatic arthritis is characterized by asymmetric arthritis in the fingers or toes. Other less frequent joint involvement includes distal interphalangeal inflammation, symmetric polyarthritis with seronegativity for rheumatoid factor, arthritis mutilans, and ankylosing spondylitis. Arthritis usually occurs after skin involvement.

I. CLASSIC DESCRIPTION (Figs. 14–14 and 14–15)

Distribution: Extensor surfaces, particularly the elbows, knees, scalp, and sacral areas, typically sparing the face; in inverse psoriasis, flexural areas, such as axillae or groin

Primary: Plaques, papules

Secondary: Erythema, scale

Well-developed lesions will have the typical thick, silvery scale characteristic of psoriasis. Peeling off this scale will reveal punctate bleeding points from capillaries close to the top layer of the skin. The presence of these areas is known as the *Auspitz* sign. With nail involvement, look for small pits or yellow-brown spots (known as *oil spots*) in the nail bed and for distal separation of the nail plate from the nail bed (onycholysis), with accumulation of scale beneath the nail plate (Fig. 14–16).

known to play a definite role in triggering the underlying disease process. Although psoriatic arthritis occurs in approximately 5% to 10% of patients with psoriasis, more general arthritic symptoms may occur in up to 30% of cases. Pso-

II. DIAGNOSIS

Diagnosis is based on the clinical appearance of typical erythematous papules and plaques, with a thick, silvery scale in the classic sites. A history of a preceding streptococcal throat infection is helpful in cases of guttate psoriasis; a family history of psoriasis also is helpful, especially when only early lesions are present. Look for pitting nails as an additional finding. Occasionally, a shave biopsy is necessary to differentiate this disease from other papulosquamous diseases. Obtain a biopsy specimen from the most-developed untreated lesion.

III. DIFFERENTIAL DIAGNOSIS

A. **Seborrheic dermatitis:** Seborrheic dermatitis initially may be difficult to distinguish from scalp or groin psoriasis, but the thick, silvery scales of psoriasis and nail pitting are lacking.

B. **Candidiasis:** Inverse psoriasis lacks the satellite lesions seen in candidiasis. A KOH preparation will show pseudohyphae and/or yeast.

C. **Psoriasiform drug eruptions:** Beta blockers, lithium, and gold can cause a psoriasiform drug eruption or possibly exacerbate underlying psoriasis. Historically, the onset should correlate with initi-

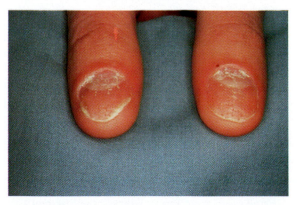

Fig. 14–16
Psoriasis. Nail involvement with pitting and separation of the distal nail plate (onycholysis). (Courtesy Marshall Guill, MD.)

ation of the drug and should resolve with drug withdrawal.

D. **Secondary syphilis:** Look for mucous membrane involvement with syphilis. The psoriatic distribution may not be present, and thick, silvery scales usually are not seen in syphilitic lesions.

E. **HIV-related psoriasis:** Individuals who are seropositive for human immunodeficiency virus (HIV) and have psoriatic-like lesions tend to have an explosive disease onset, with extensive lesions that are resistant to treatment. Look for other signs and symptoms of HIV infection.

F. **Cutaneous T-cell lymphoma:** The thick, silvery scales, nail involvement, and classic distribution are absent, and many psoriatic therapies will not be effective.

IV. TREATMENT

A. **Emollients:** Useful in all cases (e.g., Eucerin Plus lotion or cream, Lubriderm Moisture Plus, Moisturel).

B. **Keratolytic agents:**
1. Useful in conjunction with topical corticosteroids, tar, anthralin, or light therapies, especially when the scales are thick.
2. Scalp: If the scale is very thick, use P & S Liquid (OTC). Massage the preparation into the scalp at bedtime and wash it out in the morning.
3. Body and extremities: Use 2% to 10% salicylic acid in petrolatum. Apply once or twice daily to the thickest scaling areas.

C. **Topical therapy for involvement of 20% or less of the body surface** (Box 14–7):
1. *Topical steroids:* Use as first-line therapy.
   a. *Face and groin:* Start with low-potency agents (e.g., *hydrocortisone* 1% cream or *desonide* 0.05% cream or lotion) 2 or 3 times daily.
   b. *Scalp:*

BOX 14–7.

Topical Therapy for Psoriasis: Involvement of Less Than 20% of body surface*

1. Emollients
2. Keratolytic agents
3. Topical corticosteroids: Use lowest potency to control disease
4. Calcipotriene ointment: Vitamin D analogue
5. Anthralin: Use as short-contact therapy
6. Coal tar: Use in conjunction with topical steroids or anthralin
7. Medicated shampoos: Useful for scalp psoriasis, in conjunction with topical steroids and other treatments

*Agents listed in descending order of preference. If disease is not controlled with first agent, then a trial of an alternative agent is warranted.

(1.) Start with medium- to high-potency agents (e.g., *betamethasone valerate* 0.1% solution [20, 60 ml], *fluocinolone acetonide* 0.01% solution or shampoo [20, 60 ml], or *triamcinolone* 0.1% lotion [15, 60 ml]) to affected areas 2 or 3 times daily.

(2.) If no improvement after 2 weeks, consider a higher-potency lotion (e.g., *fluocinonide* 0.05% solution [20, 60 ml] 2 or 3 times daily or *betamethasone dipropionate* 0.05% lotion [30, 60 ml] twice daily), but use for 2 weeks only, then switch back to a medium-potency preparation.

(3.) Alternatively, try using a medium-potency topical steroid oil, (Derma-Smoothe) under occlusion with a shower cap, at bedtime to increase the penetration.

(4.) Medicated shampoos are useful for helping to control scalp psoriasis in conjunction with topical corticosteroids. Use one that contains a keratolytic agent, such as salicylic acid (e.g., P & S or T/Sal), tar (e.g., Ioni T, T/Gel, Denorex), or combinations (e.g., Ionil T Plus, T/Sal).

c. *Body and extremities:*

(1.) Thick plaques require at least a medium-potency preparation (e.g., *triamcinolone* 0.1% cream) 2 or 3 times daily.

(2.) If no response after 2 weeks, increase the potency to class I or II topical corticosteroids, such as *betamethasone dipropionate* 0.05% cream or ointment (15, 45 g) twice a day for 2 weeks.

(3.) Return to using a medium-potency agent after 2 weeks, although high-potency agents can be used on weekends as "pulse" therapy, if necessary, to control lesions.

(4.) Hands and feet tolerate increased potency with topical agents under occlusion with plastic wrap, applied nightly, with caution regarding thinning of the skin and systemic absorption.

(5.) Isolated stubborn plaques may be injected with *triamcinolone* 5 mg/ml intralesionally with 5 mg for a 2 x 2-cm plaque. Side effects of atrophy and telangiectasia should be noted.

d. *Follow-up should be based on therapeutic response* and the strength of the topical agents used. For example, if there is no response to therapy after 2 or 3 weeks or if the patient is using potent topical corticosteroids, follow up within several weeks to evaluate the need for alternative therapies. Monitor for side effects every 2 to 3 months.

2. *Calcipotriene:* 0.005% ointment or cream (30, 60, 100 g)
   a. A synthetic vitamin D analog, calcipotriene is usually as effective as medium-potency topical steroids, but the effect is more variable. Calcipotriene is also useful as a rotational therapy, in addition to primary therapy. The ointment is more effective than the cream.
   b. Apply sparingly to affected areas bid for at least 6 weeks, avoiding use on the face and groin because of possible irritation.
   c. Side effects of burning, itching, and skin irritation may occur in 10% to 15% of patients. The medication is contraindicated in patients with hypercalcemia or Vitamin D toxicity. Systemic absorption can occur when the medication is used over extensive body areas.
   d. Does not cause skin atrophy or hypothalamic-pituitary-adrenal axis suppression.
   e. Cost is about $1 per gram, comparable to class I topical steroids.
3. *Topical anthralin:* An antimitotic and reducing agent.
   a. *Short-contact therapy:* Start with 0.1% concentration *Drithocreme* (0.1%, 0.25%, 0.5%, 1% or *Micanol* 1% available in 50-g tubes) to chronic, thick plaques for 15 to 60 minutes, then shower with soap and cool or lukewarm water.
   b. Increase daily exposure duration to a maximum of 1 hour, as tolerated. Apply only to plaques; burning, irritation, and purple-brown staining may occur wherever the anthralin contacts the skin (less likely with *micanol* 1% cream).
   c. If no irritation occurs after daily contact for 1 hour, repeat the process with increasing strengths of anthralin. If irritation occurs, interrupt therapy and restart at a lower concentration. Use daily, until the skin is smooth. Skin staining will resolve in 1 to 3 weeks.
4. *Coal tar:* Useful as an antimitotic agent.
   a. Most commonly used in conjunction with ultraviolet B light therapy and other topical treatments.
   b. Apply T-Derm Tar Oil (4 oz), Estar Tar Gel (90 g), or Fototar Tar Cream (85 g, 1 lb) (OTC) to affected areas 10 to 15 minutes before bedtime, or use Balnetar bath oil (8 oz) (OTC) bathtub soak for 10 to 20 minutes. Instruct patients that staining and photosensitization may occur, and therefore patients should avoid direct sunlight after application.
   c. Folliculitis as a side effect also may occur, requiring discontinuation of the agent.
D. **Greater than 20% of body involved**: (Box 14–8). Refer to a dermatologist for consideration of alternative therapies.
   1. **Light therapy** can be done with ultraviolet A or B. UVB light therapy often is used in combination with other ther-

---

BOX 14–8.

Topical Therapy for Psoriasis: Involvement of Greater Than 20% of body surface*

1. Emollients
2. Keratolytic agents
3. Ultraviolet B light therapy*: Use in combination with tars or anthralin
4. Ultraviolet A light therapy: Use with oral or topical psoralens (PUVA)
5. Methotrexate
6. Etretinate/acitretin
7. Low-dose cyclosporine
8. Sulfasalazine (Azulfidine)

*Agents listed in descending order of preference.

apies, such as tar or anthralin. Home units are also available. UVA light therapy with oral or topical psoralens as photosensitizing agents is known as PUVA therapy. Long-term side effects of PUVA therapy include a possible increased risk for developing cutaneous squamous cell carcinomas. Hand and foot units often are used when disease is limited.

2. ***Etretinate or acitretin are synthetic retinoids*** that may be used as single agents, most predictably effective in pustular or erythrodermic psoriasis but also when used in combination with PUVA (Re-PUVA).

3. ***Low-dose cyclosporine or azulfidine*** are being used in very recalcitrant cases unresponsive to other therapies. Serious potential side effects should limit use of these drugs to experienced clinicians.

E. **Stress monitoring and control:**

1. **Both physical and emotional stress** play direct roles in causing flare-ups of psoriasis. Look for signs of infection, such as a streptococcal throat infection or a urinary tract infection.

2. Emotional issues that cause flare-ups should be addressed and psychologic consultation obtained as needed.

a. Assist patients in learning coping techniques, such as stress reduction with meditation, progressive muscle relaxation, or biofeedback, or in developing a lifestyle that includes regular exercise.

b. Address issues of altered body image, if appropriate, considering whether the condition is severe or persistent.

c. If cost is a major concern, consider first treating areas that are exposed to public view.

V. **PATIENT EDUCATION**

A. Explain that the treatment goal is control, rather than cure, of the disease.

B. Educate patients about the role of stress in causing flare-ups. Discuss lifestyle issues (e.g., exercise, avoidance of excess alcohol) and stress recognition.

C. Explain that careful and gradually increasing amounts of sun exposure may help with control, but emphasize avoidance of sunburn and use of sunscreen on uninvolved sun-exposed skin (e.g., face).

D. Teach patients to gradually discontinue topical medication once the involved areas have cleared up and to switch to the lowest-potency agent(s) that will control the outbreak of new lesions.

E. Give patients the address for the National Psoriasis Foundation, which prints many educational materials and may be a valuable resource and support service.*

SEBORRHEIC DERMATITIS ICD-9 (690.10)

Seborrheic dermatitis is a common, chronic, erythematous scaling eruption of unknown cause that affects all age groups (infancy, pubertal), but usually affects adults age 20 to 50 or older. Scalp involvement is commonly known as *dandruff* in adults and *cradle cap* in infants. Adult involvement tends to be recurrent but usually is easily controlled. *Pityrosporum ovale,* a normal yeast flora, is thought to play a role in seborrheic dermatitis. A severe and rare form of seborrheic dermatitis can occur in children with a functional complement (C5) deficiency. Severe, recalcitrant seborrheic dermatitis may be an early cutaneous sign of HIV infection.

*National Psoriasis Foundation, 6600 S.W. 92nd Ave., Ste. 300, Portland, OR 97223-7195; 503-244-7404, FAX: 503-245-0626. Web site: http://www.psoriasis.org/

I. CLASSIC DESCRIPTION (Figs. 14–17 and 14–18)

Distribution: *Infants:* Scalp, diaper area
Adults: Scalp, eyebrows, paranasal, nasolabial fold, external auditory canal, chest, groin
Primary: Plaques
Secondary: Erythema, scale, fissures, exudate; symmetric eyelid involvement in adults may occur as blepharitis

II. DIAGNOSIS

The diagnosis is based clinically on the recognition of erythematous, often greasy, scaling plaques in the characteristic distribution.

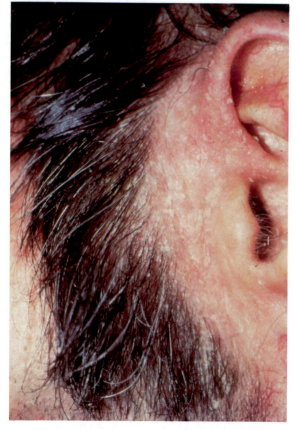

Fig. 14–17
Seborrheic dermatitis. Note prominent scaling. (Courtesy Department of Dermatology, University of North Carolina at Chapel Hill.)

III. DIFFERENTIAL DIAGNOSIS

A. **Psoriasis:** Psoriasis, especially of the scalp, may be difficult to differentiate from seborrhea. Look for the thick, silvery scales, nail pitting, and lesions on the elbows or knees that are typical for psoriasis. Facial involvement is less common in psoriasis.

B. **Tinea capitis/faciale:** In children with scalp scaling, a KOH and/or fungal culture should be performed to rule out fungal infections, such as tinea capitis, a more likely diagnosis in this age group. Look for the presence of a dermatophyte when treating "resistant seborrheic dermatitis." Tinea faciale tends to be unilateral.

C. **Tinea cruris:** Look for the well-demarcated borders of tinea cruris. KOH preps will demonstrate hyphae.

D. **Candidiasis:** Beefy red plaques are present, along with satellite lesions that are KOH-positive for yeast.

E. **HIV disease:** Extensive or treatment-resistant seborrheic dermatitis should alert the clinician to look for other signs of HIV disease.

F. **Acne rosacea:** Look for central facial erythema. Some scaling may be present, and the two diseases may exist simulta-

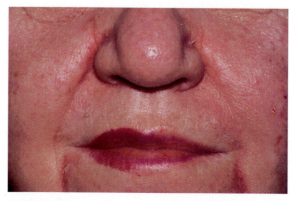

Fig. 14–18
Seborrheic dermatitis. Note paranasal and infraoral erythematous scaling plaques.

neously in adults. Acne rosacea typically has a significant flushing component. Telangiectasia and inflammatory papules may also be present.

G. **Histiocytosis X:** A rare malignancy in infants, with skin findings similar to seborrheic dermatitis. Purpura is usually seen in seborrheic lesions.

H. **Lupus erythematosus:** Systemic findings and photosensitivity are absent in seborrhea. Look for scalp and ear involvement of seborrhea.

I. **Pityriasis rosea:** Facial involvement is rare. Acute onset of herald patch is followed by oval scaling papules and plaques that resolve over several months. Look for scalp and ear involvement of seborrhea.

J. **Zinc deficiency and glucagonomas** are quite rare and can present with periorificial erythematous scaling plaques.

IV. TREATMENT

A. **Medicated shampoos:** Become familiar with two or three preparations and use based on experience (See Box 14–9).
  1. Active ingredients include coal tar, salicylic acid, sulfur, zinc pyrithione, and selenium sulfide, either separately or in combination.
  2. Instruct patients to apply the shampoo to affected hair-bearing areas and leave on for 5 to 10 minutes before rinsing.
  3. Ketoconazole shampoo (available only by prescription) used 2 or 3 times

a week for 1 month is effective in some cases. Use once a week to maintain effects.
  4. Corticosteroid shampoo: *Fluocinolone acetonide* 0.01% 2 to 3 times a week for 1 month, then monthly. Educate patients that the shampoo does not lather.

B. **Topical corticosteroid lotions or solutions:** Use in combination with a medicated shampoo if the medicated shampoo fails to control the disease after 2 to 3 weeks or for severe initial disease.
  1. *Scalp:*
    a. With adults, start with a medium-potency agent (e.g., *betamethasone valerate* 0.1% lotion [20, 60 ml]) twice daily. If not effective after 2 weeks, may increase to *flucinonide* 0.05% solution (20, 60 ml) twice a day or *fluocinolone acetonide* 0.01% oil (120 ml) nightly, with a shower cap, but try to decrease to the mildest agent that will control scaling and pruritus.
    b. Try to decrease to *hydrocortisone* 1% to 2.5% lotion (60, 20 ml) once or twice a day, if possible.
    c. Use only on involved areas, not diffusely, for control, and avoid the face.
  2. *Face or groin:* Use low-potency agents (e.g., *hydrocortisone* 1% cream or *desonide* 0.05% cream [15 g]) once or twice a day, as necessary, to control erythema and scale. If the eyebrows are involved, consider a lotion rather than a cream for easier application.
  3. *Chest:* Use *triamcinolone* 0.1% lotion 2 or 3 times a day to control erythema, scale, and pruritus. Men can use medicated shampoo in this area as well.

BOX 14–9.

Seborrheic Dermatitis: Topical Shampoos

Coal tar: Denorex, T/Gel, Pentrax, Tegrin
Salicylic acid: Ionil Plus, P & S
Sulfur: Sulfoam
Zinc pyrithione: Zincon
Selenium sulfide: Exsel, Selsun blue
Ketoconazole: Nizoral
Combinations: T/Sal (coal tar and salicylic acid); Sebulex (salicyclic acid and sulfur)

C. Recalcitrant disease:

1. In cases that remain unresponsive, consider using *ketoconazole* 2% cream (15, 30, 60 g) daily to affected facial areas to address a possible yeast component. Often used in conjunction with a topical corticosteroid cream but applied at a different time during the day, although it may be effective as a single agent.

2. Sodium sulfacetamide 10% and sulfur 5% lotions (25 g) are additional treatment alternatives for resistant facial seborrheic dermatitis. Apply a thin layer once or twice a day, alone or in conjunction with other topical therapies.

D. Cradle cap: For infants, apply warm

mineral oil, massaging it into the scalp, or use, sparingly, a medicated shampoo containing salicylic acid and sulfur. Look for and treat any secondary infections. If recurrent, consider using medicated shampoos 3 times a week and/or *hydrocortisone* 1% lotion for control.

V. PATIENT EDUCATION

(See patient education handout in Appendix M.)

A. Educate patients about control, rather than cure, of seborrheic dermatitis.

B. Emphasize the importance of leaving medicated shampoos on for a minimum of 5 to 10 minutes before rinsing.

C. Educate patients about using topical corticosteroids as necessary to control erythema, scale, or pruritus.

SUGGESTED READING

Botella-Estrada R et al: Erythroderma: a clinicopathological study of 56 cases, *Arch Dermatol* 130:1503–1507, 1994.

Drake LA et al: Guidelines of care for atopic dermatitis, *J Am Acad Dermatol* 26:485–488, 1992.

Drake LA et al: Guidelines of care for psoriasis, *J Am Acad Dermatol* 28:632–637, 1993.

Drake LA et al: Guidelines of care for contact dermatitis, *J Am Acad Dermatol* 32:109–113, 1995.

Drake LA et al: The antipruritic effect of 5% doxepin cream in patients with eczematous dermatitis, *Arch Dermatol* 131:1403–1408, 1995.

Dubin DB, Dover JS: Making methotrexate therapy more palatable, *Fitzpatrick's J Clin Dermatol* 3:48–53, 1995.

Eisen D: The vulvovaginal-gingival syndrome of lichen planus, *Arch Dermatol* 130:1370–1382, 1994.

Greaves MW, Weinstein GD: Drug therapy: treatment of psoriasis, *N Engl J Med* 332:581–588, 1995.

Halbert AR, Weston Wl, Morelli JG: Atopic dermatitis: is it an allergic disease? *J Am Acad Dermatol* 33:1008–1018, 1995.

Kanj LF, Phillips TJ: Management of leg ulcers, *Fitzpatrick's J Clin Dermatol* 2:52–60, 1994.

Lynch PJ, Edwards L: *Genital dermatology,* New York, 1994, Churchill Livingstone.

Meffert JJ, Davis BM, Grimwood RE: Lichen sclerosus, *J Am Acad Dermatol* 32:393–416, 1995.

Morren AA et al: Atopic dermatitis: triggering factors, *J Am Acad Dermatol* 31:467–473, 1994.

Paller AS: Childhood atopic dermatitis: update on therapy, *Clin Cases Dermatol* 2:9–14, 1990.

Phillips TJ, Dover JS: Recent advances in dermatology, *N Engl J Med* 326:167–178, 1992.

Rietschel RL, Fowler JF Jr: *Fisher's contact dermatitis,* ed 4, Baltimore, 1995, Williams and Wilkins.

Rothe MJ, Grant-Kels JM: Atopic dermatitis: an update, *J Am Acad Dermatol* 35:1–13, 1996.

Ruzicka T: Psoriatic arthritis, *Arch Dermatol* 132:215–219, 1996.

Taylor JS, Praditsuwan P: Latex allergy: review of 44 cases, including outcome and frequent association with allergic hand eczema, *Arch Dermatol* 132:265–271, 1996.

Weinstein GD, Gottleib AB: *Therapy of moderate-to-severe psoriasis,* Stamford, Conn, 1993, Haber and Flora.

CHAPTER 15

Sexually Transmitted Diseases

CHANCROID ICD-9 (099.0)

Chancroid is a sexually transmitted disease (STD) that results in genital ulcers. The disease gets its name from its superficial resemblance to the chancre of syphilis. Although relatively uncommon in the United States, chancroid is commonly found in many areas of the world. Caused by a gram-negative coccobacillus, *Haemophilus ducreyi*, chancroid affects males 10 times more frequently than females. Epidemics are most often linked to multiple cases in males, resulting from sexual contact with a few infected female prostitutes. Lesions appear after a 3- to 5-day incubation period, although carriers may be asymptomatic.

In patients with genital ulcers, 3% to 10% will have coinfection with another STD, such as syphilis, herpes, or HIV disease.

I. CLASSIC DESCRIPTION

Distribution: *Males:* Penis shaft, most often
Females: Labia, posterior fourchette; less often, vagina or cervix
Primary: Papules, pustules
Secondary: Ulcers, exudate, erythema, edema
Single or multiple papules or pustules break down into shaggy, ragged-edged ulcers that often are quite painful (Fig. 15–1). There is surrounding erythema and associated edema. Painful adenopathy may be unilateral or bilateral, with suppuration of nodes in severe cases.

II. DIAGNOSIS

Diagnosis is based on the history of a recent sexual encounter with an infected carrier, the clinical appearance of one or more painful genital ulcers with ragged edges, and associated adenopathy, particularly suppurative adenopathy of the inguinal nodes. Be particularly suspicious of any genital ulcer in a patient who recently has traveled outside of the United States or who has had sex with a prostitute. A properly done Gram's stain of the lesion may

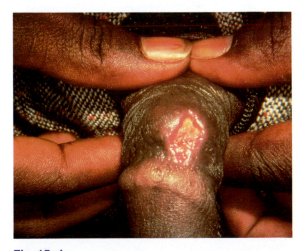

Fig. 15–1
Chanchroid. Note shaggy, ragged-edged ulcer with edema and exudative base. (Courtesy Beverly Sanders, MD.)

demonstrate (50%) the characteristic property of *H. ducreyi* to appear as a "school of fish" or "railroad tracks" on the slide. Roll a cotton swab in one direction on the base of the ulcer, then roll again in the same direction onto a glass slide. This technique will preserve the organism's agglutination properties. *H. ducreyi* is extremely difficult to grow, and the special media required is not widely available; therefore routine bacterial cultures are not helpful.

III. DIFFERENTIAL DIAGNOSIS (Table 15–1)

A. **Herpes simplex:** Herpes simplex infections may be difficult to distinguish from chancroid if the characteristic vesicles are not present. A prodrome history, previous similar infections, and the presence of multiple, grouped, shallow erosions are helpful in making the diagnosis of herpes simplex. In addition, Tzanck smear, culture, and/or smears for direct antigen testing will help differentiate the two disorders.

B. **Granuloma inguinale:** A rare cause of genital ulcers, this disease is characterized by beefy red lesions that resemble granulation tissue; tender adenopathy is not a predominant feature. Culture may be helpful (see Ch. 22).

C. **Syphilis:** Syphilitic chancres in primary syphilis are characteristically painless, and adenopathy is not so symptomatic. Syphilitic lesions are usually well demarcated, have a cleaner base than those of chancroid, test positive for *T. Pallidum* by darkfield examination, and have a positive serologic test 7 days after the onset of ulcers.

IV. TREATMENT

A. **Antibiotics:**

1. First-line therapy: *Azithromycin* 1 g PO once, *ceftriaxone* 250 mg IM, or *erythromycin* 500 mg PO 4 times daily for 7 days.
2. Alternative therapy: *Amoxicillin/ clavulanic acid* 500 mg PO tid for 7 days or *ciprofloxacin* 500 mg PO bid for 3 days (contraindicated in pregnant or lactating women and in children).
3. If the patient is HIV positive, *erythromycin* is the preferred therapy.

B. **Treatment of fluctuant nodes:** Try antibiotic therapy first, avoiding incision and drainage, if possible, to prevent delay in healing and the formation of sinus tracts. Aspirate through normal-appearing skin only if the nodes are unresponsive to antibiotic therapy.

TABLE 15–1.
Genital Ulcer Diseases

	Primary Syphilis	Chancroid	Herpes Simplex	Lymphogranuloma Venereum
Ulcers	Single or multiple, classically painless, well-circumscribed	Single or multiple, painful, shaggy border, exudative	Grouped, multiple, painful, vesicles may be present	Single or multiple, painful
Adenopathy	Usually painless	Marked, may be fluctuant	Tender and marked	Marked, with "groove" sign
Features	Signs of secondary syphilis may be present	Cases usually occur in clusters; painful	Prodrome history	Primary lesion may be missed, adenopathy prominent
Diagnosis	Darkfield, serology	Gram's stain with attention to technique	Tzanck smear, antigen smear, culture	LGV titers, culture of nodal aspirate

C. Local ulcer care:
  1. Clean gently with dilute hydrogen peroxide (1:1 with tap water) twice a day.
  2. Topical antibiotic ointments (e.g., Polysporin, bacitracin) may be soothing but are not otherwise useful in treating the infection.
D. Screen for other sexually transmitted diseases, particularly HIV disease. Patients with chancroid often have coinfections with other organisms. Other screening laboratory tests include rapid plasma reagin (RPR) and gonococcal and chlamydial cultures. Even if screening results are negative, counsel all patients about HIV and other sexually transmitted diseases, because the presence of a genital ulcer indicates ongoing risky behavior and provides a direct portal of entry for other diseases.
E. Partner notification and treatment are essential, even if the partner has no symptoms. All sex partners within 10 days preceding the onset of lesions should be treated. Notify the county health department or other appropriate health authority about positive cases.

F. Follow-up:
  1. Follow-up at 1 week should reveal resolution of the ulcer and improvement but not resolution of the lymphadenopathy.
  2. Observe until the ulcer has completely healed (may require 2 to 3 weeks in large ulcers).
  3. Consider repeating serologic testing for syphilis 1 to 3 months after completion of therapy.
  4. If the ulcer is unresponsive, consider an alternative antibiotic regimen or the possibility of coinfection, including HIV.

V. PATIENT EDUCATION
  A. Emphasize abstinence from sexual intercourse until the lesion has healed completely.
  B. Explain the need and importance of partner identification and notification.
  C. Emphasize the need and rationale for using barrier methods (e.g., condoms).
  D. Review risk factors for HIV disease. Explain that an open sore puts the patient at a much greater risk for other infections.

CONDYLOMA ACUMINATA ICD-9 (078.11)

Condyloma acuminata, also known as *genital* or *venereal warts,* is infection of the genitalia and surrounding skin by the human papillomavirus (HPV). The virus invades and infects skin, leaving intact virions present in the skin's granular layer. HPV infections may be clinical, subclinical, or, as recent evidence demonstrates, latent, with intact virus in normal surrounding skin. Considering all forms of infection, condyloma acuminata is probably the most common sexually transmitted disease in teenagers and young adults, with 1% to 2% of those sexually active having genital warts and an additional 10% to 20% having latent infection.

There is a 50% chance of transmission after a single sexual contact with an infected partner. The incubation period for clinically apparent lesions typically ranges from 1 to 6 months, but in some people may be much longer. Lesions may persist, resolve spontaneously (20% to 30%), or progress. With the recent concept of latency, it is thought that recurrences may be more likely than reinfection.

A primary concern in the treatment of condyloma acuminata is the presence of specific HPV types being associated with dysplasia and carcinoma, particularly of the female genitalia. However, *the HPV types associated with the great majority of condylomas, types 6 and 11, are usually not associated with dysplasia.* HPV types 16, 18, 31, 33, 34, 35, 39, and 48 have been more commonly associated with genital and cervical carcinoma. Most patients are infected with only one strain. Laryngeal papillomas have been associated with infants delivered of mothers infected with HPV. Immunosuppressed patients tend to have lesions that progress more rapidly and frequently into carcinoma. Condylomas also grow more rapidly during pregnancy.

I. CLASSIC DESCRIPTION

Distribution: Vulva, cervix, vagina, penis, perianal/anal regions
Primary: Papules, plaques, nodules
Secondary: Typically flesh-colored; erythema present if lesion is irritated
Lesions may be exophytic, "cauliflower-like" (Fig. 15–2).

II. DIAGNOSIS

Diagnosis is based on the clinical appearance of flesh-colored lesions in the characteristic location. Biopsy is rarely indicated for diagnosis but may be useful in treatment of resistant lesions, particularly for exophytic cervical lesions, to rule out dysplasia. HPV subtyping, although available by polymerase chain reaction, is not routinely indicated at this time, because the clinical use-

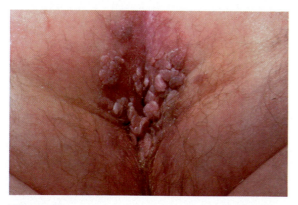

Fig. 15–2
Condyloma acuminatum. Note multiple exophytic perineal warts. (Courtesy Department of Dermatology, University of North Carolina at Chapel Hill.)

fulness of the test for patient management is not known.

A simple test sometimes used to detect subclinical lesions is to apply 3% acetic acid on a washcloth (dilute white vinegar from the grocery store, which is 5%) to an area for 8 to 10 minutes, then examine with a magnifying lens or colposcope. Areas of abnormal epithelium will become white (called *acetowhitening*). However, this test is not highly specific, and false positive results are not uncommon, because any abnormal epithelium will acetowhiten. The clinical usefulness of this test has decreased because of the recommendation to avoid unnecessary treatment of subclinical disease in the absence of significant dysplasia.

III. DIFFERENTIAL DIAGNOSIS

A. **Condyloma lata:** Condyloma lata are flesh-colored papules of secondary syphilis located in the genital-perianal region. There usually is an associated generalized exanthem; lesions are smooth, not exophytic; and serology and darkfield examination from the exudate of an open lesion are positive.

B. **Bowenoid papulosis:** These lesions are found on the genitalia and present as erythematous papules, leukoplakia, or, more commonly, as hyperpigmented papules or plaques and also are associated with HPV type 16. Bowenoid papulosis lesions are resistant to therapy, and female contacts have an increased risk for cervical carcinoma.

C. **Molluscum contagiosum:** Molluscum are characterized by pearly, smooth, umbilicated papules. A stain for "molluscum bodies" or biopsy will readily distinguish the two conditions but usually is not necessary.

D. **Acrochordons:** These easily can be mistaken for venereal warts, although skin tags are less frequently found on the genitals. Smooth contour and biopsy, if necessary, usually will differentiate.

E. Squamous cell carcinoma: Squamous cell carcinoma may present as an ulcer or an erosion *de novo* or in a previously diagnosed genital wart. A rare form of anogenital squamous cell carcinoma may present as a verrucous mass. Biopsy any lesions that are recalcitrant to therapies.

IV. TREATMENT

A. Treatment of HPV is controversial because currently there is inadequate knowledge on the epidemiology and clinical course of the disease. Because HPV has been demonstrated in adjacent normal skin after extensive laser therapy, it is likely that no current therapy totally eradicates HPV. In addition, recurrences are common, regardless of the treatment method. However, general agreement exists that clinicians should:

1. Confirm the diagnosis and screen for underlying coinfections (e.g., syphilis, HIV disease).
2. Establish wart therapy goals that attempt to:
   a. Remove exophytic warts, particularly when they are symptomatic and distressful to a patient.
   b. Induce wart-free periods.
   c. Use therapy that is not worse than the disease.
   d. Identify lesions that may be associated with cancer, especially cervical cancer.
3. Monitor immunosuppressed patients because of an increased risk of squamous cell carcinoma.
4. Treatment of subclinical disease is indicated only if there is coexistent significant dysplasia.

B. Liquid nitrogen therapy:

1. Best used on "dry" areas (e.g., shaft of penis, external female genitalia, upper thighs). Avoid use in the vagina. If used properly, liquid nitrogen therapy will not cause scarring.
2. Do a 10- to 30-second freeze, with repeated freeze–thaw cycles, depending on the size of the lesion. Let patients know that the procedure usually causes pain during and after freezing.
3. Educate patients on the possibility of blistering, including a "blood blister," and postinflammatory hypopigmentation, particularly in black patients.
4. Repeat as necessary at 7- to 14-day intervals. If warts persist beyond three treatment cycles, alternative therapies or diagnoses should be considered.
5. Expect cure rates of 63% to 88% and recurrence rates of 21% to 39%.

C. *Podophyllin* resin: Podoyphyllin comes in a variety of strengths, from 10% to 25%, in tincture of benzoin. Limit the volume used at any one treatment session to 0.5 ml and treat an area of less than 10 cm^2 per treatment session.

1. Best used with lesions in areas of moisture or occlusion (e.g., perianal, mucosal, or inguinal folds, rather than the penis shaft).
2. Apply the medication to lesions, allowing it to dry completely.
3. Instruct the patient to leave the preparation on for 4 to 12 hours, then wash off thoroughly with soap and water.
4. Expected reactions include localized pain, burning, inflammation, or erosions. Sitz baths twice daily are helpful if erosions are severe.
5. Repeat therapy at 7- to 10-day intervals. If warts persist beyond six treatment cycles, alternative therapies should be tried.
6. Podophyllin is contraindicated in pregnant women. Systemic toxicity, especially to nonintact skin or in children, if large volumes are used, also has been reported.

7. Expect cure rates of 32% to 79% and recurrence rates of 27% to 65%.
8. Stool softeners may be helpful if treated lesions involve the anus.

D. *Podofilox* 0.5%: (Condylox, 3.5 ml)
1. Available by prescription for at home treatment ($50 to $60 for 4 weeks of therapy).
2. Apply twice daily for 3 days, omit for 4 days; repeat the cycle for 3 to 4 weeks until lesions are gone. Unlike podophyllin, Podofilox does not need to be washed off.
3. The medication is contraindicated in pregnant women.
4. Patients should return for evaluation if any lesions fail to resolve after four cycles of treatment.
5. Expect cure rates of 45% to 88% and recurrence rates of 33% to 60%.

E. *Trichloroacetic acid* 80% to 90%:
1. Apply for a few seconds, only to warts. Apply sodium bicarbonate (baking soda) to neutralize unreacted acid.
2. Repeat applications as needed at weekly intervals.
3. No advantage over other treatments, although sometimes it is useful for small warts.
4. If no improvement is seen after six applications, alternative therapies should be employed.
5. Expected cure and recurrence rates have not been fully determined, but are probably similar to podophyllin.

F. Snip excision and electrodessication: Although not recommended as first-line therapy, surgery may be useful for recalcitrant disease, particularly for large or pedunculated lesions.
1. Anesthetize with *lidocaine* 1% (2 to 3 minutes before) or *EMLA* cream (1 to 2 hours before) before the procedure, then do a snip excision of lesions, using aluminum chloride or electrocautery for hemostasis.

2. Suturing may be required for larger lesions.
3. Do not use this therapy proximal to the anal verge.

G. Referral:
1. Cytologic examination is indicated when cervical lesions are identified, because dysplasia must be excluded.
2. For recalcitrant lesions, refer for laser surgery, intralesional *interferon,* and/or biopsy.

H. Follow-up: Patient compliance with follow-up visits and treatment are essential for success with any treatment regimen. Initial follow-up should be at 1 to 2 weeks, regardless of therapy. The number of lesions and response to therapy will require individualizing remaining follow-up appointments. Subsequent follow-up every 6 months may be recommended.

I. Children: Lesions in children may be acquired perinatally, congenitally, from sexual abuse, or from exposure to other cutaneous warts. *Children, especially over age 3, should at least be evaluated for the possibility of sexual abuse when lesions are found in anogenital locations.* Treatment should proceed cautiously, with small amounts of podophyllin or cautious observation.

J. Cervical warts: Dysplasia must be ruled out through cytologic examination before treatment is initiated. Colposcopy and/or biopsy may be necessary, especially in exophytic lesions.

V. PATIENT EDUCATION
A. Emphasize the infectious nature of the disease, its sexual transmission, its possible long-term relationship to cancer, and the importance of compliance with therapy.
B. Explain the importance of partner notification, recognizing that established partners probably have at least subclinical infection and that clinical infection

may not be apparent or detectable in the partner for months or possibly even years.

C. Educate patients about the importance of using appropriate barrier techniques (e.g., condoms). However, because partner exposure has probably already occurred if the patient is in a longstanding monogomous relationship, condoms may not be needed.

D. Explain that the initial and subsequent treatments may not eradicate the virus and that recurrences are possible. The treatment works only on visible lesions.

E. Explain the side effects of various treatment plans. Erosions from podophyllin treatment can be severe. Sitz baths, topical antibiotics, and gentle cleansing with dilute hydrogen peroxide may be more helpful than leaving patients to their own devices to ease discomfort.

F. Have patients contact the National STD Hotline.*

HERPES SIMPLEX ICD-9 (054.10 GENITAL)

Herpes simplex virus (HSV) infections are the most common cause of genital ulcers, affecting an estimated 30 million people in the United States alone. The predominant cause of genital herpes infections, especially recurrent infections, is HSV-2, although 30% of genital infections are caused by HSV-1 (see Chapter 18 for full discussion of HSV-1 lesions). HSV infections usually occur in sexually active teenagers and young adults. The incubation period is typically 6 to 8 days, but ranges from 2 to 26 days. After the initial skin infection, the virus resides in the nerve root ganglion, remaining latent until subclinical reactivation with viral shedding or clinical recurrence with active, visible lesions.

Primary infections are characterized by generalized symptoms (e.g., fever, arthralgias, malaise, dysuria, headache, backache). Inguinal adenopathy often is quite painful. Primary infections tend to be more severe, with more lesions and edema, and last longer than recurrences. As many as 40% of infected people may have asymptomatic primary infections. Fifty percent of all herpes-infected patients will experience symptomatic recurrences. Recurrences are often characterized by a prodrome, such as a burning or tingling sensation, followed by the appearance of characteristic lesions within a few hours to days. Triggers for recurrences include emo-

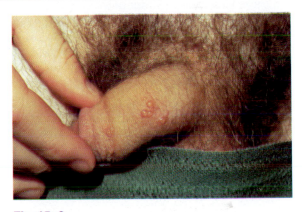

Fig. 15–3
Genital herpes simplex. Note intact, grouped vesicles on an erythematous base. (Courtesy Department of Dermatology, University of North Carolina at Chapel Hill.)

tional or immunologic stress, trauma, and menses.

I. CLASSIC DESCRIPTION (Fig. 15–3)
Distribution: *Males:* Glans, shaft, urethral canal, perianal region

*National STD Hotline: 1-800-227-8922. Operators will answer questions regarding STDs from 8:00 AM to 11:00 PM (Mon.-Fri.) Eastern Standard Time. The American Social Health Association also has a hotline and is an excellent resource for patient support: P.O. Box 13827, Research Triangle Park, NC, 27709; 919-361-8400, 8:00 AM-5:30 PM (Mon.-Fri.); FAX 919-361-8425; Web site: http://sunsite.unc.edu/ASHA/

Females: Labia, inner thighs, mucosa, cervix, perianal region
Primary: Grouped vesicles, pustules
Secondary: Erosions, erythema, edema, exudate; painful inguinal adenopathy may be present
Recurrent outbreaks may occur on the buttocks or sacral region.

II. DIAGNOSIS

Diagnosis is based on the presence of grouped vesicles or erosions on an erythematous base, that are confirmed to be herpes simplex virus through testing. A simple confirmatory test is to look for the presence of multinucleated giant cells by Tzanck smear. Unroof the vesicle, then use a no. 15 blade to scrape the floor of the vesicle. Place scrapings on a slide, air dry, and stain (see Chapter 3). Lesions should be 1 to 4 days old for the best results. Other confirmatory tests include direct viral antigen smears or viral cultures. Viral antigen smears require smearing of scraped material onto a glass slide, air drying, and transportation to a testing facility, although an in-office test is available, allowing testing directly from the swab. Viral cultures require use of Dacron swabs and special culture media, which should be provided by the testing facility.

Serology is useful in differentiating primary vs. recurrent disease. In primary disease, HSV antibodies are absent initially, then rise fourfold. Fewer than 5% of patients will demonstrate a rise in antibody titer in recurrent disease.

III. DIFFERENTIAL DIAGNOSIS

See Table 15–1.

IV. TREATMENT

A. Primary herpes simplex infections, immunocompetent host:

1. *Valacyclovir* 500 mg bid for 5 days or until lesions heal. If started as soon as symptoms appear, treatment may decrease symptom duration, decrease viral shedding, and help lesions heal faster but will not influence the incidence or severity of recurrent disease. Topical *acyclovir* is not recommended because it is substantially less effective than oral therapy.
2. Pain control: *Acetaminophen,* Sitz baths, and urination in a tub of water may decrease stinging.
3. Treat any secondary infections (e.g., *Candida*).

B. Primary infection in immunocompromised patients:

1. Intravenous *acyclovir* 5 mg/kg tid for 7 days, adjusting the dosage as needed for decreased renal function.
2. Consider consultation for severe infections, for any apparent resistant cases, and for those that occur in immunosuppressed children, particularly if encephalitis is a possible complication.

C. Recurrent herpes simplex infections:

1. *Valacyclovir* 500 mg or *famciclovir* 125 mg bid for 5 days. Beginning use at the first sign of a prodrome often helps decrease the severity of the recurrence, improves healing time, and decreases viral shedding. Such therapy is especially useful if erythema multiforme is associated with the recurrent HSV infection or if the symptoms are severe.
2. For more than five recurrences a year or when bullous erythema multiforme is associated with infection, use suppressive therapy with *valacyclovir* 500 mg 1 tablet once a day for 6 to 12 months, then try tapering the dosage to the lowest dose that will prevent recurrence. Overall, the natural history of the disease is for recurrences to become less frequent over time. With suppressive therapy, viral shedding is reduced by 95%. Discontinue suppressive therapy at the end of 1 year to evaluate need for ongoing therapy.

D. Screen for other sexually transmitted diseases: Patients with HSV may have more than one infection. Include STD counseling and testing for HIV disease in the treatment plan.

E. Provide emotional support: Empathy is important, especially at the initial visit. Consider follow-up telephone calls, patient information brochures, telephone numbers, and reassurance.

V. PATIENT EDUCATION

A. Educate patients about the infectious nature of the disease and about avoidance of sexual activity, especially while lesions are present. Emphasize condom use.

B. Explain that the disease is recurrent and sometimes unpredictable, and that viral shedding may occur, even without active lesions, during an apparent asymptomatic phase.

C. Remind patients that you will provide emotional support and continuity for them and their sexual partners.

D. Tell women of child-bearing age that during any future pregnancies they need to notify their clinicians of their history of herpes.

E. Educate patients on precipitating factors (e.g., emotional stress, trauma, fever).

F. Patients interested in immediate confidential information or support groups can contact the Herpes Resource Center Coordinator.*

LYMPHOGRANULOMA VENEREUM ICD-9 (099.1)

Lymphogranuloma venereum is a sexually transmitted genital ulcer disease caused by *Chlamydia trachomatis* (serotypes L1, L2, and L3). The disease is endemic in tropical regions, but less than 1000 cases are found yearly in the United States. After exposure to an infected person and an incubation period of 5 to 21 days, patients may exhibit papules or vesicles that rapidly break down into erosive lesions and heal, often without being seen. More than 50% of lesions may be asymptomatic and heal without scarring.

Seven to 14 days after the primary lesions heal, tender inguinal lymphadenopathy, usually unilateral, becomes the prominent feature (Fig. 15–4). Fever, headache, and arthralgias may be present. Late manifestations in both male and female patients are related to lymphatic obstruction as a result of chronic inflammation, with elephantiasis in severe cases.

I. CLASSIC DESCRIPTION

Distribution: *Males:* Penis
Females: Cervix, fourchette, labia
Primary: Papules, pustules, vesicles
Secondary: Erosion, ulcers
Unilateral or bilateral tender adenopathy

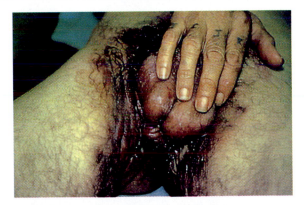

Fig. 15–4
Lymphogranuloma venereum. Note multiple buboes with exudate and ulceration. (Courtesy Beverly Sanders, MD.)

can become fluctuant buboes, with subsequent ulceration. Rectal involvement occurs primarily through anal intercourse or secondarily through spread of lesions via secretions or though translymphatics.

*Herpes Resource Center Coordinator, P.O. Box 13827, Research Triangle Park, NC 27709; 919-361-8488 (9:00 AM-7:00 PM Mon.-Fri.); or National STD Hotline, 1-800-227-8922. Web site: http://sunsite.unc.edu/ASHA/

II. DIAGNOSIS

Diagnosis is suspected by the history of recent sexual exposure and the clinical presence of inflamed and/or enlarged inguinal lymph nodes. Diagnosis is confirmed by the presence of an LGV IgM titer (usually performed in state laboratories) greater than 1:32. Culture of lymph node aspirates is highly specific but is not widely available. The "groove" sign is seen when the inguinal ligament runs prominently between enlarged femoral and inguinal lymph nodes.

III. DIFFERENTIAL DIAGNOSIS

See Table 15–1.

IV. TREATMENT

A. **Oral antibiotics:**
   1. First-line therapy: *Doxycycline* 100 mg PO twice daily for 21 days.
   2. Alternative regimens: *Erythromycin* 500 mg or *sulfisoxazole* 500 mg PO 4 times daily for 21 days.
B. **Treatment of fluctuant nodes:** Try antibiotics first. Avoid incision and drainage because this may delay healing and lead to the formation of sinus tracts. Aspirate through normal-appearing skin only if the nodes are unresponsive to antibiotic therapy.
C. **Local ulcer care:**
   1. Dilute hydrogen peroxide 1:1 with tap water; cleanse lesions gently twice a day.
   2. Topical antibiotic ointments may be soothing, but are not otherwise useful in treating the infection.
D. **Screen for other sexually transmitted diseases.** Often more than one infection is present. Include counseling and testing for HIV disease, because the presence of a genital ulcer indicates ongoing risky behavior and provides a direct portal of entry for other STDs.
E. **Partner notification and treatment are essential.** Even if the partner has no symptoms, notify the local health authority of a confirmed case.
F. **Follow-up:**
   1. Follow-up at 1 week should reveal improvement but not resolution of lymphadenopathy. Eighty percent of ulcers are healed after 2 weeks.
   2. Assess lymph nodes for need of needle aspiration.
   3. Observe for fistulas or sinus tract formation.
   4. Serologic testing for syphilis should be considered 2 to 3 months after therapy.
   5. If unresponsive, consider alternative antibiotic regimens or the possibility of coinfection, including HIV.

V. PATIENT EDUCATION

A. Educate patients to abstain from sexual intercourse until lesions have healed completely.
B. Emphasize the need for partner identification and notification.
C. Emphasize the need for future condom use.
D. Explain that open genital sores put the patient at risk for other infections (e.g., hepatitis B, HIV). Counsel about high-risk sexual behaviors.

SYPHILIS ICD-9 (091.9 BY STAGE AND SITE)

Syphilis is caused by the spirochete *Treponema pallidum* and is one of the oldest and best-studied diseases. It also remains an important worldwide source of disability. The disease gets its name from Italian pathologist Girolama Fran-castoro's sixteenth-century poem, "Syphilis sive Morbus Gallicus," in which the principal character is a shepherd named *Syphilis,* who is afflicted with a sexually transmitted disease. The importance of syphilis to the development of dermatology is evident in that the original science of the skin was referred to as *Dermatology and Syphilology,* until the advent of penicillin.

Until the last few years of the 1980s the clinical presentation and emphasis on syphilis decreased to the point at which many physicians may have gone through training without having seen or diagnosed a single case. However, over the last several years the incidence of syphilis has risen exponentially. Syphilis is no longer an infection relegated to textbooks but is a frequently seen clinical disease.

The epidemiology of the current epidemic has shifted to one found more frequently in association with the use of sex for drugs, especially crack cocaine; multiple infections occurring in one patient; and the typical manifestations altered by coinfection with HIV disease. (Special considerations for the HIV-infected population are considered in Chapter 16.) The rise of congenital syphilis is especially disheartening; infection causes fetal or perinatal death in 40% of infected infants.

The natural history of syphilis in a host with a normal immune system is typical. Following exposure, most commonly via direct sexual contact with an infected partner, there is an incubation period that averages 21 days (range: 6 to 90 days). Subsequently, single or multiple primary lesions known as *chancres* develop (Fig. 15–5).

Chancres classically are painless and there may be associated regional, relatively nontender, adenopathy. These lesions heal within 3 to 6 weeks.

In untreated people, *4 to 10 weeks after primary exposure, secondary syphilitic lesions appear, characterized by systemic infection* (e.g., malaise, fever, generalized adenopathy, gastritis, hepatitis, arthritis, uveitis, nephritis, acute meningitis, skin or mucous membrane lesions) (Fig. 15–6). The secondary stage, left untreated, typically lasts for 4 to 8 weeks. The majority of untreated infections subsequently enter a latent phase, during which there may be reactivation of secondary lesions. Latent syphilis is defined as the presence of a positive serology for syphilis in the absence of any clinical signs or symptoms of the disease.

In approximately 10% to 30% of patients with untreated syphilis, cardiovascular or central nervous system manifestations of tertiary syphilis subsequently develop, usually 7 to 30 years after the initial infection. Cardiovascular lesions include aortic aneurysm, sacular aneurysm, and aortic valve regurgitation. Neural involvement includes stroke complexes, general paresis, tabes dorsalis, Argyll Robertson pupils, delusions, and memory loss. Charcot joints and skin, bone, or visceral gummas also may develop.

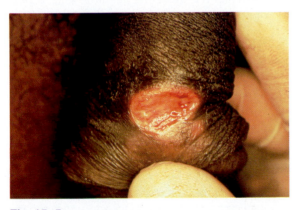

Fig. 15–5
Primary syphilis. Note well-demarcated primary chancre with clean base.

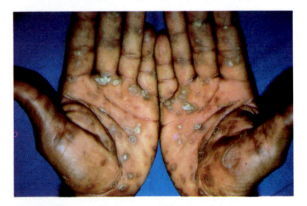

Fig. 15–6
Secondary syphilis. Note characteristic scaling palmar skin lesions. (Courtesy Beverly Sanders, MD.)

Congenital syphilis occurs after in utero infection with *T. pallidum*. If the maternal infection is treated before the sixteenth gestational week, the placenta is thought to prevent fetal infection. If appropriate treatment occurs after the sixteenth week, deafness, keratitis, and bone or joint abnormalities may be present at birth. *Early congenital manifestations* appear before age 2. Signs and symptoms include stillbirth, failure to thrive, hemolytic anemia, leukopenia, lymphadenopathy, iritis, alopecia, rhinitis, hepatosplenomegaly, jaundice, ascites, nephrosis, nephritis, osteochondritis, periostitis, and skin lesions (described below). *Late congenital syphilis* becomes apparent after age 5. Signs includes frontal bossing; saddle nose deformity; short maxilla; high, arched palate; mulberry molars; Hutchinson's teeth (peg-shaped upper central incisors); unilateral clavicular enlargement; and linear scars from the angle of the eyes, nose, and mouth, known as *rhagades*. *Hutchinson's triad* includes Hutchinson's teeth, interstitial keratitis, and eighth nerve deafness.

I. CLASSIC DESCRIPTION (Table 15–2)
II. DIAGNOSIS

The definitive diagnosis of primary syphilis is based on clinical findings, darkfield microscopy, and direct fluorescent antibody tests on lesions or tissue. Specimens for darkfield examination must be taken from moist, nonbleeding lesions, placed on a saline preparation, and promptly examined for the typical motility patterns of *T. pallidum*. Properly prepared specimens are almost always positive in primary syphilis but require experience with preparation and reading and the presence of a darkfield microscope, features that few primary care clinicians possess. Contact the local county public health authority or hospital pathologist for assistance in obtaining a specimen. Darkfield examinations should not be performed on oral lesions, because of the presence of spirochetes in the normal oral flora. Darkfield results will be negative in the face of recent effective therapy. Serologic testing

is insensitive in early primary infections and may not become positive for several weeks.

A presumptive diagnosis is possible with a positive test, using direct *T. pallidum* antigens (e.g., fluorescent treponemal antibody absorption test [FTA-ABS]), combined with a positive test using nonspecific antibodies directed against the lipoidal antigens of *T. pallidum* (e.g., Venereal Disease Research Laboratory test [VDRL], rapid plasma reagin test [RPR]). Neither test by itself is sufficient to make the diagnosis.

The direct treponemal test results are positive for life and are the tests of choice for diagnosis, whereas the nonspecific nontreponemal test results will revert to negative or persist at low titers after successful treatment. Demonstration of a fourfold rise in titer, from 1:8 to 1:32, or an increase from 1:4 to 1:16 of nontreponemal tests is consistent with reinfection. For sequential serologic tests, the same test and preferably the same laboratory should be used. The RPR is most useful as a screening test, whereas the quantitative VDRL titer is the test of choice for following therapeutic response to treatment. Rarely, false positive serologic results may be obtained with systemic diseases (e.g., systemic lupus erythematosus) or pregnancy. In some HIV-infected patients, titers alone may not be accurate and biopsy or darkfield microscopy may be required.

The diagnosis of neurosyphilis should be based on compilation of results of several tests. Perform a lumbar puncture to look for abnormal cerebrospinal fluid: pleocytosis (greater than 5 wbc/mm^3), elevated protein level, and a positive VDRL (although false negative results can occur with the VDRL). The FTA-ABS is more sensitive but less specific, thus giving more false positives but fewer false negatives.

The diagnosis of congenital syphilis is confirmed as follows: (1) Serum from the infant (not umbilical cord) should be used for testing, to prevent false positive results. (2)

TABLE 15–2.

Skin Manifestations and Diagnosis of Syphilis

	Stage			
	Primary	Secondary	Tertiary	Congenital
Distribution	At contact site, including mouth, rectum *Females:* Labia, cervix *Males:* Penis shaft, glans	Generalized, including mucous membranes; bilateral and symmetric	Generalized	Generalized
Primary lesions	Papule	Macules, papules, plaques, pustules	Nodules, tumors, or none	Macules, papules, plaques, pustules, vesicles
Secondary lesions	Erythema, "chancre," well-circumscribed single or multiple lesions with clean base and serous discharge	Scale, erythema, hyperpigmentation *Alopecia:* Moth-eaten *Mucous patches:* gray erosions on mucous membranes *Condyloma lata:* Flat-topped papules on perianal region (see Fig. 15–7)	Ulcers, exudate, or none	Scale, erythema, hyperpigmentation, alopecia Desquamation of palms and soles
Features	Classically painless, with nontender inguinal adenopathy	Skin lesions may imitate many common rashes, including pityriasis rosea, psoriasis, or tinea corporis; still highly infectious	Consider as part of workup in any patient with dementia	*Snuffles:* highly infectious mucous nasal discharge
Diagnostic tests	Darkfield examination, immunofluorescent staining of smears; VDRL positive 7–10 days after chancre; biopsy specimen for histologic study	Darkfield examination, serologic tests along with titer	*Spinal tap:* pleocytosis, elevated protein, positive serologic findings in CSF or blood	Darkfield examination from umbilical cord or mucocutaneous lesions; serologic tests positive, but may be from maternal antibodies Follow serial tests or serial titers

Serial serologic tests are performed to follow the effectiveness of treatment or the diminution of transplacentally acquired maternal antibody. (3) Specimens from the placenta and umbilical cord should be checked with darkfield microscopy, immunofluorescence, or silver stains for the presence of spirochetes in infants born to a mother with reactive serum or when the placenta is hydropic. All neonatal lesions should be examined for treponemes.

III. DIFFERENTIAL DIAGNOSIS

    A. Primary syphilis: See Table 15–1.

B. **Secondary syphilis:** (Fig. 15–7)
1. **Pityriasis rosea:** Look for the herald patch of pityriasis rosea. Palmar, plantar, or mucous membrane involvement and a recent genital lesion more likely indicate syphilis. Serology is indicated to differentiate.
2. **Tinea corporis:** The lesions of syphilis are typically bilateral and symmetric; those of tinea corporis tend to be more isolated. A KOH prep will demonstrate hyphae in tinea corporis.
3. **Drug eruption:** With the acute onset of an eruption, seek a history of recent drug ingestion and historic lack of a recent genital lesion. Lesions caused by drug eruptions tend to be monomorphic.
4. **Lichen planus:** Lesions of lichen planus tend to be located on the wrists and ankles, with associated lacelike buccal mucosa lesions; syphilitic lesions may be on the palms and soles, with associated mucous patches.

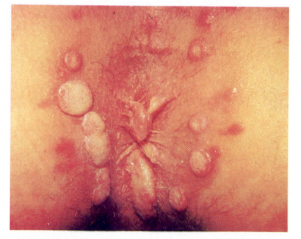

Fig. 15–7
Secondary syphilis. Note flat-topped perianal papules characteristic of condyloma lata. (Courtesy Beverly Sanders, MD.)

5. **Condyloma acuminatam** (see Fig. 15–2): Warty papules of syphilis tend to be flat-topped and associated with generalized exanthem. Condyloma acuminatam tends to be more exophytic and chronic. Condyloma lata lesions are darkfield positive for spirochetes.
6. **Viral exanthem:** Usually there is no recent history of a genital ulcer or other classic syphilitic lesions (e.g., mucous patches, palmar or plantar involvement). Tests for syphilis are negative.
7. **Psoriasis:** Psoriatic lesions usually are chronic, with a characteristic thick, silvery scale. Look for psoriatic nail changes (e.g., pitting).

C. **Congenital syphilis**
1. Hydrops fetalis: Differentiate from blood group incompatibility.
2. Rhinorrhea as a result of bacterial or viral infections: Rhinorrhea as a result of syphilis will be persistent. Look for generalized exanthem. Spirochetes are present in the nasal discharge, and maternal serum should be positive.
3. Intrauterine growth retardation as a result of other congenital infections (e.g., HSV, rubella, cytomegalovirus, toxoplasmosis): Maternal and fetal serologic studies should help differentiate these conditions.

IV. **TREATMENT**
A. **Screen all patients for HIV and other STD diseases.**
B. **Primary, secondary, and early latent syphilis of less than 1 year's duration:**
1. *Benzathine penicillin G* 2.4 million U IM in a single dose (although some experts now advocate two doses).
2. In nonpregnant, penicillin-allergic patients, choose one of the following:
   a. *Doxycycline* 100 mg PO twice daily for 2 weeks.

b. *Tetracycline* 500 mg PO 4 times a day for 2 weeks.

c. *Erythromycin* 500 mg PO 4 times a day for 2 weeks.

3. Follow-up:

   a. Reexamine at 3 and 6 months for clinical and serologic cure.

   b. HIV tests and CSF examination are indicated if the nontreponemal antibody titers (VDRL) have not declined by fourfold in 3 months in primary or secondary syphilis or by 6 months in early latent syphilis, if signs and symptoms persist after reinfection has been ruled out, or for any signs of neurosyphilis (e.g., menigitis, progressive dementia, uveitis, auditory or cranial nerve problems).

   c. HIV-infected patients should have more frequent follow-up, including serologic testing monthly for 3 months, then every 3 months for 1 year. Any fourfold rise should be followed by a CSF examination, treating with the neurosyphilis regimen unless reinfection is the cause.

C. **Late latent syphilis of more than 1 year's duration, gummas, or cardiovascular syphilis:**

1. Perform a thorough clinical examination, looking for signs of aortitis, iritis, neurosyphilis, etc.

2. Lumbar puncture is indicated in the case of any of the following:

   a. Neurologic signs or symptoms are present.

   b. There is treatment failure.

   c. The nontreponemal antibody titer is equal to or greater than 1:32 (unless the duration of infection is less than 1 year).

   d. Other evidence of active syphilis is present (e.g., iritis, gumma, or aortitis).

e. The HIV antibody test is positive.

f. Nonpenicillin therapy is planned.

3. *Benzathine penicillin G* 2.4 million U IM weekly for 3 weeks.

4. Penicillin-allergic patients:

   a. If pregnant, consider desensitization.

   b. If nonpregnant, use *doxycycline* 100 mg PO twice daily for 4 weeks or *tetracycline* 500 mg PO 4 times a day for 4 weeks.

5. Follow-up: Nontreponemal titers should be repeated at 6 and 12 months. If titers increase fourfold or fail to decrease or for continuing signs of syphilis, lumbar puncture should be performed and the patient retreated.

D. **Neurosyphilis:**

1. *Aqueous crystalline penicillin G* 2 million to 4 million U IV q4h for 10 to 14 days.

2. Alternative regimen if outpatient compliance can be ensured:

   a. *Procaine penicillin* 2.4 million U IM daily with *probenecid* 500 mg PO 4 times daily for 10 to 14 days. Consider additional treatment with *benzathine penicillin* 2.4 million U IM after completion of above therapy.

   b. Penicillin-allergic patients should be desensitized.

3. Follow-up:

   a. If initial CSF pleocytosis is present, repeat CSF examination every 6 months until the cell count is normal.

   b. Consider retreating if the cell count remains abnormal.

E. **Congenital syphilis:** (Box 15–1) Infants should not be discharged from the hospital until the serologic status of the mother is known.

1. Assess infant risk and look thoroughly for any physical signs of syphilis for infants at high risk.

BOX 15–1
Congenital Syphilis

INFANTS AT HIGH RISK

- Positive infant serum at birth to woman with untreated syphilis
- Treatment of woman less than 1 month before delivery
- Treatment with a drug other than penicillin
- Treatment with failure to document decreasing titers
- Treatment with insufficient follow-up.

PRESUMPTIVE DIAGNOSIS

- Any evidence of active disease
- Reactive CSF-VDRL
- Abnormal CSF findings (greater than 5 cells/mm^3, protein greater than 50 mg/dl)
- Quantitative nontreponemal serology titers 4 times or greater than mother's
- Positive FTA-ABS 19S IgM antibody
- Untreated maternal syphilis
- Maternal relapse or reinfection

2. Laboratory measures:
   a. Perform nontreponemal antibody titers on infant, not cord, blood.
   b. Examine the CSF for cells, protein, and perform VDRL test.
   c. Consider performing long bone radiograph studies to rule out osteochondritis, osteitis, or periostitis; check chest radiograph, CBC, and liver profile.
   d. Examine placenta or amniotic cord for specific antitreponemal antibody staining.
3. Treatment:
   a. *Crystalline penicillin G* 50,000 U/kg IV daily q12 hours on days 1 to 7, then q8 hours on days 10 to 14, *or*
   b. *Aqueous procaine penicillin G* 50,000 U/kg IM daily for a minimum of 10 to 14 days.
   c. If the mother was adequately treated during pregnancy but follow-up cannot be ensured, consider *benzathine penicillin G* 50,000 U/kg IM in a single dose.

   d. For neurologic involvement, use *aqueous crystalline penicillin G* 200 to 300,000 U/kg/day IV or IM for 10 to 14 days.
4. Follow-up:
   a. Monthly for 3 months, then at 6 and 12 months, with serologic testing, CSF examination, and clinical examination.
   b. Nontreponemal antibody titers should be decreasing by 3 months and should have disappeared by 6 months if treated appropriately.
   c. If titers are stable or increasing, or if the CSF cell count is still abnormal after 2 years, the child should be reevaluated and retreated. Treponemal tests may be positive despite effective therapy.
   d. Developmental evaluation at age 2 should be done in all children symptomatic at birth with active congenital infection.

F. **Syphilis in children** (after newborn period):
   1. Perform CSF exam to rule out neurosyphilis.
   2. Review birth and maternal records to determine if infection is congenital or acquired.
   3. Inform child protection agency of condition, for full evaluation.
   4. Treat with *benzathine penicillin G* 50,000 U/kg IM, up to 2.4 million U, in a single dose.

G. **Syphilis in HIV disease:**
   1. Treatment is the same as for adults, but multiple treatments may be needed.
   2. Examine CSF before and after therapy and for any patient that represents a treatment failure.
   3. Follow-up is needed at 1, 2, 3, 6, 9, and 12 months.

H. **Partner notification and treatment are essential, even if the partner is asymptomatic.**

V. PATIENT EDUCATION

A. Educate patients to abstain from sexual intercourse until lesions have healed completely.

B. Emphasize the need for condom use and offer instructions on usage.

C. Emphasize the need for partner identification and notification.

D. Educate patients that open sores put them at risk for obtaining other infections (e.g., hepatitis B, HIV).

E. Inform patients about the possibility of the Jarisch-Herxheimer reaction, in which any or all skin lesions may flare up within 12 hours of treatment and patient may develop fever, headache, sore throat, or myalgias. The exact mechanism is unknown, and symptoms usually resolve within 18 to 24 hours. Analgesics (e.g., acetaminophen) are indicated.

SUGGESTED READING

Centers for Disease Control: 1993 sexually transmitted disease treatment guidelines, *MMWR* 42/RR-14:1–108, 1993.

Goens JL, Schwartz RA, De Wolf K: Mucocutaneous manifestations of chancroid, lymphogranuloma venereum, and granuloma inguinale, *Am Fam Physician* 49:415–425, 1994.

Goldberg LH et al: Long-term suppression of recurrent genital herpes with acyclovir, *Arch Dermatol* 129:582–587, 1993.

Pereira FA: Herpes simplex: evolving concepts, *J Am Acad Dermatol* 35:503–520, 1996.

CHAPTER 16

Special Populations

NEWBORNS AND NEONATES

Perhaps more than any other skin lesion, a rash found on a newborn baby may provoke fear or anxiety in new parents and family members. The majority of these lesions are benign and easily treated. Reassurance often goes a long way toward dealing with any parental concerns, because many conditions of the neonatal period also resolve spontaneously. Described below are the most common dermatoses affecting newborn infants. The differential diagnoses of the most common benign neonatal skin lesions are shown in Table 16–1. Other conditions affecting young infants, such as atopic dermatitis or inherited disorders, are discussed elsewhere in this text.

The skin of neonates has the unique features of an increased ratio of surface area to volume, and under occlusive conditions, such as with the use of plastic pants, percutaneous absorption of topically applied medications is enhanced. *Therefore the use of any topical agent (e.g., corticosteroid creams) should be used cautiously in this age group.*

Seborrheic Dermatitis ICD-9 (690.12)

Seborrheic dermatitis is a nonpruritic scaling disorder of unknown cause that occurs very commonly in infants from age 2 weeks to 6 months. It typically resolves in a matter of weeks and almost always by 1 year. Scalp involvement is known commonly as *cradle cap* (Fig. 16–1). The yellow-brown scale with associated erythema is characteristic. Secondary scalp infection with *Staphylococcus aureus* can occur. Although sometimes similar to atopic dermatitis, seborrheic derma-

TABLE 16–1.

Common Benign Neonatal Skin Disorders

Condition	Clinical Features
Mongolian spots	Blue or black macules found on the lumbosacral area of most Asian, black, and Indian newborns.
Salmon patch	Erythematous macules often found on the neck.
Acne neonatorum	Papules or pustules on the face or trunk that appear after 2–4 weeks and usually resolve without treatment.
Transient neonatal pustular melanosis	Pustules, vesicles, and pigmented macules seen at birth, more often in dark-skinned infants, that resolve over days to weeks. Vesicles contain many neutrophils.
Erythema toxicum	Erythematous macules, pustules, or vesicles that appear after 24–48 hours and resolve within 1–2 weeks. Vesicles contain many eosinophils.
Milia	Multiple, small, white papules on the forehead or face, that resolve after 2–3 weeks.
Umbilical granuloma	Small granuloma appearing in umbilicus after umbilical cord detaches. Resolves with repeat silver nitrate sticks to lesion over 3–5 days.

titis in neonates does not itch and tends to resolve. Treatment involves massaging warm mineral oil daily on the affected areas to remove the scale. Daily shampooing with a mild preparation also is helpful. If the scales are thick or stubborn, use a shampoo containing salicylic acid (e.g., Sebulex). *Hydrocortisone* 1% lotion or cream (15 g) can be used sparingly once or twice a day, cautiously, in neonates. Treat any secondary infection.

Diaper Dermatitis ICD-9 (691.0)

Diaper dermatitis is the most common rash in infancy. This dermatitis is classified as an irritant dermatitis secondary to prolonged contact with ammonia, or, less commonly, is caused by residual antiseptics, soaps, or detergents in diapers. The ammonia is produced from the breakdown of urea by bacteria in fecal material. Irritation is subsequently increased by the occlusive effect of rubber or plastic diaper pants, which increase the penetration of the alkaline material into the skin. The most common predisposing factor is infrequent diaper changes. A recent course of antibiotics may also predispose an infant to develop diaper dermatitis by causing diarrhea and allowing an increased exposure to irritant material. Secondary infection with *Candida* is quite common, while staphylococcal and streptococcal infections occur less frequently.

I. CLASSIC DESCRIPTION (Fig. 16–2)

Distribution: *Diaper area:* external genitalia and buttocks; creases usually spared; may spread to abdomen

Primary: Papules, plaques; in neglected cases, vesicles and bullae

Secondary: Erythema, erosions; in neglected cases, ulcers

Secondary infection with *Candida* will have satellite beefy red papules and pustules scattered beyond the diaper area.

II. DIAGNOSIS:

Diagnosis is based on the clinical appearance. A KOH examination may confirm the presence of *Candida.*

III. DIFFERENTIAL DIAGNOSIS

A. Atopic dermatitis: The diaper area is rarely involved in atopic dermatitis. Look for signs of atopic dermatitis elsewhere, such as the extensor surfaces in infants, and a personal or family history of atopy.

B. Histiocytosis X: Look for petechial, scaling lesions in the diaper area or other areas that are unresponsive to conventional therapies. The child usually has systemic illness.

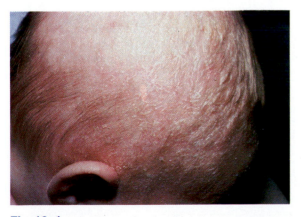

Fig. 16–1
Cradle cap. Note diffuse, greasy-looking scales on an infant's scalp. (Courtesy Department of Dermatology, University of North Carolina at Chapel Hill.)

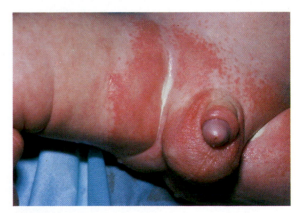
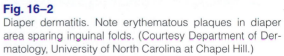

Fig. 16–2
Diaper dermatitis. Note erythematous plaques in diaper area sparing inguinal folds. (Courtesy Department of Dermatology, University of North Carolina at Chapel Hill.)

C. **Perianal cellulitis:** This rash is exclusively localized to the perianal area and may be painful. *Streptococcus pyogenes* can be cultured, when the diagnosis is strongly suspected.

D. **Psoriasis:** Psoriasis is characterized by thicker, well-demarcated areas of scaling that can also involve the creases. Look for involvement elsewhere (e.g., scalp, nails).

E. **Seborrheic dermatitis:** Seborrheic dermatitis tends to have a greasy-looking, sharply demarcated scale. Involvement of the scalp (cradle cap), posterior auricular area, and creases is also characteristic.

F. **Kawasaki syndrome:** Diffuse erythema of the perineum may be the first sign of Kawasaki syndrome. Look for other elements of the syndrome, such as high fever, conjunctivitis, lymphadenopathy, oropharyngeal involvement, and erythema or edema of the palms and soles.

IV. **TREATMENT**

A. **Prevention:** Keep the diaper area as dry as possible. Change cloth or disposable diapers frequently (e.g., every hour).

B. **Anticandidal creams:** (15, 30 g), see Table 16–2.
   1. Choose one agent and apply to affected areas if candidal infection is present.
   2. Avoid *lotrisone* and *mycolog;* both contain corticosteroid agents that are too strong for use in this age group and location.

C. **Hydrocortisone cream 1%:** Apply twice daily to decrease erythema. Limit use to less than 7 days.

D. **Barrier creams containing zinc oxide** (e.g., Desitin) may be useful. Avoid fragrance, lanolin, or combination creams.

E. **Cloth diaper laundering:** Put *washed* diapers in a washing machine half-filled with water, add 1 cup of vinegar, let soak 30 minutes, then spin dry without rinsing. Dry as usual. This will help "acidify" the diapers, producing an environment that is less conducive to the growth of ammonia-producing bacteria.

F. **Follow up:** Visits are indicated only if lesions are not responding within 4 days or clearing is not complete within 7 to 10 days. Consider bacterial cultures in recalcitrant cases.

V. **PATIENT EDUCATION**
(See patient education handout in Appendix F.)

A. Educate the caretakers and parents that frequent diaper changes (e.g., hourly during waking hours) are essential for improvement.

B. Encourage diaper changes 1 hour after the child goes to sleep for the night if the child is age 6 to 12 months.

C. Avoid unnecessary occlusion, such as rubber or plastic diaper pants.

D. Encourage periods of not wearing any

TABLE 16–2.

Anticandidal Creams

Generic Name	Brand Name	Size(g)	Dosage	Availability	Cost 15-g Tube
Ciclopirox olamine	Loprox	15, 30, 90	bid	Prescription	$18.59
Clotrimazole	Lotrimin AF	15	bid	OTC	6.34
	Lotrimin	30, 45, 90		Prescription	
Econazole	Spectazole	15, 30, 85	qd	Prescription	20.09
Ketoconazole	Nizoral	15, 30, 60	qd	Prescription	19.72
Miconazole nitrate	Monistat-Derm	15	bid	OTC	20.00
		30, 60, 90		Prescription	
Nystatin	Mycostatin	15, 30	bid	Prescription	6.49

diaper if possible (i.e., sleeping on a rubber sheet).

E. Instruct caretakers and parents to cleanse the diaper area gently with warm water after each diaper change. Avoid the use of soap, if possible, or use soap substitutes, such as Cetaphil or Aquanil. Avoid fragrance-containing diaper wipes.

F. Educate patients to alternate hydrocortisone and antiyeast creams, emphasizing that those creams should be used sparingly and rubbed in until they disappear; while barrier creams (Desitin) should be applied liberally.

Erythema Toxicum Neonatorum ICD-9 (778.8)

I. CLASSIC DESCRIPTION

Erythema toxicum neonatorum is a transient, erythematous, pustular eruption (Fig.16–3) present in almost 50% of term infants and less commonly in preterm infants. Pustules or vesicles appear at birth on the trunk, face, and proximal extremities. New lesions may continue to develop for up to 10 days, with individual lesions lasting 4 to 5 days. Pilosebaceous unit plugging is thought to be the underlying cause of these

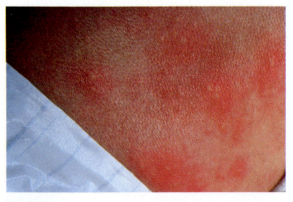

Fig. 16–3
Erythema toxicum neonatorum. Note pustules on an erythematous base involving the trunk. (Courtesy Steve Resnick, MD.)

lesions. The pustules consist of eosinophils, and blood eosinophilia is a frequent finding.

II. DIAGNOSIS

Diagnosis is based on the clinical appearance of the lesions. Wright's stain of a lesion will demonstrate the bright red-orange granules of eosinophils. Pustules or vesicles are 1 to 4 mm in diameter and have surrounding erythema.

III. DIFFERENTIAL DIAGNOSIS

A. **Transient neonatal pustulosis:** Clinically, lesions are similar, with pustules appearing on an erythematous base. Neonatal pustulosis appears more commonly in black infants and heals with characteristic hyperpigmentation. Wright's stain will demonstrate neutrophils rather than eosinophils.

B. **Folliculitis:** Erythematous areas are usually smaller in folliculitis; Wright's stain demonstrates neutrophils rather than eosinophils.

C. **Miliaria:** Erythematous areas are smaller in miliaria, and the sweat glands, not the pilosebaceous units, are involved. Miliaria is more common in preterm infants, and occurs in response to heat.

D. **Pityrosporum folliculitis:** Scrape pustules on the cheek and look for extensive yeasts on KOH exam in persistent cases.

IV. TREATMENT

No treatment is necessary other than reassurance of the parents.

Neonatal Acne ICD-9 (706.1)

Neonatal acne is a common neonatal skin disorder, usually appearing between ages 2 and 4 weeks in affected infants (Fig. 16–4). It results as a response to maternal androgen stimulation. Papules and pustules usually last from several weeks to several months. The differential diagnosis is the same as for erythema toxicum neonatorum. The condition resolves spontaneously without treatment.

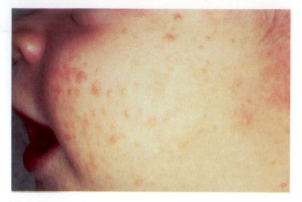

Fig. 16–4
Erythematous papules and pustules characteristic of neonatal acne. (Courtesy Marshall Guill, MD.)

Hemangiomas ICD-9 (Hemangioma, salmon patch 228.01; Port-wine stain 757.32; Sturge-Weber syndrome 759.6)

Hemangiomas are blood vessel growths, often classified as either *flat* or *raised*. Clinicians should recognize these lesions so they can reassure parents who are worried about an enlarging pigmented area that, in most cases, the lesion is benign and will likely regress with time.

There are three distinct common hemangiomas:

1. **Nevus flammeus,** also known as *port-wine stain*. (Fig. 16–5), is present at birth as a red or red-purple flat area; the pigmentation persists throughout life. Enlarged mature capillaries and dilated blood vessels may progress, with advancing age, to involve deeper layers of the dermis and manifest as dark, raised papules or nodules that develop in a previously flat lesion. *Sturge-Weber syndrome* consists of a port-wine stain involving predominantly the ophthalmologic branch of the trigeminal nerve, with associated leptomeningeal involvement. Calcified lesions in the meningeal vasculature and anomalies are associated with epilepsy, hemiplegia, and mental retardation.

2. **Salmon patches,** also known as *stork bites* (Fig. 16–6), are extremely common, oc-

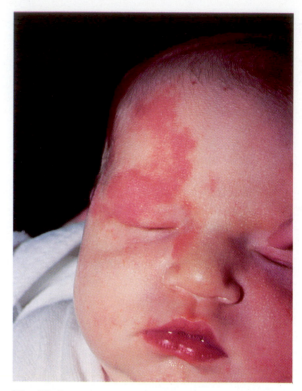

Fig. 16–5
Port-wine stain in trigeminal V1 (ophthalmic division) distribution. Workup did not reveal Sturge-Weber syndrome. (Courtesy Department of Dermatology, University of North Carolina at Chapel Hill.)

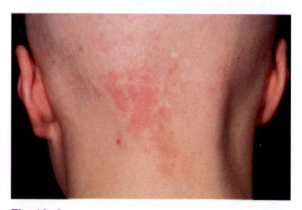

Fig. 16–6
Salmon patch. (From Habif TP: *Clinical dermatology,* ed 3, St Louis, 1995, Mosby.)

curing in 7 of 10 white infants. These lesions are present at birth and consist of mature dilated dermal capillaries that resolve rather than progress.

3. **Capillary hemangiomas,** also known as *strawberry marks* (Fig. 16–7), rarely are present at birth but usually develop within the first few days to months of life.

The lesions consist of proliferating endothelial cells; initially there are a few telangiectases, followed by development of typical lesions. Lesions usually begin to involute by age 15 months, and 50% will completely resolve by age 5 years; virtually all resolve by puberty. When these hemangiomas are located subglottically or if there are multiple head and neck hemangiomas, airway or visual obstruction may result. Occasionally, other problems may be present, such as erosion or ulceration of lesions, a consumptive coagulopathy, or high-output cardiac failure.

I. CLASSIC DESCRIPTION
Distribution: *Port-wine stain:* Localized, most frequently on face
Salmon patch: Posterior neck, glabella, upper eyelids

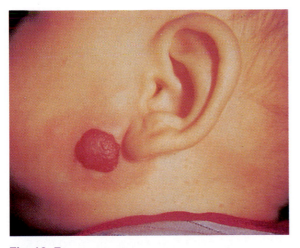

Fig. 16–7
Capillary hemangioma. Note soft, compressible, localized tumor. (Courtesy Beverly Sanders, MD.)

Strawberry hemangioma: Localized or regional
Primary: *Port-wine stain:* Macule; papules or nodules may develop with age
Salmon patch: Macule
Strawberry hemangioma: Telangiectatic macule that develops into a papule, nodule, or tumor
Secondary: Erythema, red/purple; ulceration and crusting may occur in strawberry hemangiomas

II. DIAGNOSIS
Diagnosis is based on the clinical appearance of the lesion.

III. DIFFERENTIAL DIAGNOSIS
A. Lymphangioma: Look for clear, deep-seated vesicles or lesions that present as a painless mass that gradually enlarges.
B. Cavernous hemangioma: Typically this is a soft globular tumor with texture likened to a "bag of worms." Deeper tissues are involved, and cavernous hemangiomas may be more persistent than strawberry hemangiomas, with associated arteriovenous malformation.

IV. TREATMENT
A. No treatment other than reassurance is needed for salmon patches and uncomplicated and nonfacial strawberry hemangiomas: Reassure parents that salmon patches will usually resolve and that strawberry hemangiomas will usually involute.
B. Treatment of complicated strawberry hemangiomas is imperative if consumption coagulopathy, airway obstruction, visual obstruction, or high-output cardiac failure are present. Also strongly consider early treatment for periorbital lesions to prevent ocular problems or potentially disfiguring facial lesions from developing. Treatment options include:
   1. Referral for pulsed dye vascular laser therapy. Treat lesions as early as possible, even during the neonatal period, without delay, for best results.

2. *Prednisone* 1 to 6 mg/kg/day daily or every other day for 4 to 8 weeks if there is systemic involvement. Best results are obtained if patient is younger than 8 months.
3. Instruct parents to use pressure and/or ice packs if bleeding occurs.

C. **Port-wine stain:**
1. Refer early on for pulsed dye laser therapy. The younger the patient, the better the response to treatment.
2. Evaluate patients with facial involvement for possible Sturge-Weber syndrome, especially if the lesion is bilateral or if the ophthalmic branch of the trigeminal nerve is involved. The workup includes electroencephalography, magnetic resonance imaging, cerebral angiography, and ophthalmologic examination.

D. **Cosmesis:** Specialized makeups (e.g., Covermark or Dermablend), available at most large retail stores, can provide excellent cosmetic coverage.

V. **PATIENT EDUCATION**
Suggest patients contact a support group.

DERMATOSES IN DARK-SKINNED PATIENTS

Skin disorders in dark-skinned patients are sometimes more difficult for clinicians to diagnose, because the morphologic changes, particularly secondary pigmentary changes, often are more subtle. For this reason, clinicians should remember that common rashes easily recognized in fair-skinned patients may be more challenging to diagnose when they occur in dark-skinned patients. In addition, several disorders occur more frequently in dark-skinned populations or the consequences of the disorders are more severe. These diseases are detailed below. It is important to note, however, that these skin disorders can and do occur in all populations.

Keloids ICD-9 (701.4)

The term *keloid* is derived from Greek words meaning *tumorlike*. Keloids are composed of abnormal fibroblasts present in scar tissue, and in some patients the resulting lesions are severely disfiguring. For unknown reasons, certain individuals, most commonly blacks, develop a hyperproliferation of these fibroblasts in response to trauma or, less commonly, *de novo*. Keloids may be asymptomatic, pruritic, tender to palpation, or, occasionally, the source of sharp, shooting pains. *Any skin insult* (e.g., ear piercing, lacerations, secondarily infected skin lesions, surgery) *can cause keloid formation in predis-posed people*. **Acne keloidalis nuchae** refers to inflamed pustules and papules on the posterior neck that often heal with keloid formation.

I. **CLASSIC DESCRIPTION** (Fig. 16–8)
Distribution: Ears, neck, jaw, presternal chest, shoulders, upper back
Primary: Papules, nodules, plaques, tumors
Secondary: Scar, hyperpigmentation, erythema/purplish

II. **DIAGNOSIS**
Diagnosis is based on the clinical appearance.

III. **TREATMENT**
A. **Prevention:** The best treatment is preventing unnecessary trauma, including surgery, whenever possible. Treat any skin problems (e.g., acne, infections) as early as possible to minimize areas of inflammation.
B. **For keloids that are painful or cosmetically disfiguring:**
1. **Intralesional corticosteroids:** First-line therapy.
   a. *Triamcinolone:* 10 mg/ml initial concentration for most keloids.
   b. Apply liquid nitrogen for 10 to 15 seconds before injection, for local anesthesia and as an aid to injection. Permanent hypopigmentation

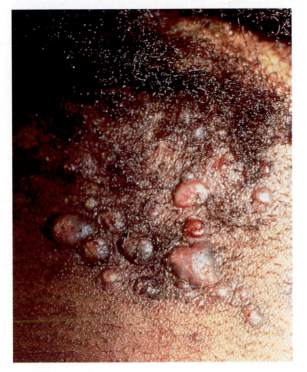

Fig. 16–8
Multiple small keloids occurring in response to inflammation. (Courtesy Marshall Guill, MD.)

may result if liquid nitrogen is used for 30 seconds or longer.

c. Using a 27- or 30-gauge needle with the bevel directed up toward the skin, inject enough medicine to make the keloid blanch (usually 0.1 to 0.5 ml). Inject into the keloid as the needle is withdrawn from the skin. Be sure that the injection occurs in the bulk of the lesion and not underneath it, or lipoatrophy may occur.

d. Use a Luer-Lok (twist on) type of syringe, because injections are often made under pressure.

e. Inject at monthly intervals, increasing the concentration by 10 mg/ml until the lesion softens and flattens, then decrease the frequency and strength of injections. Do not ex-

ceed 40 mg per visit. Atrophy and hypopigmentation may occur at higher concentrations.

f. Wear protective goggles when injecting, to avoid spraying medication or blood into your eyes.

g. Surgery is recommended if there is no response after four injections.

2. **Excision:**

a. Either scalpel excision or carbon dioxide laser excision may be indicated if injection therapy alone is unsuccessful or unlikely to give significant improvement.

b. Use with preoperative, intraoperative, or postoperative *triamcinolone* injections.

3. **Silicone gel sheeting:** Useful as an adjunct in preventing keloid formation or hypertrophic scars in new sites of injury in predisposed individuals.

a. Available by prescription; pharmacies can special-order it.

b. The sheeting is clear and sticky and should be cut to fit the size of the keloid.

c. Place sheeting on top of the keloid and tape it into place, leaving it on for 12 to 24 hours a day.

d. Wash the sheet daily and replace it every 10 to 14 days.

e. Judge effectiveness after 2 to 6 months.

4. **Cryosurgery:**

a. May be useful in combination with other modalities.

b. Use a 10- to 30-second freeze–thaw cycle, repeating up to 3 times.

c. Repeat once a month until response occurs.

d. Permanent hypopigmentation may occur.

5. **Radiation therapy:** Although this modality has been successful, the long-term risks associated with it make it not to be recommended in most cases.

C. Despite therapy, recurrences are possible.

IV. PATIENT EDUCATION
A. Advise patients to minimize skin trauma, avoid unnecessary surgery (e.g., ear piercing, elective mole removals), and make sure any skin infections are treated promptly, to avoid further keloid development.
B. Explain about the possibility of recurrence despite adequate therapy.
C. Educate that compliance for follow-up visits is essential in achieving any long-lasting response to therapy.
D. Educate that the earlier keloids are treated, the more likely it is that they will respond to therapy.
E. Document explanations on possibilities of atrophy, telangiectasia, and hypopigmentation with *triamcinolone* injections.
F. Instruct patient to avoid shaving in the neck region if the patient has acne keloidalis nuchae. Encourage patients to allow the posterior hair to only be trimmed with scissors and trimmed no shorter than ⅛ inch.

Pseudofolliculitis Barbae ICD-9 (706.1)

Pseudofolliculitis barbae occurs when the free ends of tightly coiled hairs reenter the skin, causing a "pseudofolliculitis" or a foreign body-like inflammatory reaction. (Fig. 16–9). At least 50% of black men and 3% of white men who shave have the tendency to develop these lesions, usually on the cheeks or neck. Shaving makes free ends of coiled hairs sharper, thereby predisposing individuals to the problem. Inflammation around these free ends results in papules that become repeatedly irritated by shaving. Complications include pruritus, postinflammatory hyperpigmentation, scarring, keloid formation, and secondary infection. Occupational problems may occur when an employer requires no facial hair (e.g., the military, food handlers).

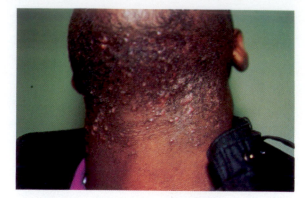

Fig. 16–9
Pseudofolliculitis barbae. Note multiple papules, pustules, and scar formation confined to the beard area. (Courtesy Beverly Sanders, MD.)

I. CLASSIC DESCRIPTION
Distribution: Any shaved area: face, posterior neck, axilla, legs
Primary: Papules, nodules, pustules
Secondary: Erythema, hyperpigmentation, scar, keloid

II. DIAGNOSIS
The diagnosis is clinical. Look for a piece of hair protruding from individual lesions.

III. DIFFERENTIAL DIAGNOSIS
Folliculitis: Folliculitis tends to produce more localized inflammation. Pseudofolliculitis tends to be a chronic problem and is "pseudofollicular" rather than follicular.

IV. TREATMENT
A. **Avoiding close shaving is essential.** This preventive therapy usually cures the disease. Work with employers, if necessary, so that patients can avoid shaving.
B. **Acutely inflamed lesions:**
   1. Use warm compresses with tap water for 10 minutes 3 times a day.
   2. Release ingrowing hairs gently, using a sterilized needle or tweezers.
   3. Use *hydrocortisone 1% cream,* as necessary, for inflammation.
   4. Antibiotics:
      a. Topical *erythromycin* twice daily for mild pustular involvement: ointment

(Akne-Mycin) or solution (A/T/S, Erymax).

b. Oral *erythromycin* or *tetracycline* 500 mg twice daily, depending on the severity of the secondary infection.

C. For those who must shave:

1. Initially, allow hairs to grow ¼ inch or more to overcome the spring effect in hairs so they will no longer become embedded. Subsequently, clip hairs no shorter than needed for maintenance. Use fine scissors or special facial hair clippers.

2. Rinse and compress the face with warm tap water for several minutes.

3. Use generous amounts of a highly lubricating shaving cream or gel (e.g., Easy Shave), and allow the cream to soften the skin for 5 to 10 minutes before shaving.

4. Only use sharp razors, shaving in the direction of hair growth.

5. Specialized guarded razors (e.g., "PFB Bump Fighter") may be found in pharmacies or are available by mail order.*

6. After shaving, rinse the face with tap water, then apply cold-water compresses for 5 minutes.

7. *Tretinoin* solution, gel, or cream, in early or mild disease, may be useful as an adjunct to shaving but also may cause stinging, burning, and peeling.

8. Depilatories: Use every 3 days.
   a. Ali, Royal Crown, and Magic Shave cream depilatories may cause severe irritation, resulting in postinflammatory hyperpigmentation.
   b. Educate patients to use a small test area first.

*Moore Innovations, Inc., P.O. Box 300445, Houston, TX 77230-0445.

c. Use *hydrocortisone 1% cream* afterward to decrease inflammation, if necessary.

D. Embedded hairs: Gently try to release, not pluck, any embedded curled hairs with a sterilized needle.

V. PATIENT EDUCATION

A. Educate patients extensively about the role of shaving.

B. Educate on shaving techniques if patients must shave.

C. Educate to use cream depilatories on a test area first.

Vitiligo ICD-9 (709.0)

Vitiligo is an acquired skin depigmentation that affects all races but is far more disfiguring in blacks. The cause, although unknown, is thought to involve an autoimmune process against melanocytes, inasmuch as, histologically, there is an absence of melanocytes, and vitiligo is sometimes seen in patients with adrenal insufficiency, autoimmune hemolytic anemia, alopecia areata. Some systemic diseases, (e.g., diabetes mellitus, thyroid disease, and pernicious anemia) also are associated with a greater incidence of vitiligo. Genetic factors seem to play a role, with 30% to 40% of patients having a positive family history.

The age of onset is variable, and the course usually is slowly progressive. Ten percent to 20% of patients may experience spontaneous repigmentation.

I. CLASSIC DESCRIPTION (Fig. 16–10)
Distribution: Predilection for acral areas and around body orifices, (e.g., mouth, eyes, nose, anus)
Primary: Macules
Secondary: Depigmentation

II. DIAGNOSIS
Diagnosis is based on the clinical presence of depigmented patches of skin.

III. DIFFERENTIAL DIAGNOSIS
A. Postinflammatory hypopigmentation: In postinflammatory hypopigmentation,

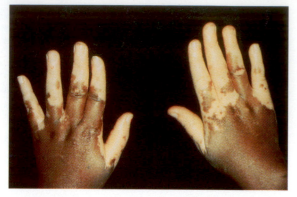

Fig. 16–10
Vitiligo. Note depigmentation of acral areas. (Courtesy Medical College of Georgia, Division of Dermatology.)

there is a decrease in pigmentation rather than absence, as in vitiligo. In addition, look for a history of antecedent trauma or inflammation. One cause is liquid nitrogen therapy.
B. **Chemically induced depigmentation:** Working with chemicals containing phenols may cause depigmentation.
C. **Piebaldism:** The lesions in piebaldism, a genetically inherited absence of pigment, are present at birth and are usually confined to the head and trunk.
D. **Morphea:** In morphea, the texture of the skin is abnormal and sclerotic.
E. **Lichen sclerosus:** The texture of the skin is thinned. There may be a follicular prominence, with complaints of burning, especially if the genitalia are involved.
F. **Leprosy:** Areas of hypopigmentation will be anesthetic in leprosy.

IV. TREATMENT
Treatment is necessary when the disease is emotionally and physically disfiguring, more likely in dark-skinned individuals. Consider contacting the National Vitiligo Foundation or contacting a dermatologist early on for treatment options.*

*National Vitiligo Foundation, P.O. Box 6337, Tyler, TX 75711; 903-531-0074.
Web site: http://pegasus.uthct.edu/Vitiligo/index.html

A. **Topical steroids may be useful with limited disease:** The success rate is about 50%.
   1. Adults and those over age 12: *Triamcinolone* 0.1% cream once a day for 4 to 6 months.
   2. Children under age 12: *Fluticasone propionate* cream (15, 30 g) or *desonide* 0.05% cream (15, 30, 60 g) once a day for 4 months.
   3. If repigmentation occurs, continue treating until no further response is noted.
   4. Follow patients every 4 weeks to avoid steroid-induced atrophy of the skin.
B. **Topical or oral psoralens plus ultraviolet light therapy** may also be useful. Refer to a dermatologist for evaluation.
C. **Screen for autoimmune diseases,** especially in children: (e.g., thyroid function, CBC, and fasting blood glucose level).
D. **Specialized makeups** (e.g., Covermark or Dermablend) are available in different shades at most large retail store cosmetic counters and provide excellent cosmetic coverage.
E. **Surgery:** Consider referral for surgery via minigrafting techniques, with or without light (PUVA) therapy, which may offer successful therapy in recalcitrant cases.
F. **Depigmentation therapy:** Consider recommending depigmentation with *hydroquinone* 20% if the vitiligo affects more than 50% of the face or body and is recalcitrant to therapy. Warn patients that this treatment is permanent, with lasting sun sensitivity. Consultation with a dermatologist is suggested.

V. PATIENT EDUCATION
A. Educate patients about sun sensitivity, the need to avoid sun exposure, and the need to use sunscreens when sun exposure is necessary.

B. Educate patients about the potential side effects of potent corticosteroid creams.

C. For more information and patient support, contact the National Vitiligo Foundation.

Postinflammatory Hyperpigmentation and Melasma ICD-9 (709.0)

Splotchy hyperpigmentation can occur as a result of several inflammatory conditions, including acne, eczema, superficial injuries, and sun exposure in combination with the effects of exogenous/endogenous hormones (melasma). Although hyperpigmentation may be disfiguring for many patients, it more often presents difficulties in patients with dark complexions. Treatment with *tretinoin* 0.05% cream nightly to the entire face for 4 to 6 months is effective in many cases. *Hydroquinone* 4% cream applied only to the darker areas once or twice daily may be used separately or in addition.

GERIATRIC DERMATOLOGY

Geriatric dermatology is important for two main reasons. First, the proportion of the population over age 65 continues to increase. Because of this expanding population and environmental changes, conditions such as skin tumors have greatly expanded in prevalence and burden of disease. Premaliganant, malignant, and benign skin tumors occur at a rate of almost 1 in 5 in people older than age 65. Common skin conditions also may be more difficult to diagnose or more resistant to treatment in elderly patients because they may be:

- institutionalized
- malnourished
- taking multiple medications
- dealing with multiple chronic diseases
- more susceptible to medication side effects

For these reasons, it is necessary to be aware of those skin conditions that most commonly affect the elderly and to concentrate on the extensive patient education necessary to successfully treat or prevent such diseases.

Quality of life issues also take on an especially important role in elderly patients. Studies in geriatric dermatology have demonstrated that concern about physical attractiveness extends beyond young adulthood to the over 65 population. Therefore even "benign," non–life-threatening skin problems in elderly patients usually influence their quality of life. Clinicians

BOX 16–1.
Common Geriatric Skin Conditions

Common dermatoses	Dermatophytosis (especially onychomycosis), seborrheic dermatitis, stasis dermatitis, contact dermatitis, malignant skin tumors, and, particularly, xerotic eczema.
Common benign tumors	Seborrheic keratosis, acrochordon, cherry hemangiomas, sebaceous hyperplasia, venous lakes, telangiectasia, epidermal inclusion cysts, milia.
Angular cheilitis	Occurs as maceration at the oral commissures, as a result of loss of alveolar bone and teeth, iron or B complex vitamin deficiency or chronic antibiotic use. *Candida* may be present in the areas. Properly fitting dentures and use of Vytone (combination low-potency steroid and antiyeast agent) or *ketoconazole* cream to the affected area twice daily may be helpful.
Generalized pruritus	Diagnostic workup of pruritus should be thorough (see Chapter 17) if there is no response to therapy after 2 to 3 weeks, because the incidence of underlying systemic disease is higher in the over 65 age group.
Drug eruptions	Elderly patients tend to take more and multiple medications.

should attempt to diagnose and treat physical and potential psychosocial disease manifestations in elderly patients. Such treatment may involve extended contact with a patient's spouse, children, or caretakers.

Skin changes associated with intrinsic aging are thinning of the dermis, more prominent vasculature, and changes in collagen, elastin, and ground substance. Such changes make the skin less stretchable and more lax and result in an increased susceptibility to trauma, with subsequent tearing. Alterations in the dermis and in skin barrier function result in poor wound healing, increased susceptibility to irritant contact dermatitis, and depot of medications in the skin, which are cleared more slowly (e.g., corticosteroids render the skin more prone to atrophy). However, most of the physical features associated with aging (e.g., pigmentary mottling, leather-like appearance, dermal atrophy) actually are the result of sun exposure and not intrinsic to aging.

BOX 16–2.
Dermatolgic Medication Use in the Elderly

1. Use lower-strength corticosteroids because of decreased metabolism, decreased cellular turnover, and increased susceptibility to depot effects, with subsequent skin atrophy.
2. Use sedating antihistamines with caution, and use lower strengths when possible (e.g., *hydroxyzine* 10 mg rather than 25 mg).
3. Use *prednisone* with caution because patients may be hypertensive or susceptible to mild changes in body fluid regulation.

Common skin disorders in geriatric populations and important diagnostic or therapeutic features are summarized in Boxes 16–1 and 16–2. Treatments are discussed under specific diagnoses. For specific resources contact the National Institute on Aging Information Center.*

HIV DISEASE

With millions of people now infected worldwide with the human immunodeficiency retrovirus (HIV) and the acquired immune deficiency syndrome (AIDS), physicians everywhere should familiarize themselves with the signs, symptoms, and treatment of this disease. Skin changes often are the first and definitely the most visible sign that the infection is present, and 80% of patients with HIV disease have skin diseases. Many skin disorders in people infected with HIV are common skin diseases (e.g., condyloma, onychomycosis, psoriasis, scabies, folliculitis, and seborrheic dermatitis) but follow a more fulminant or treatment-resistant course. A few (e.g., oral hairy leukoplakia, eosinophilic folliculitis, chronic herpes infections, treatment-resistant syphilis, or disseminated infections of cryptococcosis, histoplasmosis, or bacillary angiomatosis) are more unique to patients with suppressed immune systems.

The key to skin disorders in HIV disease is to never assume that a new papule is unimportant. Strongly consider performing a biopsy of any unknown lesion. Although a lesion may look like molluscum contagiosum, microscopic view or culture may reveal the presence of cryptococcosis. A chronic ulcer may not be a bacterial infection but rather chronic herpes simplex infection. Intractable pruritus is a common finding in HIV disease.

The earliest clinical manifestation of HIV infection, **acute retroviral syndrome,** is characterized by an acute illness that lasts approximately 8 days. Systemic complaints and findings include fever, sweats, malaise, lethargy, myalgias and arthralgias, pharyngitis, lymphadenopathy, vomiting, headache, and a skin eruption. The

*National Institute on Aging Information Center, P.O. Box 8057, Gaithersburg, MD 20898-8057; 1-800-222-2225.

skin eruption is a blanchable, erythematous macular eruption, which involves primarily the trunk and lasts about 3 or 4 days. The syndrome usually occurs 2 to 6 weeks after infection.

For information about HIV and AIDS, contact the National HIV/AIDS Hotline.*

Bacterial Infections: Staphyloccocal Folliculitis and Bacillary Angiomatosis

Like most infections in patients with HIV disease, **folliculitis** is caused by a common organism but is more fulminant and often treatment-resistant. The folliculitis is usually caused by *Staphylococcus*. Prolonged antibiotic therapy (dicloxacillin) and use of antibacterial soap (e.g., Lever 2000) may be helpful in management. The addition of *rifampin* 300 mg twice a day for 3-10 days may help eradicate the infection or chronic carrier state.

Bacillary epitheloid angiomatosis (Fig. 16–11) is an infection in individuals with HIV disease that is caused by *Bartonella henselae*. Skin lesions typically are multiple red papules or nodules and can occur on the skin, subcutaneously, and on mucous membranes. Clinically, lesions resemble pyogenic granulomas or Kaposi's sarcoma. Diagnosis is most commonly made by light microscopy of skin biopsy specimens. Treat with oral *erythromycin* 250 to 500 mg PO 4 times a day or *doxycycline* 100 mg twice a day until lesions resolve (about 3 to 4 weeks). This disease may be fatal without treatment.

Eosinophilic Pustular Folliculitis

Eosinophilic pustular folliculitis is a pruritic eruption similar in appearance to staphylococcal folliculitis, but biopsy studies reveal eosinophils rather than neutrophils. The cause is unknown. Lesions are distributed on the face, neck, trunk, and extremities. Primary pustules and secondary erythema are common. Diagnosis is based on the presence of a hair piercing the pustule, confirming the follicular location, and a 3-mm punch biopsy, showing the presence of eosinophils in the lesion. Lesions are unresponsive to antibiotic therapy. Bacterial folliculitis will typically respond to antibiotic therapy and neutrophils are present in the pustules.

Symptomatic treatment is indicated for mild to moderate pruritus with oral antihistamines (e.g., *hydroxyzine* 25 to 50 mg PO q6h, *cetrizine* 10 mg PO daily) and topical antipruritic agents. Potent topical corticosteroids, such as *betamethasone dipropionate* 0.05% bid, applied sparingly twice daily may be helpful. Oral *itraconazole* has proven helpful in some cases. Refer the patient to a dermatologist for possible *isotretinoin* or ultraviolet B light therapy if the pruritus is debilitating.

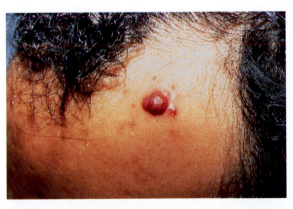

Fig. 16–11
Bacillary angiomatosis. Note erythematous, friable nodule resembling a pyogenic granuloma. (Courtesy Department of Dermatology, University of North Carolina at Chapel Hill.)

Fungal Infections: Dermatophytosis, Candidiasis, Cryptococcosis, and Histoplasmosis

Dermatophyte infections are common in HIV disease and tend to be more dramatic and treatment-resistant. Systemic therapy with *griseofulvin, terbinafine,* or *itraconazole* may be necessary if lesions are widespread or becoming

*National HIV/AIDS Hotline, 1-800-342-AIDS.

secondarily infected. Toenail involvement by itself should not be treated systemically. However, patients often are receiving oral *itraconazole* or *fluconazole* for candidiasis, and this will serve to treat the dermatophyte infection(s). Mucocutaneous candidiasis is common and may be the initial infection suggesting HIV infection. Chronic treatment with oral antiyeast agents is often required. Esophageal involvement may produce dysphagia and anorexia.

Less common fungal infections are caused by deep fungi, such as *Cryptococcus* and *Histoplasma*. Cutaneous involvement signals a systemic infection with the organism. Cryptococcal skin lesions may be dome-shaped, waxy papules and typically are multiple (Fig. 16–12). Cutaneous histoplasmosis skin lesions may be erythematous papules or cellulitis-like, ulcerative, or pustular lesions. Diagnosis sometimes can be confirmed by a touch prep of the base of a punch biopsy (not in formalin, must be fresh tissue) onto a clean glass slide and then staining for the organism. Half of the biopsy specimen should be processed and the pathologist should be alerted to the possible diagnosis. Culture of the other half of the specimen or an additional lesion also should be performed.

Viral Infections: Oral Hairy Leukoplakia, Molluscum Contagiosum, Herpes, and Human Papillomavirus

Oral hairy leukoplakia is a disorder most often seen in immunosuppressed individuals and is caused by the Epstein-Barr virus (EBV). In one series of HIV-infected patients the incidence was 8.4%. EBV may be the first manifestation of HIV infection and is predictive of progessive immunosuppression. Lesions may be asymptomatic or cause burning or other discomfort. Look on the lateral tongue margin for white plaques that do not scrape off (Fig. 16–13).

Diagnosis is based on the lesion's clinical appearance in an immunosuppressed patient. A KOH test must be performed to rule out the presence of *Candida*. However, inasmuch as coinfection is common, treat with oral *fluconazole* for 10 days to rule out or treat coexisting *Candida*. Culture for EBV with Southern blot hybridization.

If symptoms are present, *tretinoin* solution daily for 15 to 20 days may help. Alternative treatments include oral *acyclovir* 800 mg qid or *podophyllin* 25% applied sparingly (let dry for 30 seconds before allowing the tongue back into the mouth).

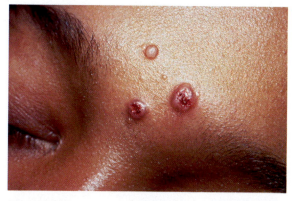

Fig. 16–12
Crusted papules of cutaneous cryptococcosis in an HIV-infected patient. (Courtesy Department of Dermatology, University of North Carolina at Chapel Hill.)

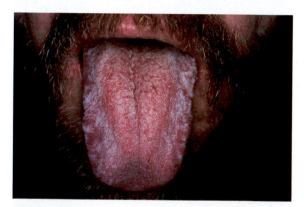

Fig. 16–13
Oral hairy leukoplakia. Note white plaques involving the lateral margins of the tongue. (Courtesy Medical College of Georgia, Division of Dermatology.)

Molluscum contagiosum is a common viral skin infection (see Fig. 18–8). However, multiple lesions that are treatment-resistant may point to T cell immunodeficiency. Treatment does not differ for immunosuppressed individuals. Cutaneous cryptococcosis may mimic molluscum, although it is rare, and a shave biopsy will differentiate the two. For rapid diagnosis, do special stains on fresh tissue. Although treatment does not necessarily vary from that of a nonimmunosuppressed individual, (see p. 245) lesions tend to be more recalcitrant and recurrent.

Herpes simplex viral infections may be signaled as chronic ulcerative lesions of the mouth or groin. Herpes ulcers that are present for more than 1 month in an HIV-positive patient are an AIDS-defining illness. The differential diagnosis includes bacterial infections and possible cytomegalovirus (CMV). Tzanck stain should reveal multinucleated giant cells, and culture will confirm the diagnosis. CMV also is a possible, although less common, viral cause of chronic cutaneous ulcers in immunosuppressed patients. Coinfections can occur; therefore biopsy is indicated in any nonhealing ulcer, particularly perianal ulcers, to identify all possible pathogens. Long-term, high-dose *acyclovir* (400 mg 5 times a day until reepithelialization occurs) therapy may be necessary to control herpes simplex infections. Intravenous *acyclovir* or *foscarnet* may be necessary in resistant or severe cases.

Herpes zoster viral infections have been noted in earlier works to be a hallmark of progression to AIDS. The outbreak in HIV-infected patients tends to be more chronic, with painful hyperkeratotic or ulcerative lesions that resolve with scarring. There may be an increased rate of postherpetic neuralgia. Treatment with high-dose *acyclovir* (800 mg PO 5 times a day, or, more rarely, intravenous) is indicated.

Human papillomavirus infections in HIV-infected patients may have an increased incidence of associated rectal carcinoma. The warts often are treatment-resistant. Therapeutic goals should include treating any visible lesions and monitoring for malignant transformation in resistant lesions. Specific treatments do not differ (See Chapter 15).

Papulosquamous Eruptions: Psoriasis, Scabies, Seborrheic Dermatitis, and Syphilis

Psoriasis in HIV-infected patients tends to be more severe, likely to be associated with arthritis, likely to be in an inverse distribution, and likely to be treatment-resistant. Exfoliative dermatitis as a result of psoriasis may develop. If possible, use *anthralin* therapy (see Chapter 14) rather than widespread topical corticosteroids, because of absorption and subsequent systemic effects. *Methotrexate* is contraindicated because of immunosuppression. Oral broad-spectrum antibiotics may be helpful, and some improvement is often seen after initiation of antiretroviral therapy. Referral for ultraviolet light or retinoid with light therapy may be useful, although there is concern about immunomodulation with light therapies. UVB may be slightly more immunomodulating (in patients with HIV disease) than psoralens with ultraviolet A therapy (PUVA) in recent series of patients followed during and after phototherapy. *Calcipotriene* 0.005% ointment (10, 30, 60 g) twice a day has a role in limited disease.

Scabies can occur as the more fulminant infestation of Norwegian scabies, with numerous mites present in the HIV-infected patient (Fig. 16–14). Crusting plaques on the genitalia or widespread lesions may be present. Typical burrows may be absent, but a scabies prep will demonstrate multiple mites and eggs. Keratolytic agents (salicylic acid 10% to 40% in petrolatum) may be necessary to remove hyperkeratotic lesions. Repeat application of a scabicide (see Chapter 6) weekly until all thickened lesions have resolved. Contacts must also be treated. Patients with scabies and AIDS who were treated with oral *ivermectin* have shown excellent success.*

*Meinking et al: The treatment of scabies with ivermectin, *N Eng J Med* 33:26–30, 1995.

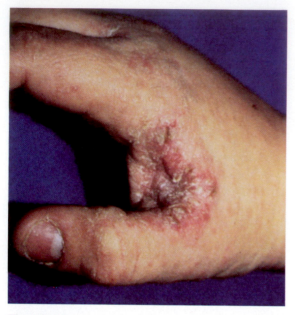

Fig. 16–14
Norwegian scabies. (Courtesy Beverly Sanders, MD.)

Seborrheic dermatitis is common (40% to 50%) in the HIV-infected population and tends to be extensive and treatment-resistant. Use a mild topical corticosteroid, such as *desonide* cream (15, 60 g) twice a day and topical *ketoconazole* 2% (15, 30, 60 g) once a day for the face. Sulfur-based lotions are useful for the face and body; medicated shampoos with mild topical corticosteroids are useful for the scalp.

Syphilis in HIV disease is unique in that the results of serologic studies may not be reliable. Patients may be seronegative on all standard tests, but spirochetes may be found on skin biopsy. Prozone phenomenon may be present if there is an excess of antibody binding to all of the antigen sites. Dilution of serum upon retesting is easily performed by most laboratories; however, no antibody may be present. Recurrences may develop, even after adequate therapy for secondary syphilis. Syphilis may also progress much more rapidly to later stages (e.g., neurosyphilis) within a matter of months.

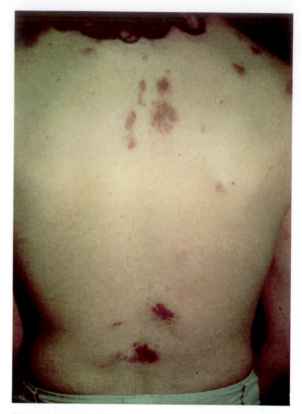

Fig. 16–15
Kaposi's sarcoma. Note multiple violet lesions in a patient with AIDS. (Courtesy Beverly Sanders, MD.)

In HIV-infected patients, when clinical findings suggest that a syphilitic infection is present but serologic tests are not helpful, alternative tests (e.g., biopsy, darkfield examination, and direct fluorescent antibody staining of lesion material) should be used. Some authorities recommend that all HIV patients with syphilis receive an evaluation for neurosyphilis via a lumbar puncture. Close follow-up is essential (e.g., monthly for 3 months, then every 3 months for 1 year).

Xerotic eczema can manifest as severe pruritus with diffuse scaling. The disorder is noted in as many as 5% of the HIV-infected population. Treatment often consists of emollients, mild soaps, antihistamines, and ultraviolet B therapy. Scabies and drug-related pruritus should be ruled out.

Malignancies: Kaposi's Sarcoma ICD-9 (176.0)

Kaposi's sarcoma was initially described in elderly men of eastern European Jewish ancestry. In 1981 the sudden epidemic outbreak of disseminated Kaposi's sarcoma helped characterize and identify AIDS. The epidemiology of disseminated Kaposi's sarcoma has changed such that the incidence has increased, it is found primarily in homosexual HIV-infected patients, and it follows a more aggressive course. Human herpes virus 8 has been identified in Kaposi's sarcoma lesions of AIDS and non-AIDS patients.

Lesions may be flat, macular, red patches or indurated plaques. Papules may develop into nodules and then tumors (Fig. 16–15). Any site may be involved, including the oral mucosa. The diagnosis is made by biopsy of suspicious lesions. The pathologist should be familiar with identifying such lesions. The differential diagnosis includes bacillary angiomatosis. For treatment updates, contact the following web site: http://cancer.med.upenn.edu/disease/kaposi/

HOMELESS

The increasing number of homeless people and their myriad medical, dental, mental, and social problems make the recognition, treatment, and prevention of illness in this diverse population an important component of the primary care clinician's knowledge base. Clinicians may see and treat homeless people in special clinics, emergency rooms, private offices, or hospitals.

Skin disorders comprise the greatest number of diseases seen in the homeless and are the source of considerable disability. Up to one fourth of homeless adults and one third of homeless children will have associated skin disease. Despite the difficulties of working with this population, clinicians can significantly improve the quality of daily life for a homeless person by the prompt recognition and appropriate treatment of a very few common dermatologic conditions. It is most important that the clinician appropriately identify a patient as truly homeless, because the ramifications for successful treatment and prevention of disease are then quite different. A small improvement in a debilitating skin disorder may be a large success when caring for a homeless person.

The most common skin disorders affecting homeless people are shown in Box 16–3. Each of these disorders is discussed in detail elsewhere in this text, but several important points are relevant to the homeless population. For instance, homeless people are particularly susceptible to developing skin disorders because of predisposing environmental factors (Box 16–4). Although diagnosis often is not difficult, effective treatment is challenging because:

- Homeless people have difficulty accessing appropriate medications.
- They may be confused about instructions or forget to take the medication.

BOX 16–3.
Common Skin Disorders Found in Homeless Patients

Infestations (scabies and lice)
Infections (impetigo, cellulitis, abscesses)
Foot problems (fungal infections, ulcers)
Venous stasis ulcers
Wound lacerations
Frost bite
Eczema
Warts

BOX 16–4.
Environmental Factors Predisposing to Skin Disorders in Homeless Populations

Sleeping outside
Sharing bedding, clothes, and brushes
Picking up discarded clothes
Poor sanitation
Prolonged standing or walking
Sleeping in a seated position or on hard surfaces
Frequent lacerations and contusions

- They may lose their medicine or it may be stolen.
- They frequently fail to have appropriate follow-up.
- Treating contacts is often difficult, so reinfestation is common.
- They may be illiterate or have other language and cultural barriers.
- Mental health problems may prevent compliance with therapy.
- Drug abuse may confound the treatment plan.

Following simple medication dispensing guidelines (Box 16–5) may help to improve compliance with therapy.

Infestations

Infestations, particularly of scabies and pediculosis (lice), are frequent causes of disease in homeless people. Scabies may present with complications resulting from secondary infections, including abscesses, pyogenic pneumonia, septicemia, or secondary impetigo with glomerulonephritis. Pediculosis corporis, or infestation by the body louse (similar in appearance to the head louse), is found with increased frequency in homeless men, on their chest, abdomen, and upper back. Pediculosis corporis is characterized by severe and generalized pruritus, especially on the trunk. Lice and their eggs (nits) are demonstrable in clothing seams, which are in contact with the body surface. Lice bite marks are usually obscured by the excoriations, and the eruption often looks eczematous (Fig. 16–16).

BOX 16–5.

Medication Guidelines for Homeless People

Write simple, detailed instructions, including the patient's name, on how to take medications.
Give samples, if available.
Place all medications in waterproof containers.
Avoid giving any medications with an alcohol base.
Avoid giving refills on potentially toxic medications.
Consider using antibiotics prophylactically in wound infections.

The appropriate treatment for most infestations involves choosing the appropriate medication and following medication dispensing guidelines (Box 16–5). Infested clothing worn over the preceding 3 days must be laundered with hot water and dried in a hot dryer (20 minutes at least) and also may be treated with a pediculocide spray. Alternatively, the old clothes may be disposed of and new clothes obtained. Treat any secondary infections. Finally, attempt to alleviate predisposing environmental conditions (e.g., overcrowded shelters, poor sanitary conditions) known to increase infestations and notify shelter personnel in any dwelling in which the patient may be staying about the infestation so that potential contacts also can be treated.

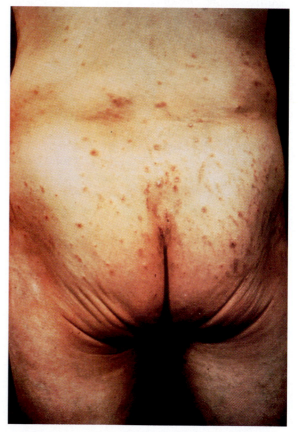

Fig. 16–16
Pediculosis corporis. (Courtesy Department of Dermatology, University of North Carolina at Chapel Hill.)

Ulcers and Foot Problems

Venous stasis ulcers and generalized foot problems frequently are seen in homeless populations because of the tendency of homeless people to spend prolonged time on their feet, including walking, often without proper sanitary services or sufficient clothing to maintain healthy feet. Exposure to cold and water and repeated trauma are other predisposing factors. *Always examine the feet of homeless patients.* Look for signs of swelling, rashes, blisters, toe and ankle ulcers, fungal infection, eczema, or phlebitis. Examine the shoes for rocks or nails coming through the sole.

Effective treatment relies on preventing more serious disorders by paying attention to and treating the early signs of venous insufficiency (e.g., ankle swelling, dermatitis eczema). While awake, patients should wear stockings if possible. Stockings should be removed when asleep, and patients should sleep with their legs elevated. Assess the condition of the patient's shoes and if needed, assist them in obtaining new shoes.

For early lesions, instruct patients to use simple hygiene measures, such as washing daily with soap and water, followed by a dressing change. Topical antibiotic therapies should be applied twice daily. Consider using an Unna's boot for more serious venous stasis ulcers and arrange for follow-up in 1 week. *For more advanced lesions,* consider, in addition to the above treatment, wound debridement, bed rest, and systemic antibiotics. Consider the possibility of underlying systemic disease (e.g., diabetes, deep venous thrombosis). In diabetic homeless patients with foot lesions, refer immediately to a hospital setting for appropriate treatment to prevent extremity loss.

Wounds

Wound infections in homeless patients are important because of the frequency with which they occur, combined with the increased tendency for them to become secondarily infected as a result of poor sanitation. These wounds may come from lacerations, abrasions, contusions, or infected bug bites or because of secondary infection from infestations such as scabies or lice. A homeless patient may receive sutures to repair a laceration and then lack resources to have appropriate follow-up for suture removal or to keep the lesion clean.

Appropriate treatment once again emphasizes good preventive measures, patient education, and compliance with therapy. Provide instructions for proper medication use (Box 16–5). Consider early use of topical and systemic antibiotics, for treatment or prophylactically, to prevent more serious infections. Lesions should be cleaned frequently with soap and water, and special arrangements may need to be made with a shelter. Tetanus toxoid and/or immune globulin should be given in most cases, because documentation or memory of immunization usually is poor. Close follow-up within 2 to 3 days usually is indicated.

DERMATOSES OF PREGNANCY

Chloasma/Melasma ICD-9 (709.0)

Chloasma/melasma is a common disorder of hyperpigmentation in pregnancy found in 70% of pregnant women and in women taking oral contraceptives (although it may occur in the absence of both). It is thought to be the result of increased levels of a melanocyte-stimulating hormone (estrogen or possibly progesterone) and is exacerbated by sun exposure. Gestational melasma usually regresses, whereas that related to oral contraceptives or *de novo* tends to be more persistent.

I. CLASSIC DESCRIPTION
Distribution: Face
Primary: Macules

Secondary: Hyperpigmentation that is blotchy and irregular

II. DIAGNOSIS

Diagnosis is based on clinical appearance (Fig. 16–17).

III. DIFFERENTIAL DIAGNOSIS

Postinflammatory hyperpigmentation: A history of inflammatory lesions and no increased prominence with sun exposure are suggestive of postinflammatory hyperpigmentation.

IV. TREATMENT

A. **No treatment is advised during pregnancy,** other than avoiding sun exposure.

B. **Bleaching agents for nonpregnant patients:**

1. *Hydroquinone* 2% (Solaquin) available OTC or 4% cream or gel (with sunblock: Solaquin Forte or Eldopaque Forte; without sunblock: Eldoquin Forte or Melanex) available by prescription.
   a. Apply to a test area for two or three applications before using broadly on involved areas, because of potential allergic or irritant reactions.
   b. Apply once or twice daily for 2 to 4 months.
   c. Prolonged use of OTC preparations has been associated with cutaneous ochronosis.

2. *Tretinoin* 0.05% cream at bedtime. Test on small areas for two or three applications; warn patients that it also may cause irritation. Use for at least 4 to 6 months before judging effectiveness.

3. Daily use of broad-spectrum sun protection (e.g., sunblock for babies spf 30 by Johnson and Johnson) is crucial during and after therapy to prevent new lesions and to maintain improvement.

V. PATIENT EDUCATION

A. Emphasize the importance of daily sunscreen use and sun protection, regardless if sun exposure is intended.

B. Educate about the need to continue sun protection, even after improvement has been achieved with topical medications.

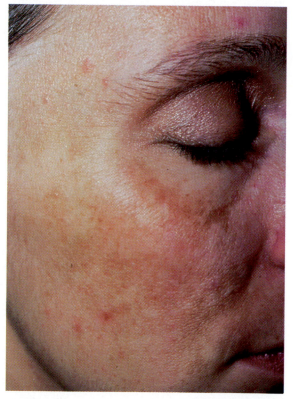

Fig. 16–17
Chloasma/melasma. Note mottled hyperpigmentation. (Courtesy Department of Dermatology, University of North Carolina at Chapel Hill.)

Herpes Gestationis ICD-9 (646.8)

Herpes gestationis is a very rare, intensely pruritic, recurrent, autoimmune bullous disease that can occur at any time during pregnancy, immediately postpartum, or with the use of oral contraceptives postpartum. The relationship to pregnancy and oral contraceptive use also points to a hormonal influence on the disease. Herpes is a misnomer, because the disease is not caused by the herpes virus, although some patients have associated systemic complaints of malaise, fever, nausea, and headache as a prodrome. The typical course is one of exacerbations and remissions during pregnancy, and the disease usually resolves 3 months after delivery. Recurrences in subsequent pregnancies may occur earlier and be more severe.

I. CLASSIC DESCRIPTION (Fig. 16–18)

Distribution: Periumbilically initially, then spreading to the rest of the trunk; may involve extremities, even palms and soles; typically spares mucous membranes

Primary: Papules, vesicles, plaques, bullae

Secondary: Erythema, edema, excoriation Circinate, or ring-shaped, configurations are classic.

II. DIAGNOSIS

Diagnosis is based on the appearance of intensely pruritic lesions that start in the periumbilical region during pregnancy. True vesicles may not be seen in many cases. A 3- to 4-mm punch biopsy of perilesional skin will reveal linear deposits of C3, with or without IgG, by direct immunofluorescence.

III. DIFFERENTIAL DIAGNOSIS

A. Pruritic urticarial papules and plaques of pregnancy: Onset is usually confined to the third trimester. Vesicles and bullae are absent, lesions tend to originate in striae rather than periumbilically, there is no exacerbation postpartum or with oral contraceptives, and immunoflourescence stains are negative.

B. Scabies: Look for a history of other family member involvement. Lesions should include excoriated papules or pustules between the finger webs or on the wrists, groin, or feet.

C. Bullous pemphigoid: Bullous pemphigoid is a disease of older adults and has a predilection for flexural areas.

D. Erythema multiforme: Targetlike lesions do not necessarily involve the trunk and may be associated with a recent herpes simplex outbreak. Lesions typically are not intensely pruritic and can be differentiated histologically.

E. Bullous drug eruption: A history of recent drug exposure coinciding with the onset of an eruption should be present.

F. Pemphigus vulgaris: Pemphigus vulgaris is typically a disease of older adults, frequently with mucous membrane involvement.

IV. TREATMENT

A. Mild cases:
1. Topical corticosteroids: *Triamcinolone acetonide* 0.1% in sufficient quantity (½ to 1 lb) to cover the involved areas 2 or 3 times a day.
2. Antihistamines: *Diphenhydramine* (25 to 50 mg) or *hydroxyzine hydrochloride* (10 to 50 mg) 4 times daily, as necessary.

B. Severe cases: *Prednisone* 40 mg/day in divided doses. Taper after delivery.

C. Consultation with a dermatologist and obstetrician is recommended because there may be an increased risk of prematurity associated with the disease and, occasionally, newborn infants may have transient lesions similar to those of affected mothers.

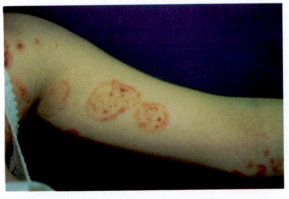

Fig. 16–18
Herpes gestationis with erythematous, circinate papules and vesicles. (Courtesy Beverly Sanders, MD.)

Pruritic Urticarial Papules and Plaques of Pregnancy ICD-9 (708.9)

Pruritic urticarial papules and plaques of pregnancy (PUPPP) is a pruritic disorder of unknown cause that occurs most commonly during the third trimester in primigravidas. PUPPP is not likely to recur with subsequent pregnancies and has no association with fetal morbidity. Resolution of symptoms occurs with delivery.

I. CLASSIC DESCRIPTION

Distribution: Begins in striae, then generalizes to rest of trunk and proximal extremities

Primary: Papules, plaques

Secondary: Erythema

Individual lesions may have a pale halo with erythema that blanches easily with pressure (Fig. 16–19 *A, B*).

II. DIAGNOSIS

The diagnosis is clinical. However, if herpes gestationis is a possible diagnosis, biopsy with direct immunofluorescence may be necessary to differentiate the two diseases.

III. DIFFERENTIAL DIAGNOSIS

A. Drug eruption: Usually, few medications are taken in pregnancy, so a relationship to recent medication use probably will be present.

B. Herpes gestationis: Herpes gestationis is quite rare. Lesions typically begin in the periumbilical region, are vesiculobullous, have excoriations, and were present in previous pregnancies or occurred earlier in the pregnancy. Biopsy with direct immunoflourescence will differentiate in difficult cases.

C. Urticaria: Individual lesions in urticaria last less than 24 hours and usually are not particularly localized periumbilically. Mucous membranes can be involved.

D. Viral exanthem: Systemic complaints may be present, with a recent history of viral symptoms. The rash tends to be more morbilliform.

E. Cholestasis of pregnancy: Look for intense, generalized pruritus, without associated lesions. Patients may have elevated bilirubin levels and develop jaundice.

F. Scabies: Look for the typical distribution and involvement of other family members.

G. Contact dermatitis: Look for sharply demarcated, even linear lesions that may vesiculate. History should reveal possible sources (e.g., poison ivy, perfumes).

IV. TREATMENT

Treatment is centered around relief of pruritus; cure usually comes only with delivery.

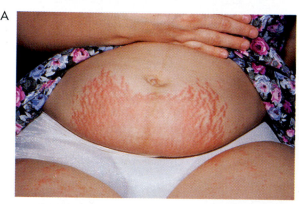

Fig. 16–19
A, Pruritic urticarial papules and **B,** plaques of pregnancy. Note involvement of striae, with extension onto proximal thighs. (Courtesy Department of Dermatology, University of North Carolina at Chapel Hill.)

A. Topical corticosteroid creams:
   1. *Triamcinolone acetonide* 0.1% cream or *hydrocortisone* 1% cream 2 or 3 times a day.
   2. Use the least-potent agent that will control the disease.
   3. Prescribe sufficient quantity (½ to 1 pound).

B. Oral corticosteroids: Prednisone
   1. Indicated only in rare, severe cases unresponsive to topical corticosteroids.
   2. Use tapering dosages (e.g., 40 mg for 2 days, then decrease by 5 mg every 1 or 2 days); consider alternate-day dosing if several weeks of treatment are necessary.

   3. Consultation with a dermatologist or obstetrician is recommended.

C. Antihistamines: *Diphenhydramine* (25 to 50 mg) or *hydroxyzine hydrochloride* (10 to 50 mg) 3 or 4 times a day, as necessary.

V. PATIENT EDUCATION
  A. Reassure patients that the rash and itching will resolve with delivery.
  B. Educate patients that warmth only makes itching worse (e.g., avoid hot showers).
  C. Emphasize taking cool baths with baking soda or Aveeno.

SUGGESTED READING

Berman B, Bieley HC: Adjunct therapies to surgical management of keloids, *Dermatol Surg* 22:126–130, 1996.

Buchness MR: Treatment of skin diseases in HIV-infected patients, *Dermatol Clin* 13:231–238, 1995.

Cohen PR, Scher RK: Geriatric nail disorders: diagnosis and treatment, *J Am Acad Dermatol* 26:521–531, 1992.

Coopman SA et al: Cutaneous disease and drug reactions in HIV infection, *N Engl J Med* 328:1670–1674, 1993.

Elmets CA: Management of common superficial fungal infections in patients with AIDS, *J Am Acad Dermatol* 31:S60–63, 1994.

Garden JM, Bakus AD, Paller AS: Treatment of cutaneous hemangiomas by the flashlamp-pumped pulsed dye laser: prospective analysis, *J Pediatr* 120:555–560, 1992.

Gastel B: Working with your older patient: a clinician's handbook, *J Geriatr Dermatol* 4:103–118, 1996.

Glenn MJ, Bennett RG, Kelly AP: Acne keloidalis nuchae: treatment with excision and second intention healing, *J Am Acad Dermatol* 33:243–246, 1995.

Gold MH: Topical silicone gel sheeting in the treatment of hypertrophic scars and keloids, *Dermatol Surg* 19: 912–916, 1993.

Grimes PE: Melasma, *Arch Dermatol* 131:1453–1457, 1995.

Montagna W, Prota G, Kenney JA Jr: *Black skin,* San Diego, 1993, Academic Press.

Moy JA, Sanches MR: The cutaneous manifestations of violence and poverty, *Arch Dermatol* 128:829–839, 1992.

Powell FC, Daniel Su WP, Perry HC: Pyoderma grangrenosum: classification and management, *J Am Acad Dermatol* 34:395–409, 1996.

Nemeth AJ: Keloids and hypertrophic scars, *J Dermatol Surg Oncol* 19:738–746, 1993.

Sahn EE: Vesiculopustular diseases of neonates and infants, *Curr Opin Pediatr* 6:442–446, 1994.

Schwartz R: Kaposi's sarcoma: advances and perspectives, *J Am Acad Dermatol* 34:804–814, 1996.

Shornick JK, Black MM: Fetal risks in herpes gestationis, *J Am Acad Dermatol* 29:545–549, 1993.

Usantine R: Skin diseases of the homeless. In Wood D, ed: *Delivering health care to homeless persons: the diagnosis and management of medical and mental health conditions,* New York, 1992, Springer.

CHAPTER 17

Urticaria

URTICARIA ICD-9 (708.9; ALLERGIC 708.0; IDIOPATHIC 708.1; CAUSED BY COLD AND HEAT 708.2; DERMATOGRAPHIA 708.3; CHOLINERGIC 708.5; CHRONIC 708.8)

The term *urticaria* is derived from the Latin word *uro*, meaning *to burn*, and the nettle *Urtica*, the leaves of which produce a stinging sensation when touching the skin. Urticaria is a common condition characterized by pruritic transient hives or wheals as a result of vasodilation and subsequent fluid leakage into the dermis (Fig. 17–1). Along with intense itching, the often recurrent nature and frequently unknown cause of the disease make urticaria a very debilitating skin condition for millions of people every year.

Urticaria can occur as a result of circulating antigens (e.g., drugs, inhalants) or, rarely, immune complexes that result in release of histamine or alterations in the arachidonic pathway (e.g., nonsteroidal antiinflammatory drugs [NSAIDs]). Other causes include physical or environmental exposure, such as in cold urticaria, which occurs on exposure to rewarming, or in pressure urticaria, which occurs 3 to 6 hours after sustained pressure to a body part. Lesions last less than 24 hours and can occur in virtually any distribution.

The underlying cause is identifiable in fewer than 25% to 50% of cases. In some people, stress may precipitate urticaria. However, regardless of the underlying cause, stress decreases the patient's tolerance of pruritus and its unpredictable nature. Twenty percent of the population will

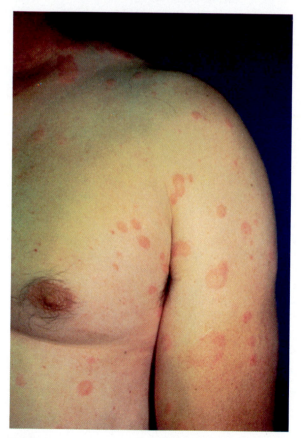

Fig. 17–1
Multiple erythematous wheals of urticaria. (Courtesy Department of Dermatology, University of North Carolina at Chapel Hill.)

228

have urticaria at one time or another in their lifetime.

Acute urticaria is defined as lesions that are present for less than 6 weeks and *chronic urticaria* as those lasting longer. *Angioedema* describes involvement of deeper tissues, with predilection for those involving the mucous membranes, including the larynx and gastrointestinal tract (see Fig. 9–4). Extensive generalized urticaria may be life-threatening, with involvement of major organ systems, including cardiovascular collapse.

I. CLASSIC DESCRIPTION

Distribution: Generalized; lesions change in size and shape; individual lesions last less than 24 hours; can be oval, arciform, annular, and, as they coalesce, polycyclic or even serpiginous

Primary: Wheal

Secondary: Erythema, edema

Angioedema lesions may not be erythematous because of their deeper location.

II. DIAGNOSIS

Diagnosis usually is not difficult, but identifying a specific precipitating agent is often time-consuming and it may be impossible to pinpoint the agent with certainty. The most important consideration is to take a careful and meticulous history. This history should include questions concerning time of onset, medications, environmental changes, foods, and chronic and acute illnesses (Table 17–1 and Box 17–1). The drug history should include drugs the patient may have taken for some time, because the offending drug does not have to be a new drug. For instance, a patient taking ibuprofen or hydrochlorothiazide can become sensitized even after prolonged use of the medication. The physical examination should include a search for active sources of infection or for underlying systemic diseases.

III. DIFFERENTIAL DIAGNOSIS

A. Erythema multiforme: Erythema multiforme has central clearing and lesions that are targetlike; individual lesions last longer than 24 hours. It is typically not pruritic.

B. Insect bites: Lesions usually have a central punctum and excoriations; lesions last longer than 24 hours.

C. Dermatographism: Wheals only occur *after* the skin has been scratched.

TABLE 17–1.

Urticaria: Common Causes and Findings

Etiology	Common Examples
Medications[1]	Antibiotics, aspirin, NSAIDs, narcotics, radiocontrast dyes
Foods[1,2]	Chocolate, shellfish, nuts, berries, spices
Stings[1,2]	Bees, wasps
Inhalants[1,2]	Animal dander, pollen
Physical[3]	Pressure, cold, heat, exercise, sun exposure, dermatographism
Infections[4]	Viral (e.g., hepatitis B, respiratory syncytial virus, etc.), chronic sinus or dental conditions, streptococcus, parasites
Systemic[4]	Thyroid, autoimmune, cancer, blood product reaction
Contact[5]	Chemicals, perfumes, dyes, soaps, lotions, latex gloves

1. May find increased blood eosinophilia.
2. Symptoms usually appear within 2 hours of exposure.
3. Symptoms occur after environmental exposure.
4. Look for physical or laboratory findings consistent with the underlying disease.
5. Symptoms appear within minutes of exposure.

BOX 17–1.

Urticaria Patient History Recording Form*

Date_____Pt. name_____Chart #_____

I. General features:
  A. Date of onset of hives_____
  B. Frequency of attacks (daily, weekly)_____
  C. Time of day when symptoms most severe_____

II. Medications:
  A. List all medications, both prescription and over-the-counter, taken by mouth or put on the skin, in the eyes, and so on, up to 1 month preceding onset of symptoms. List the dates these were taken.

  _____
  _____
  _____

  B. List any recent vaccines or diagnostic tests (e.g., x-ray with contrast media).

  _____

III. Infections:
  A. List any recent (1 month before symptoms) infections (e.g., sore throat; sinus infection; yeast infection; fungal infection of skin, hair, or nails; colds; flu; mononucleosis; tooth abscess; urinary tract infection); include dates.

  _____
  _____

IV. Systemic complaints:
  A. Do you ever have swelling of the lips or tongue, nausea, adominal pain, or difficulty in breathing, especially associated with hives?_____
  B. Do you have any other symptoms (e.g., joint pain, muscle ache, fever, or pain in the skin lesions?

  _____
  C. Do any of the hives last longer than 24 hours?_____
  D. Do any of the hives leave a stain on your skin?_____
  E. Do you have a history of lupus erythematosus, vasculitis, serum sickness, thyroid disease, or cryoglobulinemia?

  _____
  F. Are you pregnant?_____

V. Physical urticaria:
  Do the hives appear related to any of the following?
  Cold_____Heat_____Bathing_____Physical pressure_____
  Exercise_____Sunlight_____Rubbing or scratching_____Stress_____
  Vibration_____Other (e.g., animals, soaps)_____

VI. Allergies:
  List any known allergies (e.g., food, medications, insect bites, other).

  _____

VII. Occupational/recreational:
  A. Do hives appear to occur in relation to any of the following?
    1. Any specific location (indoors/outdoors, work/home)?_____
    2. During work week or weekends predominantly?_____
    3. Do they improve while you are away on vacation?_____
    4. Are they related to any recreational activities?_____

*Modified from Gross AS, LaTour DL, King LE Jr: Chronic urticaria: a model questionnaire for patient screening, *Cutis* 46:421–424, 1990.

D. Angioedema: Deeper, subcutaneous tissue is involved, including the eyelids, tongue, lips, larynx, and gastrointestinal tract, sometimes with nausea and abdominal pain. Angioedema may be life-threatening. A hereditary form exists in which attacks are precipitated by minor trauma (e.g., dental work).

E. Urticarial vasculitis: Wheals last longer than 24 hours and leave purpuric staining on the skin; may be associated with systemic vasculitis.

F. Contact dermatitis: Wheals may be the initial lesion with contact dermatitis, but they will last longer than 24 hours, often evolving into vesicles.

G. Mastocytosis/urticaria pigmentosa: Look for collections of mast cells in the dermis that are typically red/brown and urticate after rubbing or stroking. Systemic manifestations may occur.

IV. TREATMENT

A. Discontinue precipitating agents.

1. Stop using any drug suspected of causing urticaria. Although the etiologic agent is most typically a new one, long-standing medications may also be the cause.

2. Avoid any suspect foods or drinks.
3. Avoid aspirin and other NSAIDs.
4. Avoid alcohol, excessive heat, and exertion.

B. Acute urticaria: Identify etiologic agent if possible and keep the patient comfortable with antihistamines.

1. H_1 blockers: See Table 17–2.
2. H_2 blockers may be useful in recalcitrant cases, in addition to H_1 blockers: *cimetidine* 300 mg qid, *ranitidine* 150 mg bid, *famotidine* 20 mg once a day, or *nizatidine* 150 mg bid.
3. *Prednisone:*
   a. Useful in cases of acute urticaria that are unresponsive to antihistamines.

TABLE 17–2.

Antihistamines for Urticaria

Agent	Brand Name	Adult Dose	Pediatric Dose
Nonsedating H₁ blockers: Preferred[1]			
Astemizole[2]	Hismanal	10 mg qd	Not available
Cetrizine[3]	Zyrtec	10 mg qd	5 mg/5 ml 5-10 ml qd (6-11 y/o)
Loratidine	Claritin	10 mg qd	10 mg/10 ml 10 ml qd (6-11 y/o)
Terfenadine[2]	Seldane	60 mg bid	Not available
Sedating H₁ blockers: Alternative[4]			
Hydroxyzine	Atarax	25-50 mg qid	10 mg/5 ml 50 mg/d divided q6h (<6 y/o) 50-100 mg/d in divided q6h (6-11 y/o)
Chlorpheniramine (OTC)[5]	Chlor-Trimeton	4 mg qid	2 mg/5 ml 1.0 mg q6h (2-6 y/o) 2.0-3.0 mg q6h (6-11 y/o)
Diphenhydramine (OTC)	Benadryl	25-50 mg qid	12.5 mg/5 ml 5 mg/kg/d divided q6h (<6 y/o) 12.5-25 mg q4-6h (6-11 y/o)
Cyproheptadine	Periactin	4-8 mg qid	2 mg/5 ml 0.25 mg/kg/d divided q8h (2-11 y/o)
Clemastine fumarate (OTC)	Tavist	1.34-2.68 mg tid	0.5 mg/5 ml 10-15 ml bid (6-11 y/o)

1. Nonsedating antihistamines are considerably more expensive than sedating antihistamines.
2. Be aware of possible drug interactions with *erythromycin, ketoconazole terfenadine, cyclosporine, astemizole, cisapride,* and *alprazolam.*
3. Ten to 50% may initially find this drug to be mildly sedating, but tolerance develops rapidly.
4. A single nightly dose may be effective in some patients, particularly if sleep disturbances are prominent.
5. Least expensive OTC-nonprescription-agent.

TABLE 17–3.

Chronic Urticaria: Screening Tests

General	Symptom-Directed
CBC with differential	Thyroid tests
Sedimentation rate	Complement levels
Urinalysis	Antinuclear antibodies
Chemistry profile	Cryoglobulins
Liver profile	Stool for ova and parasites
	Dental or sinus radiographs
	Chest radiograph
	Hepatitis profile

    b. 0.5 to 1.0 mg/kg/day, tapered over 10 to 15 days.

    c. Oral corticosteroids are not indicated in the control of chronic urticaria.

C. Acute anaphylaxis: 1:1000 *epinephrine* 0.3 to 1.0 ml SC or IM (see Chapter 9).

D. Chronic urticaria:

1. A general screen is indicated for underlying abnormalities, reserving more specialized tests as symptoms indicate (Table 17–3).

2. Use antihistamines as described above for symptom relief.

3. For refractory chronic urticaria, consider *doxepin* 10 to 100 mg as a single dose at bedtime.

4. Consider an elimination diet. In patients with aspirin sensitivity, use a tartrazine-free diet. Be suspicious of a particular food that produces symptoms within 2 hours of ingestion.

E. Biopsy: If the lesions last longer than 24 hours and leave a purpuric stain, obtain a biopsy specimen to rule out vasculitis.

F. Referral: Allergy testing may be helpful in chronic urticaria that is unresponsive to conventional treatment. If control is difficult, consider referral to a dermatologist or an allergist.

V. PATIENT EDUCATION

(See patient education handout in Appendix W.)

A. Educate patients about possible etiologic agents (e.g., drugs, infections, foods) and their avoidance.

B. Consider asking the patient to keep a log of all foods and drugs, including eyedrops, chewing gum, and nonprescription medications. Attempt to correlate this log with outbreaks.

C. Educate the patient about the symptoms of anaphylaxis.

D. Emphasize symptom control with round-the-clock (vs. prn) antihistamine use.

E. Remind patients of the sedating effects of some antihistamines.

F. Provide emotional support for what can and often is a very debilitating condition. *Follow-up phone calls and appointments are important.*

G. Inform patients that they should tell their provider which treatments work best and which are ineffective. Because there are many agents, often it is a matter of trial and error before the best treatment(s) for a patient is found.

H. Information for patients may be obtained on the World Wide Web.*

SUGGESTED READING

Cooper KC: Urticaria and angioedema: diagnosis and evaluation, *J Am Acad Dermatol* 25:166–175, 1991.

Mahmood T: Urticaria, *Am Fam Physician* 51:811–816, 1995.

Ormerod AD: Urticaria: recognition, causes, and treatment, *Drugs* 48:717–730, 1994.

*http://www.derm-infonet.com/urticaria.html

CHAPTER 18

Viral Diseases

ERYTHEMA INFECTIOSUM ICD-9 (057.0)

Erythema infectiosum, also known as *slapped-cheek disease* or *fifth disease*, is caused by parvovirus B19. The virus is thought to be spread by respiratory secretions and most commonly occurs in children age 5 to 15 during late winter and early spring. The disease is characterized by a prodromal illness with mild fever, sore throat, and malaise that precedes the onset of erythema of the cheeks by 1 to 4 days (Fig. 18–1). This is followed by the diffuse reticulate pattern of erythema on the trunk and extremities. Recurrences for several weeks may occur following changes in temperature, exposure to sunlight, or emotional upset.

A symmetric peripheral polyarthropathy occasionally occurs, usually in adults. In pregnant women there is a possible association with spontaneous abortion and stillbirth. The parvovirus infection also has been implicated in transient aplastic crises in patients with hemolytic anemias and with chronic anemias in immunosuppressed patients.

I. CLASSIC DESCRIPTION
Distribution: Bilateral cheeks, followed by truncal and extremity involvement
Primary: Macules, papules, plaques
Secondary: Erythema
Pruritus may be a feature of the eruption.

II. DIAGNOSIS
The diagnosis usually is made clinically in a patient with a recent prodromal illness, followed by the appearance of diffuse erythematous plaques on both cheeks and the reticulate, blanchable truncal or extremity erythema. The IgM antibody assay is the most sensitive test for detecting recent infection and is positive in 90% of the cases by 3 days after the onset of symptoms. IgG is present by day 7 and persists for years, although it may not be detectable in patients with chronic B19 infection.

III. DIFFERENTIAL DIAGNOSIS
(Table 18–1)
A. **Erysipelas:** Patients with erysipelas are toxic, with severe fever; involvement is unilateral.
B. **Rubella:** The eruptions and fever are similar to those of erythema infectiosum, and the rash also begins on the face but is not confined to the cheeks. Truncal and extremity eruption of rubella is not lacelike, and the rash fades in 1 to 2 days in the order it occurred, followed by fine desquamation.
C. **Roseola (exanthem subitum):** The eruption of roseola occurs as the fever

subsides, initially on the neck and trunk, then the arms, face, and legs, rather than beginning on the cheeks.

IV. TREATMENT AND PATIENT EDUCATION

A. **Reassure worried parents** that the child's illness is benign.

B. **No treatment is necessary,** except control of pruritus, if present.

C. **Pruritus may be controlled with antihistamines,** such as *hydroxyzine hydrochloride* and topical agents containing *menthol, phenol,* or *pramoxine* (e.g., Sarna, Prax) (OTC) or by prescription (Cetaphil) with 0.5% *menthol* and/or 0.5% *phenol.*

D. **Attempt to prevent infections in high-risk groups** (e.g., patients with hemolytic anemia, pregnant women, immunodeficient patients) by preventing contact with known carriers. The greatest risk, however, occurs before symptoms are present. When the rash appears, the condition probably is no longer infectious.

A

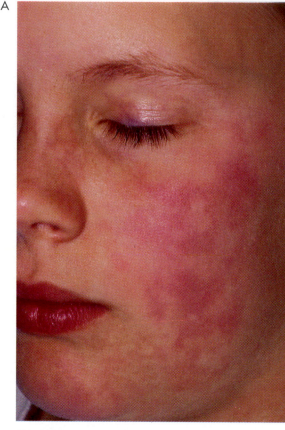

B

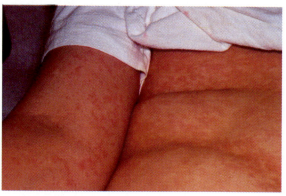

Fig. 18–1
Erythema infectiosum. **A,** Note diffuse erythema and characteristic distribution on cheeks. **B,** Note reticular and lacelike erythema of extremities. (Courtesy Department of Dermatology, University of North Carolina at Chapel Hill.)

TABLE 18–1.

Differential Diagnosis of Childhood Exanthems

Disease	Typical age	Characteristics
Erythema infectiosum (fifth disease)	5–15years	Usually late winter and early spring; prodromal illness with mild fever, sore throat, and malaise that precedes onset of erythema of cheeks by 1–4 days, followed by diffuse reticulate erythema on the trunk and extremities.
Kawasaki syndrome (mucocutaneous lymph node syndrome)	Children younger than age 5 years	Characterized by 5 or more days of fever that is poorly responsive to antipyretics; skin findings involve red lips and tongue and a generalized exanthem that may be discrete, morbilliform, scarlatiniform, or even urticarial. Generalized macules and papules may coalesce into plaques, with erythema and desquamation of the hands, feet, and perineal region occurring 10–14 days after disease onset.
Measles (rubeola)	Children and young adults	Prodrome is characterized by the "three C's": cough, coryza, and conjunctivitis. The fever is high for 1–2 days, returns to normal for 1 day, and then becomes elevated with the onset of erythematous macules, first on the upper neck, then the face, and finally to the upper extremities and trunk. A petechial eruption may appear on the soft palate before the rash, followed 1–2 days later by *Koplik's spots,* blue-white macules seen on the buccal mucosa adjacent to the second molars (Fig. 18–7)
Roseola (exanthema subitum)	6 months to 3 years	Abrupt onset of fever, with few other symptoms; persists for 3 to 5 days. Defervescence is followed by an exanthem on the neck and trunk, followed by arms, face, and legs. The rash is characterized by bright, circular, rosy rings of blanching erythema that last 1 to 2 days.
Rubella (German measles, 3 day measles)	Children and young adults	The rash begins on the neck or face as the fever is subsiding, spreading rapidly (hours) to the trunk and extremities. The rash fades in 1–2 days in the order it occurred, followed by fine desquamation. Systemic symptoms of fatigue, headache, and fever (mild) precede the onset of the rash.
Scarlet fever	Children	Caused by a streptococcal toxin, the fever and sore throat may be associated with an erythematous eruption involving the face and neck with circumoral pallor; a fine erythematous papular eruption then spreads to the trunk within 1–2 days. Sandpaper-like feel to the rash is typical. Petechiae may be seen in skin folds (Pastia's lines). Strawberry tongue may be evident, along with typical findings of pharyngitis. Desquamation may be dramatic, especially on the hands and feet (Fig. 18–15).

HAND, FOOT, AND MOUTH DISEASE ICD-9 (074.3)

Hand, foot, and mouth disease is caused by the coxsackievirus, most commonly A16. Sporadic cases are caused by other strains (A7, A9, A10, B2, B5), and epidemic cases are associated with strains A16, or enterovirus 71. After exposure through an enteric route (oral-oral or oral-fecal), the virus has an incubation period of 3 to 5 days. Viral replication occurs in the buccal mucosa and ileum and then the lymph nodes; within 72 hours a viremia is present. Children most commonly are affected. The prodrome occurs as a low-grade fever, malaise, and abdominal pain. Other associated systemic complaints include sore throat, cough, coryza, diarrhea, nausea, and vomiting. The disease most commonly occurs in late summer through early fall, with epidemics occurring horizontally (e.g., in a day care center) or vertically (e.g., in a family). Rare complications include myocarditis, meningitis, or encephalitis. In immunocompromised patients, the disease can be recurrent.

I. CLASSIC DESCRIPTION (Fig. 18–2)
   Distribution: Mouth (90%) and acral locations; less commonly, involvement of the legs, arms, and face
   Primary: Macules that evolve into papules and vesicles
   Secondary: Erythema, erosion, mouth ulcers
   Look for oval, gray lesions on an erythematous base. Cervical or submandibular adenopathy may be present.

II. DIAGNOSIS
   Diagnosis is based on the clinical appearance of oval lesions in the characteristic distribution. Culture or serologic testing rarely, if ever, is indicated to diagnose this type of coxsackievirus infection and is available only through specialized laboratories.

III. DIFFERENTIAL DIAGNOSIS
   A. Varicella: Vesicles typically are more scattered and predominantly truncal rather than confined to the acral areas. Tzanck prep will demonstrate multinucleated giant cells.
   B. Herpes simplex: Vesicles are grouped in herpes simplex, and usually there is not widespread acral involvement.
   C. Aphthae: The lesions in hand, foot, and mouth disease tend to be more uniform, smaller, and more shallow. Aphthae tend to be recurrent.
   D. Insect bites: A central punctum often is seen in insect bites, and there are no oral lesions.
   E. Herpangina: A viral infection caused by

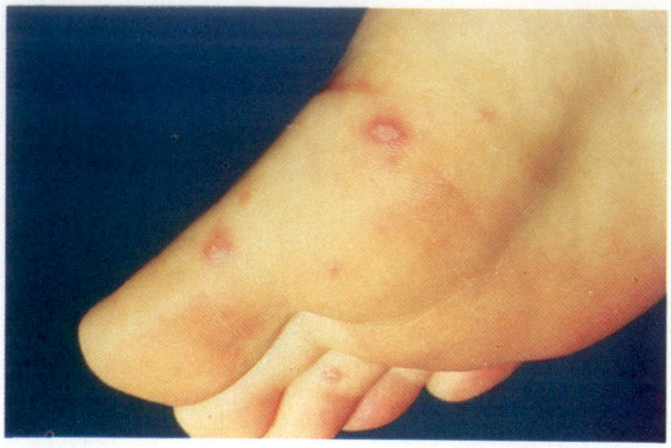

Fig. 18–2
Hand, foot, and mouth disease. Note oval lesions on an erythematous base. (Courtesy Marshall Guill, MD.)

another coxsackievirus or enterovirus, in which lesions are confined to the oral cavity and tonsillar pillars. There is no specific treatment.

IV. TREATMENT AND PATIENT EDUCATION
   A. Reassure parents about the systemic symptoms, especially the natural course of the fever, malaise, and oral pain.
   B. Pain control for oral lesions:
      1. *Adults:* Viscous *lidocaine* 2% swish and spit. Do not use immediately before lying down.
      2. *Adults and children:* diphenhydramine elixir 1:1 with *aluminum hydroxide/magnesium hydroxide* swish and spit.
   C. Maintain adequate fluid intake (e.g., use Popsicles and cold drinks).
   D. Use antipyretics (e.g., *acetaminophen*) at regular intervals.

HERPANGINA ICD-9 (074.0)

Herpangina traditionally refers to an infection by group A coxsackieviruses but probably is caused by many enteroviral infections, not only coxsackievirus. The disease most commonly affects children and adolescents in the summer and early fall. The onset is a relatively mild febrile illness with or without oral lesions. An incubation period of approximately 4 days is followed by the sudden onset of fever, which lasts 1 to 4 days. Headache, myalgias, and sore throat occur more commonly than vomiting or abdominal pain. The virus has been demonstrated in oropharyngeal secretions and feces.

I. CLASSIC DESCRIPTION
Distribution: Soft palate, tonsillar pilar, fauces
Primary: Papules, vesicles
Secondary: Erosions, ulcers, erythema
Look for gray-white papulovesicular lesions 1 to 2 mm in diameter that break down into shallow ulcers with a surrounding zone of erythema (Fig. 18–3).

II. DIAGNOSIS
Diagnosis is based on the clinical appearance of lesions localized to the oral mucosa. Culture of the oral lesions and serologic testing are rarely indicated and available only in specialized laboratories.

III. DIFFERENTIAL DIAGNOSIS
A. **Herpes simplex virus infection:** In herpes simplex infections the onset is typically more gradual, and the prodrome may be more severe in primary infection. A Tzanck prep will demonstrate multinucleated giant cells, and a viral direct antigen smear and/or culture will confirm the diagnosis in early lesions.
B. **Hand, foot, and mouth disease:** Look for acrally distributed, oval, gray, papulovesicular lesions.
C. **Herpes zoster infection:** The unilateral location of herpes zoster lesions is diagnostic.
D. **Aphthae:** Painful single or multiple oral lesions with a gray base; may look similar to the lesions of herpangina. The his-

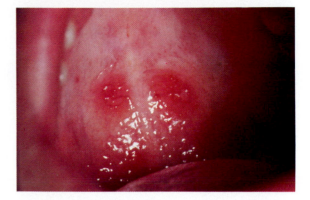

Fig. 18–3
Herpangina with shallow ulcers in the roof of the mouth. (Courtesy of Marshall Guill, MD.)

tory of recurrent disease is consistent with aphthae.
E. **Behçet's disease:** There are recurrent oral and genital ulcers and uveitis, arthritis, and vasculitis.

IV. TREATMENT AND PATIENT EDUCATION
A. **Pain control for oral lesions:**
1. *Adults:* Viscous *lidocaine* 2%, swish and spit. Do not use before lying down.
2. *Adults and children:* Diphenhydramine elixir 1:1 with *aluminum hydroxide/magnesium hydroxide,* swish and spit.
B. **Maintain adequate fluid intake** (e.g., use Popsicles and cold drinks).
C. **Use antipyretics** (e.g., *acetaminophen*) at regular intervals.
D. **Reassure parents** and support their role in caring for an ill-feeling child with systemic symptoms.

HERPES SIMPLEX ICD-9 (LABIALIS 054.9; WHITLOW 054.6)

Herpes simplex virus (HSV) infections are acute, painful, recurrent, vesicular eruptions caused by the DNA viruses herpesvirus types I and II. The incubation period is approximately 4 to 10 days, followed by development of the *classic lesions of grouped vesicles on an erythematous base.* HSV is highly contagious, and the infection occurs after direct contact with the skin. The virus subsequently spreads to involve autonomic and sensory nerve endings, remaining latent in neural ganglia. Recurrent disease occurs with reactivation of latent virus. Precipitating factors for recurrent disease include emotional stress, ultraviolet radiation, trauma, fatigue, and fever.

Primary HSV infections most commonly occur as a gingivostomatitis, usually caused by HSV-1, affecting children age 6 months to 6 years. Primary infections are more severe than recurrent infections and may be accompanied by fever, malaise, headache, and significant adenopathy. Gingivostomatitis also may cause sore throat and decreased oral intake because of pain.

Recurrences are seen in approximately 45% of people with herpes simplex gingivostomatitis, occurring in HSV-1 with a frequency of approximately two outbreaks per year. Recurrent disease often is characterized by a prodrome of tingling, burning, or even itching, followed by the outbreak of fewer and less symptomatic lesions than in the initial infection. The natural history of HSV is for the number of recurrences to decrease over time. (HSV-2, the most common cause of genital herpes simplex infections, is discussed fully in Chapter 15.) A rare, disseminated form of HSV, known as **Kaposi's varicelliform eruption,** may occur in some patients with an underlying skin disease, such as atopic dermatitis.

Herpetic whitlow (Fig. 18–4, *A*) refers to fingertip infection with HSV, often the result of thumbsucking in infants or young children.

I. CLASSIC DESCRIPTION (Fig. 18–4B, 18–5)

Distribution: Any skin site; mouth most commonly, including tongue, palate, buccal mucosa, gingiva; recurrent disease occurs most commonly on lips and face; fingertips

Primary: Vesicles, pustules, papules

Secondary: Erythema, edema, exudate, crust, erosions, ulcers

Look for grouped vesicles or erosions on an erythematous base. Adenopathy frequently is present, and chronic ulcers may develop in immunocompromised patients.

II. DIAGNOSIS

Diagnosis of HSV usually is based on the clinical appearance of the lesions in characteristic locations. An easy confirmatory test is the identification of multinucleated giant cells by Tzanck smear. Remove the top of the vesicle, letting off the fluid. Then scrape the vesicle floor with a no. 15 blade, place the specimen on a slide, spray with cytology preparation, and air dry as described in Chapter 3. Lesions should be 1 to 3 days old for best results.

A commercially available office test is based on a monoclonal antibody filtration

A 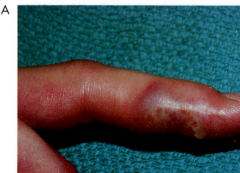 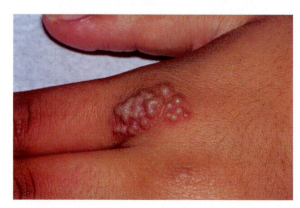 B

Fig. 18–4
A, Herpetic whitlow. Note edematous index finger with draining vesicle. (Courtesy Department of Dermatoiogy, University of North Carolina at Chapel Hill.) **B,** Herpes simplex. Note grouped vesicles on an erythematous base.

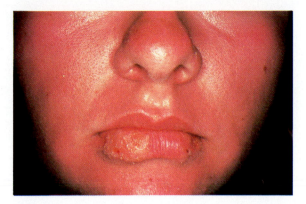

Fig. 18–5
Herpes simplex. Note grouped vesicles on an erythematous base and subsequent edema. (Courtesy John Cook, MD.)

type of enzyme immunoassay for HSV.* The test is rapid (less than 15 minutes), simple to use, and has 100% sensitivity for HSV vesicular lesions and 75% sensitivity for other types.

Other confirmatory tests include direct viral antigen smears or viral cultures. Viral antigen smears require smearing the scraped material onto a glass slide, air drying, and transporting it to a testing facility or using recently developed office tests. Viral cultures require the use of Dacron swabs inoculated into special culture media also provided by the testing facility.

III. DIFFERENTIAL DIAGNOSIS

A. **Hand, foot, and mouth disease:** Look for a few scattered lesions and the characteristic oval vesicles on the hands and/or feet.

B. **Erythema multiforme:** Exclusive oral involvement may evolve as bullae, then erosions. Look for target lesions elsewhere. Erythema multiforme can occur secondary to HSV infection, appearing several days after the onset of the viral lesions.

C. **Varicella:** Look for scattered, broad le-

sions, as opposed to the isolated, grouped vesicles of HSV.

D. **Herpes zoster:** Unilateral, dermatomal distribution can be helpful in differentiating herpes zoster from HSV; however, at times only culture, typing, and/or the presence of recurrent disease can differentiate the two.

E. **Herpangina:** Lesions tend to be more shallow. Recurrent HSV occurs primarily on the lips and skin, rather than on the inner oral mucosa.

IV. TREATMENT

A. **Mild HSV gingivostomatitis, first episode:**
1. Children: *Acyclovir* 200 mg/5 ml 5 mg/kg/day in five divided doses for 7 days.
2. Adults: *Valacyclovir* 500 mg twice a day for 5 days.
3. Consider pain-control measures (e.g., *acetaminophen* with or without *codeine,* drinking cold fluids, sucking on Popsicles, using topical anesthetic agents, such as *diphenhydramine* elixir mixed 1:1 with *aluminum hydroxide/magnesium hydroxide* swish and spit or viscous *lidocaine* in adults).
4. Adjust doses in patients with renal failure.

B. **Primary HSV-2 genital infections or severe HSV-1:**
1. Immunocompetent host: *Valacyclovir* 500 to 1000 mg twice a day for 7 days may help lesions heal faster and decrease viral shedding but will not influence the incidence of recurrent disease. The medication must be given within 24 to 48 hours of the onset of vesicles.
2. Immunocompromised host: Consider hospitalizing patient and using intravenous *acyclovir* 5 mg/kg q8h for 7 days or *acyclovir* 400 mg PO q8h for 14 to 21 days; adjust dosage for renal

*Kodak SureCell Herpes Test Kit.

function. Use *valacyclovir* with extreme caution, if at all, with immuncompromised patients because of reports of thrombotic thrombocytopenic purpura and hemolytic uremic syndrome in up to 3% of patients. Resistant cases may respond to *foscarnet*.

C. **Recurrent herpes simplex infections, Immunocompetent:**

1. Use pain-control measures.
2. Treat any secondary infection.
3. *Valacyclovir* 500 mg twice a day for 5 days or *famciclovir* 125 mg PO bid for 5 days at the first sign of a prodrome often helps decrease the severity of the recurrence, improves healing time, and decreases viral shedding. Such therapy is especially useful if erythema multiforme is associated with the recurrent HSV infections. No data is available on the effectiveness of the medication if it is given more than 1 to 2 days after the outset of the recurrence. Intermittent therapy does not influence the rate of recurrences.
4. For more than six recurrences a year, if the episodes have involved the eye or if bullous erythema multiforme was

associated with infections, use suppressive therapy with *valacyclovir* 500 mg PO once a day for 6 to 12 months, then try discontinuing the medication to find the lowest dose that will prevent recurrences.

D. **Urgent opthalmologic consultation** is required **with ocular involvement** in primary and recurrent disease, because corneal ulceration and keratitis can be severe.

E. **HSV encephalitis**: Use intravenous *acyclovir* 10 mg/kg every 8 hours for 14 to 21 days.

V. PATIENT EDUCATION

A. Educate on the infectious and recurrent nature of the disease. Viral shedding may occur, even in the absence of active lesions in the genital region, including when on antiviral therapy.

B. Emphasize good handwashing techniques, and other hygiene practices such as not sharing towels or drinking glasses.

C. Educate about physical or emotional precipitating factors and prevention (e.g., ultraviolet radiation, use of lip balm with sun protection, chemical peels, chemotherapy, and emotional stress).

HERPES ZOSTER ICD-9 (053.9)

Herpes zoster virus (HZV) infections, more commonly known as *shingles,* occur as reactivation of the chicken pox virus, varicella, from the nerve root ganglia. Three quarters of all cases occur in patients over age 50, and 25% of the population will have had HZV by the age of 75. The acute infection often starts with neuralgia in the affected dermatome, followed by the outbreak of characteristic skin lesions. Less than 1% of all cases is bilateral. Most patients have increasingly localized pain, often with associated systemic complaints of myalgia and fever. In immunocompromised patients, dissemination and recurrence of disease are major concerns.

After the skin lesions heal in 2 to 3 weeks, clinicians must remain alert to the possibilities of *postherpetic neuralgia,* defined as *pain lasting longer than 6 weeks after infection.* This complication occurs relatively frequently, especially with advancing age, and is quite debilitating.

There is no significant association of HZV with a specific underlying malignancy, although patients who are generally immunocompromised have a predilection for the disease. The presence of herpes zoster in patients with human immunodeficiency virus (HIV) infection is noteworthy, and clinicians should inquire about HIV risk factors when zoster is diagnosed in a young adult or when a case is protracted, recurrent, or involves multiple dermatomes.

Ramsay Hunt syndrome is the zoster involvement of the geniculate ganglion, characterized by unilateral loss of taste on the anterior two thirds of the tongue; ear pain, including vesicles on the pinna; hearing deficits and/or vertigo; and possible facial palsy.

I. CLASSIC DESCRIPTION (Fig. 18–6)

Distribution: Dermatomal, unilateral; two thirds occur on trunk
Primary: Vesicles, pustules, papules
Secondary: Erythema, edema, erosions, ulcers, crust
A few scattered lesions outside of the dermatome do not necessarily indicate dissemination.

II. DIAGNOSIS

Diagnosis is most often made clinically by the appearance of *grouped vesicles on an erythematous base in a dermatomal distribution* (Fig. 18–6). The appearance of unilateral disease and a history of prior varicella infection is classic. Prodromal symptoms and complaints of pain will assist in diagnosis. A Tzanck smear will demonstrate multinucleated giant cells. Lesions should be 1 to 3 days old for best results. Other confirmatory tests include direct viral antigen smears or viral cultures.

III. DIFFERENTIAL DIAGNOSIS

A. **Herpes simplex infections:** Both HSV and HZV occur as grouped vesicles on an erythematous base and have multinucleated giant cells on Tzanck smear. Look for one group of vesicles with HSV, whereas HZV usually consists of several groups of vesicles in a dermatomal distribution. A history of prior HSV infection or viral typing through direct antigen smears or culture usually will differentiate the two conditions.

B. **Contact dermatitis:** Contact dermatitis typically itches rather than causes pain. HZV lesions are grouped vesicles, whereas contact dermatitis lesions usually are linear or bizarre in configuration.

C. **Cellulitis:** Both HSV and cellulitis can start as edematous, erythematous areas, but in cellulitis the distribution is not dermatomal and in HZV there usually is a prodrome.

IV. TREATMENT

A. **Which patients to treat:**
  1. Patients with a rash that is less than 72 hours old.
  2. Patients with a rash more than 72 hours old but who are still developing new lesions.
  3. All patients over age 50.
  4. Immunosuppressed patients.

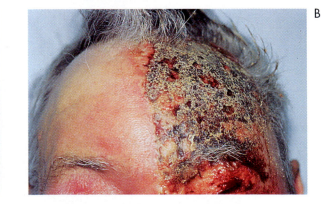

Fig. 18–6
Herpes zoster. **A,** Typical unilateral, dermatomal involvement of trunk. **B,** Severe herpes zoster with trigeminal (V1) distribution. (Courtesy Medical College of Georgia, Division of Dermatology.)

B. Medications:
1. *Valacyclovir* 500-mg tablets 1 g PO 3 times a day for 7 days or *famciclovir* 500-mg tablets 500 mg PO 3 times a day for 7 days. Use *acyclovir* 800-mg tablets 800 mg PO 5 times a day for 7 days *in immunosuppressed patients* because of reports of thrombotic thrombocytopenic purpura and he-molytic uremic syndrome in some im-munocompromised patients treated with the newer agents. Intravenous *acyclovir* may be required if dissemi-nation is of concern, more than one dermatome is involved, or the trigemi-nal nerve is affected.
2. Take each dose with 8 oz water; ad-just dosage for abnormal renal function.
3. Treatment will slow or prevent the de-velopment of new lesions, but will not influence the incidence of posther-petic neuralgia.
4. Cost of medication is approximately $125.00 to $165.00.

C. Prednisone:
1. Reliable research has not shown that prednisone is helpful in preventing postherpetic neuralgia, and the ad-verse side effects from *prednisone* are higher in the elderly.
2. Although the use of prednisone may result in improvements in the quality of life during the acute phase of infec-tion, patient selection is critical.

D. Pain control:
1. Start with *ibuprofen* or *aceta-minophen.*
2. Use narcotics (e.g., *acetaminophen* or *aspirin with codeine,* or *oxycodone with aspirin* or *acetaminophen*) on a short-term basis to control pain unre-sponsive to *ibuprofen* or *aceta-minophen.* Inasmuch as patients often are elderly, explain the possibilities of unsteadiness and constipation and

the importance of not driving while taking these medications.

E. Topical care:
1. For symptomatic relief, use cool soaks with Burow's solution, 3 times a day for 20 minutes.
2. To prevent secondary infections, apply *bacitracin* or Polysporin 3 times daily.

F. Ocular involvement: Gross eye involve-ment and/or involvement of the nasal tip (Hutchinson's sign), indicating involve-ment of the nasociliary branch of the ophthalmic nerve, should be managed with urgent ophthalmologic consultation.

G. Postherpetic neuralgia: Chronic pain persisting 1 month after lesions have healed.
1. Close follow-up for pain management and emotional support is an essential part of care for all HZV-infected patients.
2. First-line therapy includes NSAIDs.
3. Narcotics are frequently necessary for pain relief in the *acute* phase when other medications do not effectively relieve the pain or are not tolerated.
4. *Capsaicin* (Zostrix; available OTC) works by depleting substance P in the nerve endings. Do not use on open lesions.
   a. Use *capsaicin* 5 times a day for 3 to 4 weeks before deciding it does not work. If applied less often, it may cause stinging and burning.
   b. *Capsaicin* is most practical for fa-cial or neck involvement, where in-fection is localized, because of the expense of using it over a wider area.
   c. Instruct patients to avoid getting the medication in the eyes and to wash their hands immediately after using.
5. *Lidocaine* 5% ointment (35 g) or *lidocaine-prilocaine* cream *(EMLA)*

5, 30 g. Apply generously under occlusion with plastic wrap (Saran). A 1–2 day trial is necessary to determine effectiveness.

6. *Amitriptyline:*
   a. Doses of 10 to 25 mg at bedtime, increasing by 25 mg per week, up to 75 mg/day, may be helpful in some patients.
   b. Watch for anticholinergic side effects (e.g., blurred vision, dry mouth, etc.) and excessive sedation.
   c. Other antidepressants may be equally effective but with different side effect profiles.
7. *Carbamazepine:*
   a. Initiate at 100 mg PO twice a day increasing at 100 to 200 mg every 1 to 2 days to a maximum of 1200 mg per day.
   b. Titrate the dose up slowly over several weeks to avoid side effects.
8. Surgical intervention or referral to a pain clinic for alternative modalities, such as TENS (transcutaneous electrical nerve stimulation) may be necessary with severe, intractable neuralgia.

H. **Follow-up:**
   1. Many elderly patients are stoic and may not readily admit the great degree to which HZV infection is affecting activities of daily life, including sleep, sexual relations, eating, etc.
   2. Follow up patients initially 2 to 3 days after diagnosis, then again at 7 to 10 days. Continue to see the patient on a weekly basis if pain-control measures require narcotics or if the infection is disrupting sleep or other daily routines.

V. **PATIENT EDUCATION**
   A. Explain about the possibilities of post-herpetic neuralgia, emphasizing that pain management is a realistic goal.
   B. Educate patients that they can potentially infect immunocompromised patients or those who have not had chickenpox; therefore they must pay attention to routine hygiene measures (e.g., careful handwashing, not sharing towels).

MEASLES ICD-9 (055.9)

Measles, or *rubeola,* is a contagious viral infection caused by a paramyxovirus. Recent increases in measles cases emphasize the importance of clinicians becoming thoroughly familiar with the epidemiology and skin manifestations of measles. After an incubation period of 8 to 13 days, the typical measles prodrome is characterized by the "three C's": cough, coryza, and conjunctivitis, associated with a high fever. The fever course is characterized by temperature elevation for 1 or 2 days, then return to normal for 1 day, followed by elevation coinciding with the presence of the exanthem. Two weeks after exposure, *while the fever, cough, and coryza are still present, the erythematous macules appear,* first on the upper neck, then involving the face.

Extension then proceeds to the upper extremities and trunk. Early in the disease, before the onset of the rash, a petechial eruption may appear on the soft palate, followed 1 to 2 days later by *Koplik's spots,* blue-white macules with surrounding erythema that are seen on the buccal mucosa adjacent to the second molars.

Complications from measles include neurologic toxicity with encephalitis or myeloencephalitis in 0.1% of patients; rarely, subacute sclerosing panencephalitis years later; and viral pneumonitis, which may develop into a secondary bacterial infection. Atypical measles occurs primarily in those who were immunized with the killed vaccines administered between 1963 and 1967. It is also characterized by a 2- to

3-day prodrome of cough, fever, headache, myalgia, or abdominal pain, with an atypical rash typically appearing first on the distal extremities, sparing the face. Viral pneumonitis may also occur.

I. CLASSIC DESCRIPTION (Fig. 18–7)

Distribution: *Enanthem:* Koplik's spots adjacent to second molars

Exanthem: Forehead, posterior auricular area, then rest of face, finally trunk and extremities

Primary: Macules, papules

Secondary: Dull erythema; heals with hyperpigmentation and scale

With atypical measles, look for erythematous macules and papules that spread peripherally and associated edema.

II. DIAGNOSIS

Diagnosis is based on a history of exposure and presence of cough, coryza, and conjunctivitis, with fever preceding and occurring with the exanthem or the presence of Koplik's spots followed by the classic exanthem. IgM antibodies or a fourfold increase in acute and convalescent titers of IgG antibodies will confirm the diagnosis. A fluorescent antibody test may be done on nasal secretions.

III. DIFFERENTIAL DIAGNOSIS (See Table 18–1)

A. Drug eruption: The absence of cough, coryza, and conjunctivitis and the history of a suspected inciting drug will help differentiate a drug eruption from measles.

B. Other viral exanthems: Other viral exanthems lack the presence of the three C's, Koplik's spots, and the eruption pro-

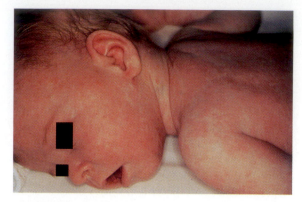

Fig. 18–7
Measles. Note diffuse erythematous involvement of face and trunk. (Courtesy Department of Dermatology, University of North Carolina at Chapel Hill.)

gression that heals with hyperpigmentation and fine scaling.

IV. TREATMENT

A. Immunoglobulin within 3 days of exposure for individuals at high risk (e.g., children less than age 12 months, pregnancy, immunocompromised) may attenuate the infection.

B. Treat any secondary infections (e.g., bronchopneumonia) with appropriate antibiotics.

C. Epidemics: Vaccination within 72 hours of exposure may provide protection.

D. Vitamin A: A dose of 200,000 U PO for 2 days may decrease morbidity and mortality in some cases of severe measles.

E. *Ribavirin:* Intravenous use of 20 to 35 mg/kg/day for 7 days may decrease severity of illness in adults.

MOLLUSCUM CONTAGIOSUM ICD-9 (078.0)

Molluscum contagiosum is a common viral skin infection caused by a pox virus. It usually occurs in young children and is quite contagious, as suggested by its name. The incubation period varies between 4 and 8 weeks. Genital lesions in teenagers or adults may be sexually transmitted.

Extensive, treatment-resistant lesions can occur in immunocompromised patients, such as those with acquired immune deficiency syndrome (AIDS). Spontaneous resolution can occur but it may take 2 or more years.

I. CLASSIC DESCRIPTION (Fig. 18–8)
 Distribution: Face, extremities, and trunk, with sparing of mucous membranes
 Primary: Papules, firm and smooth-surfaced, with central umbilication
 Secondary: Erythema, if irritated
 Lesions usually are only a few millimeters in diameter, but a rare "giant" lesion of 0.5 to 1.0 cm may occur. Lesions usually are multiple.

II. DIAGNOSIS
 The diagnosis is based on the *clinical appearance of lesions with central umbilication.* A magnifying hand lens may be helpful in observing this characteristic feature in very small lesions.

III. DIFFERENTIAL DIAGNOSIS
 A. Verruca: Verruca plana (flat warts) may look similar but do not have the central umbilication of molluscum and are not dome-shaped.
 B. Varicella: Closer inspection of varicella lesions will reveal blisters and vesicles, as opposed to the firm papules of molluscum.
 C. Basal cell carcinoma: There are usually multiple lesions with molluscum. In addition, look for telangiectasia of basal cell carcinomas typically in older patients.

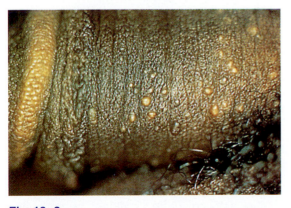

Fig. 18–8
Molluscum contagiosum. Note pearly papules with central umbilication.

 D. Folliculitis: Folliculitis lesions have a hair piercing the pustule or papule and no central umbilication.

IV. TREATMENT
 A. Base the treatment on the patient's age, the number of lesions, expectations for regression, and patient preference. (See Table 18–2.)
  1. With younger patients or when multiple lesions are present, use the least-painful method initially.
  2. Consider the option of watching for spontaneous resolution if the lesions are small, asymptomatic (not irritated), or not bothersome to the patient. However, multiple new lesions may also develop during such waiting periods.
  3. To assist in anesthesia for treating lesions in children or for treating multiple lesions in adults, consider using combination *prilocaine* 2.5% with *lidocaine* 2.5% cream (EMLA) before any procedure (see discussion of this procedure in Chapter 3).
 B. Curettage of the central core is useful when few lesions are present.
  1. A small curette (no. 2, 3, or 4) is used to scrape off the superficial lesions.
  2. Hemostasis (e.g., aluminum chloride solution) may be used if necessary.

TABLE 18–2.

Treatment for Molluscum

Molluscum type/ population	Modality
Small, asymptomatic; not spreading	Observation for spontaneous resolution
Few lesions	Curettage of the central core or liquid nitrogen therapy in combination with curettage
Younger patients	Salicylic acid, cantharidin, tretinoin gel
Older patients	Liquid nitrogen therapy in combination with curettage

3. Anesthesia may not be necessary but can be easily achieved with EMLA cream, liquid nitrogen application, or injections of bacteriostatic normal saline solution (injected to raise a wheal).

C. **Liquid nitrogen therapy may be used in combination with curettage.**
1. Because the molluscum are very superficial lesions, only a small freeze ball should be obtained.
2. This therapy is particularly effective in older patients.

D. *Cantharidin* 0.7%: An extract from a blister-causing insect, this blistering agent is applied carefully to individual lesions.
1. Cover with clear tape. Use of Mastisol will help secure the tape, increasing the potency and preventing medication from touching normal skin.
2. Blistering occurs within 2 to 24 hours, after which time the tape should be removed and the medication washed off with soap and water.
3. Use *bacitracin* or Polysporin twice daily to open areas.
4. Blistering may be very uncomfortable, and the response is extremely variable. Avoid using on the face, if possible, and only with great caution.

5. *Ibuprofen* is suggested for pain relief from blisters; however, the application of *cantharidin* itself is painless.

E. *Salicylic acid* 16.7% with lactic acid 16.7% (Duofilm 15 ml or Viranol solution 10 ml) or without lactic acid 17% (Occlusal-HP 10-ml liquid, Duoplant 7.5-ml gel, Compound W 9.3 ml-liquid or 7.5-g gel) (available OTC).
1. Use at bedtime. Instruct patients to remove dead skin gently with a nail file or washcloth before reapplying preparation to individual lesions.
2. Irritation should occur; this is necessary for the warts to peel off.

F. *Tretinoin* 0.01%, 0.025% gel, (15 g):
1. Apply sparingly at bedtime to lesions (avoiding the eyes), continuing the medication despite an expected irritation reaction.
2. Use petroleum jelly to protect the surrounding skin.

G. **STD screening:** Look for other sexually transmitted diseases in teens and adults who present with genital molluscum.

V. **PATIENT EDUCATION**
A. Explain about the mode of molluscum transmission and the contagious nature of the lesions.
B. Explain that new lesions may develop and require (re)treatment.

ROSEOLA ICD-9 (056.9)

Roseola (meaning *rosy*), also known as *exanthema subitum,* is a common, contagious viral exanthem caused by the human herpes virus 6. It usually occurs in patients age 6 months to 3 years and is *characterized by the abrupt onset of fever, with few other symptoms, that persists for 3 to 5 days. Defervescence is followed by an exanthem,* characterized by bright, circular, rosy rings of erythema, which lasts 1 to 2 days (Fig.18–9). The fever with roseola is sometimes associated with febrile seizures, although cerebrospinal fluid exams usually are normal. Rare complications include hepatitis, hemophagocytosis, and a mononucleosis-like syndrome.

I. **CLASSIC DESCRIPTION**
Distribution: Neck and trunk initially, followed by arms, face, and legs
Primary: Macules
Secondary: Erythema
The rash is discrete, confluent, and may be annular. Look for blanching erythema. Lymphadenopathy may be present, especially suboccipitally.

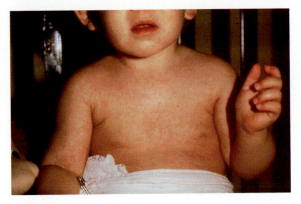

Fig. 18–9
Roseola. Note blanching, faint, confluent macules and erythema. (Courtesy Department of Dermatology, University of North Carolina at Chapel Hill.)

II. DIAGNOSIS

Diagnosis is based on the clinical history and typical disease course. Look for a history of a fever followed by a pale, erythematous, macular eruption in the appropriate age group.

III. DIFFERENTIAL DIAGNOSIS (See Table 18–1.)

A. **Rubella:** As in roseola, the exanthem appears as the fever is decreasing, but in rubella there are other systemic complaints; in roseola, there is usually only fever.

B. **Measles:** The exanthem of measles occurs along with cough, coryza, and conjunctivitis. Exanthems of measles heal with hyperpigmentation and fine scaling.

IV. TREATMENT AND PATIENT EDUCATION

No treatment, other than antipyretics, is necessary. Many parents or day care centers appropriately will be concerned about the possibility of measles because of heightened publicity about measles outbreaks; they should be reassured that the child has roseola and given an explanation of the difference between the two diseases.

VARICELLA ICD-9 (052.9)

Varicella, or chickenpox, is a primary infection caused by the DNA virus *herpesvirus varicellae,* the same agent that, when reactivated in an appropriate host, causes herpes zoster. Although varicella commonly occurs in winter, cases are reported in all seasons, with most cases diagnosed in children. After an incubation period of 10 to 20 days, patients have a febrile illness of abrupt onset, associated with malaise. Varicella is quite infectious and is spread by an airborne route. In children it often is self-limiting, with occasional scarring. Rare complications include encephalitis and *Reye's syndrome,* usually associated with salicylate use. Adults tend to be more systemically ill, with smokers, in particular, having an increased risk for significant pneumonitis. Pregnant women or immunocompromised patients need special consideration and precautions. A live, attenuated vaccine is now available and recommended for use in patients age 12 to 15 months.

I. CLASSIC DESCRIPTION

Distribution: Trunk, face, proximal extremities, mucous membranes
Primary: Vesicles, papules
Secondary: Erythema, edema, crust, excoriations
Look for crops of lesions in all stages occurring at the same time. The classic description of a vesicle on an erythematous base is a "dewdrop on a rose petal" (Fig. 18–10).

II. DIAGNOSIS

Diagnosis is made on the basis of the clinical appearance of vesicular lesions in varying stages on an erythematous base, usually in a mildly febrile patient. Tzanck smear will demonstrate multinucleated giant cells.

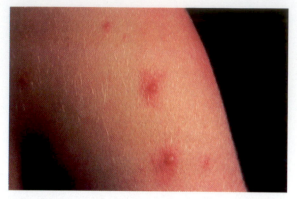

Fig. 18–10
Varicella with vesicles on an erythematous base on the left shoulder. (Courtesy John Cook, MD.)

Lesions should be 1 to 3 days old for best results. Other confirmatory tests, including direct viral antigen smears or viral cultures, rarely are necessary. *Pregnant or immunocompromised patients who are exposed to a patient with varicella and who have never had the disease themselves should immediately be tested for prior latent varicella exposure and, if negative, given varicella zoster immune globulin.*

III. DIFFERENTIAL DIAGNOSIS

A. Hand, foot, and mouth disease: Oval lesions are isolated to the extremities and, rarely, the buttocks, as opposed to vesicles on an erythematous base. Mouth lesions, however, may be difficult to distinguish, in which case a Tzanck smear will demonstrate multinucleated giant cells in varicella infections.

B. Herpes simplex: Herpes lesions occur as grouped vesicles in a localized area, whereas varicella vesicles occur as individual scattered vesicles. In primary gingivostomatitis, it may be difficult to differentiate these conditions early in the disease process. Recurrent HSV infections will be preceded by a prodrome and a history of previous infection.

C. Insect bites: In addition to a history of bites, there are no systemic manifesta-

tions, such as malaise and fever. Look for the oral lesions of varicella.

D. Pityriasis lichenoides et varioliformis acuta: This rare disease occurs as recurrent crops of papules with a purpuric center or as necrotic papules. Consider the disease if the lesions suspect for varicella last for weeks to months. Mucous membrane involvement is unusual in this disease.

E. Impetigo: Impetigo, with its honey-colored crusts, may occur as a secondary infection of varicella lesions. In varicella, look for typical malaise, fever, and possible oral involvement.

IV. TREATMENT

A. Acetaminophen for systemic complaints and fever. *Avoid salicylates.*

B. Treat any secondary bacterial infection.

C. Pruritus control:
   1. Topical agents containing *menthol, phenol, camphor, or pramoxine* (e.g., Sarna, Prax, Itch X; or by prescription, Cetaphil with ½% menthol and/or ½% phenol) can be soothing. Apply as necessary.
   2. *Hydroxyzine hydrochloride:* 10 mg/ml; 10-, 25-mg tablets.
      a. Children younger than age 6: Up to 50 mg/day in four doses; hold for somnolence.
      b. Children older than age 6: 50 to 100 mg/day in four doses.
      c. Adults: 25 to 50 mg q6h.

D. Oral involvement:
   1. Use either *diphenhydramine* elixir mixed 1:1 with *aluminum hydroxide/magnesium hydroxide* or viscous *lidocaine* 2% swish and spit for pain control.
   2. Consider the use of Popsicles to help with fluid intake.

E. For varicella in immunocompetent adults or teenagers, especially smokers, consider *valacyclovir* 500 mg 2 PO 3 times a day with a large glass of water for 7 days; adjust for renal function.

F. For varicella in immunocompromised or pregnant patients, intravenous *acyclovir* 10 to 12 mg/kg intravenously 3 times a day for 7 to 10 days; either use cautiously or avoid *valacyclovir* because of reports of thrombotic thrombocytopenic purpura and hemolytic uremic syndrome in up to 3% of patients in immunocompromised patients treated with *valacyclovir*. Although *acyclovir* remains a pregnancy category C drug, first-trimester infections may cause severe congenital defects; morbidity and mortality are higher during pregnancy. Consultation with an obstetrician or infectious disease specialist regarding use of intravenous *acyclovir* may be helpful in these cases.

G. For children on chronic salicylate therapy or with chronic cutaneous or pulmonary conditions, use oral *acyclovir* 200 mg/5ml 20 mg/kg per dose 4 times a day for 5 to 7 days for children less than 40 kg. Start within 24 hours of rash onset. Intravenous therapy may be necessary in severe cases.

H. Varicella-zoster immune globulin should be given to susceptible patients within 96 hours of exposure to modify the illness course (e.g., neonates born to mothers with varicella less than 6 days before or 2 days after delivery, premature infants, pregnant women, immunocompromised adults, smokers).

I. Lesions are infectious until crusting has occurred.

J. Scarring from lesions can be treated with various procedures, including punch excision, dermabrasion, lasers, or collagen injection. Inform patients that it takes at least 4 to 6 months for all healing to occur.

V. PATIENT EDUCATION

A. Explain about when lesions are infectious and when children can return to school (when all lesions have crusted).

B. Encourage fluid intake; use acetaminophen for fever control.

C. Explain the relationship between salicylate use and Reye's syndrome.

D. Teach adults to recognize symptoms of pneumonia, because prompt intervention is essential.

VERRUCA (WARTS) ICD-9 (078.19)

Verruca (meaning *steep places*) are so named because warts resemble small hills on the skin. Verruca can have several different forms, based on location (*genital, plantar,* and *palmar* warts) and morphology (*flat, mosaic,* and *filiform* warts). All warts are caused by the human papillomavirus (HPV), with more than 50 genetically distinct types identified. Certain types, in particular types 16 and 18, are associated with cervical cancer and, along with condyloma acuminata, are discussed in Chapter 15. Other sites for warts, including those on the digits, rarely have HPV-associated carcinomas.

Verruca occur most commonly in children and young adults, and have an incubation period of approximately 2 to 6 months. Infection occurs by skin-to-skin contact with maceration or sites of trauma (Koebner's phenomenon) predisposing patients to inoculation. There is evidence, however, of latent HPV infection possibly occurring in normal skin. Predisposing conditions for either more extensive or recalcitrant involvement may include atopic dermatitis and any condition in which there is decreased cell-mediated immunity (e.g., AIDS, organ transplantation).

I. CLASSIC DESCRIPTION

Distribution: *Common warts/verruca vulgaris:* Hands, sites of trauma (Fig. 18–11) *Plantar* and *palmar warts:* Soles, palms (Fig. 18–12)

Flat warts/verruca plana: Face, hands (Fig. 18–13)

Filiform warts: Nares, eyelid region

Primary: Papules, nodules

Secondary: Hyperkeratosis

Lesions can occur singly, in groups, or as coalescing lesions forming plaques. *Mosaic warts* are plaques of coalescing plantar or palmar warts.

II. DIAGNOSIS

Diagnosis is based on clinical appearance. If in doubt, use a no. 15 blade to scrape off any hyperkeratotic debris to reveal thrombosed capillaries, often called *seeds*. The wart also will obscure normal skin markings. Rarely, a shave biopsy may be indicated to confirm the diagnosis.

III. DIFFERENTIAL DIAGNOSIS

A. **Lichen planus:** The flat-topped papules of lichen planus may be confused with verruca plana (flat warts). Look for the oral lacy lesions of lichen planus, symmetric distribution, and Wickham's striae.

B. **Seborrheic keratosis:** Seborrheic keratoses have a stuck on appearance, with horn cysts visible on close examination. They are often pigmented.

C. **Acrochordon:** Acrochordons, or skin tags, are pedunculated flesh-colored papules that lack the roughness of warts. Filiform verruca may be pedunculated but have a characteristic filiform appearance.

D. **Clavus:** Clavus may obscure normal skin lines but lacks evidence of thrombosed capillaries, or "seeds," after scraping with a no. 15 blade.

E. **Squamous cell carcinoma:** With irregular growth, ulceration, or refractoriness to therapy, consider this diagnosis, especially in sun-exposed areas or in immunosuppressed individuals.

F. **Traumatic black heel:** Plantar warts will have black dots in the epidermis that appear similar to those of traumatic black heel, but the black specks of black heel can be removed with paring and will not bleed. Look for disruption of skin lines in plantar warts.

G. **Amelanotic melanoma:** Although extremely rare, lesions, especially on the

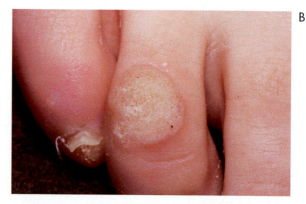

A

B

Fig. 18–11

Common warts. **A,** Periungual. (Courtesy Medical College of Georgia, Division of Dermatology.) **B,** Close up view of verruca involving dorsum of toe.

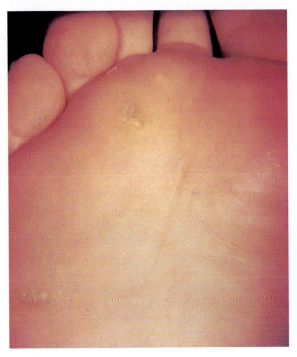

Fig. 18–12
Plantar warts. Note disruption of skin lines. (Courtesy Beverly Sanders, MD.)

palms or soles, that are treatment-resistant or atypical should be monitored closely. A biopsy may be required.

IV. TREATMENT

A. General considerations:

1. *The type and aggressiveness of therapy will depend on the type of wart, its location, and the patient's cooperation and immune status* (see Table 18–3). There are currently no specific wart therapies for treating HPV. All treatments work by being tissue-destructive, the goal being to destroy the virus-containing epidermis and preserve as much uninvolved tissue as possible. The least-painful methods should be used initially, especially in young children. More destructive therapies should be reserved for areas where scarring is not a consideration or for recalcitrant lesions.

2. Spontaneous regression may occur in as many as two thirds of warts within 2 years. However, it is far easier to treat smaller, fewer warts early on than to wait until lesions enlarge or

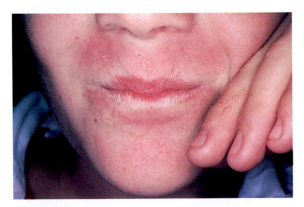

Fig. 18–13
Verruca plana. Note multiple, flesh-colored flat warts involving the fingers and perioral region. (Courtesy Medical College of Georgia, Division of Dermatology.)

TABLE 18–3.

Treatments for Warts

Indication	Modality
Common, plantar, and palmar warts in older children and adults	Liquid nitrogen, salicylic acid, bichloroacetic acid
Common, plantar, and palmar warts in young children	Observation, salicylic acid, cantharidin, bichloroacetic acid
Flat warts	Cryotherapy, 5-Fluorouracil, tretinoin
Filiform warts	Snip excision
Resistant warts	Cantharidin, in conjunction with salicylic acid, curettage and electrodessication (not plantar)
Recalcitrant warts	Referral for immunotherapy, intralesional bleomycin, or laser therapy

multiply. New warts may also appear while others are regressing, and most patients desire treatment.

3. Remember when treating verruca that the virus is microscopic and, although the skin may look normal after treatment, there often is virus still present in the remaining tissue. Unless that tissue also is removed, a few months later the warts will recur. Therefore all treatments should attempt to remove several layers of skin beyond the first signs of normal skin.

4. Therapy may take several weeks or even months, but patience and perseverance are essential. Never guarantee patients that the initial removal of a wart will be the definitive treatment.

5. Plantar warts should be treated with nonscarring methods if at all possible, because a scar on the sole of the foot can be quite painful and is irreversible. Therefore only severe, recalcitrant plantar lesions should be considered for possible surgical treatment and usually then in consultation.

B. **Liquid nitrogen therapy is useful in older children and adults but can be quite uncomfortable for younger children.**

1. Apply liquid nitrogen (anesthesia with *lidocaine* 1% may be helpful in some cases) so that there is a freeze ball of the lesion and 2 mm of surrounding normal tissue, usually 30 to 60 seconds for common, plantar, or palmar warts and 10 seconds or less for flat warts. Repeat for a total of three applications if the lesion is very thick. This therapy may be used in combination with curettage, using the liquid nitrogen as an anesthetic agent.

2. Warn patients about the normal blistering reactions and the possibility of long-lasting hypopigmentation. Use *bacitracin* or Polysporin after the blister pops.

3. Use cautiously on the digits, especially where nerves are located, to prevent severe pain and possible neuropathy.

4. After healing occurs in 4 to 7 days, apply salicylic acid for at least 7 more days (see **C,** below) to peel off a few more layers of skin, in an attempt to prevent recurrences.

5. Schedule patients for a return visit in 2 to 3 weeks to assess therapy. Consider repeating with a lighter application of liquid nitrogen to treated sites, even if normal tissue is present.

C. *Salicylic acid:* Useful agent for most warts, particularly those that are thick or multiple.

1. General patient instructions:
   a. Apply at bedtime, after soaking the affected area in warm water for 10 to 20 minutes.
   b. Remove dead skin between treatments with a nail file or pumice stone (or even a scalpel blade in reliable patients), then reapply the preparation to the warts.
   c. Irritation should occur and is necessary for the warts to peel off.
   d. Use medication less often in very painful areas. Balancing therapeutic responses and patient discomfort can be difficult.
   e. Assess response to therapy after 2 to 3 weeks.

2. All salicylic acid preparations (See Table 18–4) are available without a prescription (OTC). Stronger preparations, such as 40% plasters, usually are reserved for thicker areas (e.g., palms, soles, extremities) and lesser strengths for the digits of young children. Choose one or two forms and become thoroughly familiar with them. Products come with instructions for application, and each is slightly different. Such preparations should not be used in patients with neuropathies be-

TABLE 18–4.
Salicylic Acid Preparations

Preparation	Brand Name	Indications
Salicylic acid 17%	Occlusal HP Duoplant Compound W Duofilm Wart-Off	Liquid form allows easy application on multiple areas; useful for common, plantar, palmar, and flat warts.
Salicylic acid 16.7% and lactic acid 17.7%	Viranol	Liquid form allows easy application on multiple areas; useful for common, plantar, palmar, and flat warts.
Salicylic acid 15% in karaya gum base patches	Trans Ver Sal: 40 patches of 6 mm or 12 mm diameter, with 42 securing tapes and 1 emery file	Useful for isolated thicker lesions that allow for secure overnight taping of discs into place; instruct patients to trim patch to a size slightly larger than the lesion.
Salicylic acid 21%	Trans Plantar: 25 patches of 20 mm diameter, with 25 securing tapes and 1 emery file	Useful for isolated thicker lesions that allow for secure overnight taping of discs into place; instruct patients to trim patch to a size slightly larger than the lesion.
Salicylic acid 40%	Mediplast: 25 per box, usually available by sheet; Duofilm Patch	Especially useful for plantar warts; best applied to the wart and a few millimeters of surrounding skin, taped into place and kept dry for 48–72 hours; remove, pare down, and repeat. Tape the patch securely in place because it destroys all skin it contacts; if it gets wet, it must be reapplied.

cause of inability to judge extent of therapy and/or poor healing.

D. *Cantharidin* **0.7%:** An extract of a blistering insect; consider using in resistant cases in conjunction with or before salicylic acid preparations.

1. Apply carefully in the office to individual lesions
2. Cover with clear tape (e.g., Blenderm). Use of Mastisol to help secure the tape increases the potency and prevents the medication from touching normal skin.
3. Blistering will occur within 2 to 24 hours, after which time the tape should be removed and the medication washed off with soap and water. Use *bacitracin* or Polysporin to open areas twice daily.
4. Blistering may be very uncomfortable, and the chemotoxic response varies among patients; some have swelling with significant pain, while others may have no response at all. Although the application itself is painless, *ibuprofen*

is suggested for pain relief from the blisters that form, and stronger medications, including narcotics, may be needed.

5. After healing has occurred in 5 to 10 days, it is imperative to treat the base of the lesion with a salicylic acid preparation for an additional 5 to 7 days to prevent recurrences around the edges.
6. Preparations: (See Table 18–5) Some preparations are no longer commercially available, however the individual ingredients may be ordered and mixed either by a pharmacist or physician.*

E. *Bichloroacetic acid:* **Useful for warts on the palms or the soles.**

1. Apply to pared warts with a wooden toothpick every 7 to 10 days.
2. Use salicylic acid preparations between visits to quicken the response time.
3. At the end of therapy, when lesions

*Delasco 1-800-831-6273.

TABLE 18–5.

Cantharidin Preparations

Preparation	Indications
Cantharidin 0.7%	Useful for multiple lesions and in young children, because application is painless in the office; however, it may be painful 2–24 hours after application, and repeat applications in 10–14 days are sometimes necessary.
Cantharidin 1%, podophyillin 5%, and salicylic acid 30%	Useful for thickest lesions; use with caution on digits.

are thin, the medication may cause burning and stinging.

4. Pretreatment with EMLA can be helpful in thin lesions.

F. Curettage and desiccation are not necessarily more effective than other methods.

1. Curettage and desiccation may be useful for isolated lesions. The major problems are pain from anesthetic injection (pretreatment with EMLA cream may be helpful to ease the pain of the injection) and scarring.

2. Numb the area with *lidocaine* 1% plain if the warts are on the digits, *lidocaine* 1% with *epinephrine* 1:100,000 if elsewhere.

3. Desiccate verruca, scrape with a no. 3, 4, or 5 curette, then desiccate the base. May repeat curettage and desiccation twice.

4. Give wound care education and explain about recurrence and scarring.

5. Never perform as first-line therapy or, if possible, at all on the soles of the feet.

G. *5-Fluorouracil* (Efudex 5% cream [25 g]; Fluoroplex 1%, [30 g]): Useful for flat warts.

1. Apply to affected areas twice daily for 3 to 5 weeks.

2. Sun protection is essential.

H. *Tretinoin* (0.5%, 0.1% cream [20 g]; 0.01%, 0.025% gel [15 g]): Useful for flat warts, but improvement may take several weeks.

1. Apply once or twice a day, with a goal of mild scaling.

2. Use the highest strength that the skin will tolerate.

3. Sun protection is important.

I. Snip excision: Useful for filiform warts.

1. Anesthetize with lidocaine 1%, then snip excise.

2. Hemostasis with either cautery or aluminum chloride.

J. *Cimetidine therapy* (30 to 50 mg/kg/day in four divided doses for up to 3 months) may be useful in selected cases of recalcitrant warts. One controlled trial has not confirmed previous reports.[1]

K. Referral: Refer patients with recalcitrant warts for possible immunotherapy, intralesional *bleomycin,* or laser therapy (carbon dioxide or pulsed dye vascular).

V. PATIENT EDUCATION

(See patient education handout in Appendix X.)

A. Explain the microscopic, viral, and infectious nature of the wart.

B. Inform patients of the high rate of recurrence and the importance of following instructions carefully.

C. Educate patients thoroughly about the possible need for multiple treatments.

D. Educate about the importance of treating beyond the initial wart removal because the virus still may be present in the skin.

E. Warn patients about scarring or hypopigmentation that may occur as a result of some treatments.

F. If a young patient is having severe difficulty cooperating with or tolerating the chosen therapy, consider using occlusion therapy by applying salicylic acid to the wart, applying tape securely, and removing it every 7 days. Repeat occlusion therapy until the wart is no longer visible.

G. In patients with flat warts, discourage shaving, until warts are no longer visible for several months.

VIRAL EXANTHEMS (057.9)

Viral exanthems are a nonspecific classification of monomorphic erythematous eruptions that can occur secondary to various viral infections. The eruption itself is not unique to viral infections but may be seen in drug eruptions as well. Viruses that most commonly cause macular and papular eruptions are listed in Box 18–1.

I. **CLASSIC DESCRIPTION** (Fig. 18–14)
Distribution: Generalized and symmetric
Primary: Macules, papules
Secondary: Erythema that blanches with pressure

II. **DIAGNOSIS**
Diagnosis is based on the clinical appearance of blanchable, erythematous macules and papules in a symmetric distribution with associated systemic complaints, either occurring along with or preceding the eruption.

III. **DIFFERENTIAL DIAGNOSIS**
A. **Drug eruptions:** It may be impossible to differentiate eruptions secondary to viral infections from a drug eruption. A history of a new agent started 7 to 10 days before onset of the eruption may be more consistent with a drug eruption. Fever and systemic complaints may be present in both. Conjunctivitis, coryza, or sore throat may be more consistent with viral infections.

B. **Scarlet fever:** The rash of scarlet fever (Fig. 18–15) typically occurs with high fever and pharyngitis or skin infection (Table 18–1).

IV. **TREATMENT**
A. **Reassurance:** No treatment other than reassurance is necessary in most cases.
B. **In severe or chronic reactions, biopsy sometimes is helpful to determine whether the eruption is viral or drug-related.** Eosinophils in the skin usually are more consistent with an allergic drug reaction than a viral infection. Often the histopathologic findings are nonspecific.
C. **Pruritus control:** When present, pruritus usually can be controlled with topical agents containing *menthol, phenol, camphor,* or *pramoxine* (e.g., Sarna, Prax, Itch X), or with *hydroxyzine* 10 to 50 mg 4 times a day in adults and 5 to 10 mg 4 times a day in children.

BOX 18–1.
Viruses that Commonly Cause Exanthems

Adenovirus
Coxsackievirus A and B
Echovirus
Herpesvirus 6 and 7 (roseola)
Infectious mononucleosis
Paramyxovirus (measles)
Parvovirus (erythema infectiosum)
Togavirus (rubella)

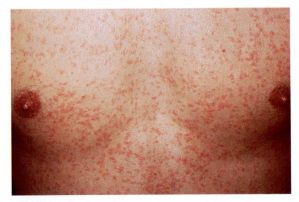

Fig. 18–14
Viral exanthem. Note diffuse morbilliform eruption. (Courtesy Department of Dermatology, University of North Carolina at Chapel Hill.)

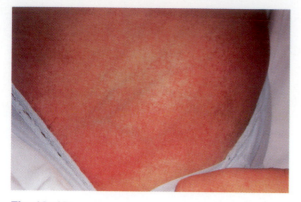

Fig. 18–15
Scarlet fever. Note fine erythematous eruption of trunk.

V. PATIENT EDUCATION

A. Reassure patients about the self-limiting nature of the illness.

B. Warn patients to avoid getting over-heated (e.g., from a hot shower), because this will cause the rash to look worse and to itch.

C. Educate patients to seek therapy if they develop significant systemic involvement (e.g., prolonged nausea, jaundice, change in urination, bruising, etc.).

SUGGESTED READING

Butner KR, Friedman DJ, Forszpaniak C: Valacyclovir compared with acyclovir for improved therapy for herpes zoster in immunocompetent adults, *Antimicrob Agents Chemother* 39:1546–1553, 1995.

Committee on Infectious Diseases: vitamin A treatment of measles, *Pediatr* 91:1014–1015, 1993.

Drake LA et al: Guidelines of care for warts: human papillomavirus, *J Am Acad Dermatol* 32:98–103, 1995.

Hall CB et al: Human herpesvirus 6 infection in children, *N Engl J Med* 331:432–438, 1994.

Herne K et al: Antiviral therapy of acute herpes zoster in older patients, *Drugs and Aging* 8:97–112, 1996.

Janniner CK, Schwartz RA: Molluscum contagiosum in children, *Cutis* 52:194–196, 1993.

Kost RG, Straus SE: Postherpetic neuralgia-pathogenesis: treatment and prevention, *N Engl J Med* 335:32–42, 1996.

Memar O, Tyring SK: Cutaneous viral infections (periodic synopsis), *J Am Acad Dermatol* 33:279–287, 1995.

Mooney MA, Janninger CK, Schwartz RA: Kaposi's varicelliform eruptions, *Cutis* 53:243–245, 1994.

Moy R, Eliezri YD: Significance of human papillomavirus-induced squamous cell carcinoma to the dermatologist, *Arch Dermatol* 130:235–238, 1994.

Parish LC, Millikan LE, eds: Contemporary tropical dermatology, *Dermatol Clin* 12:611–816, 1994.

REFERENCE

1. Bauman et al: Cimetidine therapy for multiple viral warts in children, J Am Acad Dermatol 35:271-272, 1996.

PART THREE

Cutaneous Manifestations of Systemic Disease and Miscellaneous Disorders

CHAPTER 19

Connective Tissue Diseases

The dermatologic manifestations of connective tissue diseases may be difficult and challenging to even the most experienced clinicians. What makes these disorders so complex for physicians is the tremendous diversity in signs and symptoms. In addition, it is difficult to establish clear-cut rules for workup and treatment because much about these diseases remains unknown, despite all that has been written.

Such diagnostic challenges and therapeutic unpredictability underlie our recommendations for clinicians to work together in multidisciplinary approaches to define optimal patient care. Appropriate patient education is integral to this care, because many patients have their own set of fears and misperceptions about these diseases.

DERMATOMYOSITIS ICD-9 (710.3)

Dermatomyositis is a rare (5 in each million people) inflammatory muscle disease with characteristic associated skin and connective tissue manifestations. Thought to have an autoimmune cause, it occurs twice as often in females as in males and more commonly in adults over age 40. Childhood dermatomyositis tends to be chronic and more severe, with muscle contractures. Calcium deposition in the subcutaneous tissue and fascial planes, known as *calcinosis cutis,* occurs in 40% of children and may be severely debilitating. Children also may have a systemic necrotizing vasculitis, particularly involving the gastrointestinal tract. A history of a recent upper respiratory tract infection preceding the onset of the symptoms is not uncommon.

Adults with dermatomyositis may have significantly more underlying systemic diseases, such as other connective tissue diseases or malignancy. The most common malignancies are breast, lung, ovary, stomach, colon, uterus, and nasopharynx. The rash and muscle weakness may resolve with treatment of the malignancy.

Musculoskeletal involvement is heralded by symmetric proximal muscle weakness (e.g., difficulty in climbing stairs, rising from a chair, getting out of bed, brushing the hair or teeth). Dysphagia, myalgias, arthralgias, malaise, and fever also may be present. Younger patients more frequently have overlap syndromes, with the myositis occurring in conjunction with other connective tissue diseases (e.g., systemic lupus erythematosus, Sjögren's syndrome, progressive systemic sclerosis). Polymyositis is muscle involvement without skin findings.

Classic Description

Characteristic skin findings may precede or follow the musculoskeletal symptoms (Box 19–1).

BOX 19–1.

Skin Findings in Dermatomyositis

Specific
   Periorbital heliotrope eruption
   Gottron's papules and sign
Nonspecific
   Periungual telangiectasia with ragged-edged cuticles
   Photosensitive eruption on sun-exposed areas
   Poikiloderma: hypopigmentation–hyperpigmentation
      with telangiectasia and atrophy

Findings specific for dermatomyositis include a periorbital heliotrope (violaceous) eruption with associated edema (Fig. 19–1); Gottron's erythematous to violaceous papules, occurring classically over the knuckles, elbows, and knees (Fig. 19–2); and Gottron's sign of symmetric, violaceous, erythematous, scaling eruptions on the forehead, knuckles, knees, elbows, and medial malleoli. Less specific features include photosensitivity, mottled hypopigmentation and hyperpigmentation, periungual telangiectasia, and diffuse alopecia.

Diagnosis

The diagnosis is suspected from the clinical history and physical examination demonstrating proximal muscle weakness and characteristic skin findings. Look for elevations of muscle enzymes (creatine phosphokinase [CPK], aspartate aminotransferase, aldolase, and lactic dehydrogenase). Early in the disease a 24-hour urine CPK analysis may be helpful in making the diagnosis if serum enzyme levels are normal. If enzyme levels are normal and the diagnosis is still suspected, consider obtaining an electromyogram, ultrasound, or muscle biopsy specimen from involved muscles. Use of magnetic resonance imaging may be helpful in directing a best site for muscle biopsy in subtle cases.

   Some patients with associated connective tissue diseases will have a positive antinuclear antibody (ANA) or rheumatoid factor. The presence of anti-Jo-1 or Mi-2 antibodies may help confirm the diagnosis if positive, but a negative test result

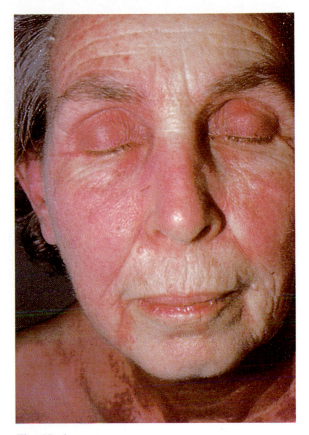

Fig. 19–1
Periorbital edema, erythema, and facial photosensitivity in an elderly woman with dermatomyositis. (Courtesy Department of Dermatology, University of North Carolina at Chapel Hill.)

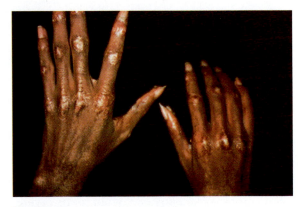

Fig. 19–2
Gottron's papules. Scaling papules over metacarpal and interphalangeal joints. (Courtesy Medical College of Georgia, Division of Dermatology.)

does not rule out the disease. Other serologic studies, such as anti-Ro/SSA, anti-La/SSB, and anti-RNP, should be performed to evaluate for other possible connective tissue diseases, especially in patients with Raynaud's phenomenon (see Table 19–3).

Approximately 10% of patients with dermatomyositis present as *amyopathic dermatomyositis.* Patients have the associated skin findings but have normal muscle enzymes and normal muscle function. The full spectrum of disease may eventually develop in such patients.

Evaluate patients over age 40 for an internal malignancy (15% to 25% incidence) by history; physical examination; routine laboratory studies; such cancer screenings as a testicle examination in males and a mammogram, pelvic ultrasound, and Papanicolaou smear in women; chest radiograph examination; and stool check for occult blood or other gastrointestinal examinations. Follow up screens at 6-month intervals.

Differential Diagnosis

Although lesions may appear similar to *psoriasis, eczema,* or a *photosensitive skin eruption,* findings in dermatomyositis have a unique distribution and heal with mottled hypopigmentation or hyperpigmentation, telangiectasia, and atrophy known as *poikiloderma.* Poikiloderma also occurs in chronic sun-damaged areas and several rare skin disorders. Findings both clinically and histologically can resemble *lupus erythematosus.* However, patients with lupus erythematosus typically will have a positive anti-DNA antibody test, which is negative in dermatomyositis.

Treatment

The mainstay of treatment is oral corticosteroid therapy coupled with rest, photoprotection, adequate protein nutrition, and physical therapy, with appropriate dermatologic and rheumatologic consultation. Start *prednisone* therapy, 0.5 to 1.5 mg/kg/day; taper gradually as symptoms allow. Other immunosuppressants, such as *methotrexate* or *azathioprine* may be necessary in unresponsive cases. The skin should be protected from sunlight with clothing, sun avoidance, and use of a broad-spectrum sunscreen (e.g., UVA guard). Topical corticosteroids, such as *hydrocortisone* 1% cream, applied topically twice daily to affected areas on the face may help with the erythema. Antimalarials, such as *hydroxychloroquine,* may be used to control skin disease in some patients.

Monitor all patients for respiratory or upper digestive tract involvement (difficulty in swallowing) and gastrointestinal vasculitis in children. Use of *aluminum hydroxide* gel 3 times daily may reduce the severity of calcinosis cutis in children. Creatine phosphokinase is the most sensitive test used to gauge the clinical response to treatment or flaring.

LUPUS ERYTHEMATOSUS ICD-9 (LOCAL/DISCOID 695.4; SYSTEMIC 710.0; DRUG-INDUCED 695.4)

Lupus erythematosus is a multisystem, chronic autoimmune disease with protean manifestations. *Lupus* refers to something that has the appearance of being gnawed at by a wolf. Lupus erythematosus was distinguished from lupus vulgaris, caused by tuberculosis, almost 150 years ago. Chronic cutaneous or discoid lupus erythematosus can cause severe disfigurement if left untreated, thus the name *lupus.* Ten to 50 cases occur per 100,000 in the United States.

The spectrum of lupus erythematosus ranges widely from isolated chronic skin lesions to fulminant renal disease. The cause is thought to be autoimmune, heralded by the production of diverse autoantibodies. Any classification system is fraught with difficulties because patients often do not fit neatly into one particular lupus category. Their disease may be confined to one organ system for long periods before a well-defined syndrome is characterized or they may have a broad spectrum of connective tissue diseases (i.e., overlap syndrome, mixed connective tissue disease).

Diagnosis and Classification

Lupus erythematosus is classified to aid in initial evaluation, diagnosis, follow-up, treatment, and especially prognosis (Tables 19–1 to 19–3, Box 19–2, and Fig. 19–3). Initially the skin is involved in 70% to 85% of patients, second only to joint disease in incidence (Figs. 19–4 to 19–6). A positive antinuclear antibody test (ANA) is found in almost all patients with systemic disease. Antiphospholipid antibodies are present in 30% of patients with systemic lupus and may be responsible for the thromboembolic manifestations (e.g., thrombophlebitis, stroke, pulmonary embolism, and abortion).

BOX 19–2.

American Rheumatism Association Criteria for Classification of Systemic Lupus Erythematosus*†

1. Malar rash
2. Discoid rash
3. Photosensitivity
4. Oral ulcers
5. Arthritis: painful, swollen, nonerosive, involving peripheral joints
6. Serositis: pleuritis, pericarditis
7. Renal disorders: proteinuria (3+) or >0.5 g/day persistent proteinuria or characteristic cellular casts
8. Neurologic disorders: seizures or psychosis in the absence of other causes
9. Hematologic disorders: hemolytic anemia, leukopenia, lymphopenia, or thrombocytopenia
10. Positive lupus erythematosus cell preparation, anti-DNA antibody, anti-Smith antibody in abnormal titers, or a false positive syphilis serologic result
11. Antinuclear antibody in an abnormal titer in the absence of any drugs associated with drug-induced lupus erythematosus

*From Tan EM, et al: *Arthritis Rheum* 25:1271–1277,1982.
†The presence of four or more criteria serially or simultaneously is consistent with the diagnosis of systemic lupus erythematosus.

Treatment

Systemic Lupus Erythematosus

Aspirin and nonsteroidal antiinflammatory agents are used for isolated arthritis or serositis. *Prednisone* 0.5 to 1.0 mg/kg/day is the mainstay of treatment for patients with multiple organ involvement or compromised function, the goal being to achieve normalization of markers for active disease (i.e., anti-ds DNA antibody, urinary sediment, sedimentation rate, complement levels, and hypertension). Use of prednisone for longer than 6 months apparently does not improve survival and increases the incidence of corticosteroid-induced side effects. Azathioprine and other immunosuppressants sometimes are used in unresponsive cases, but consultation is advised. For skin lesions, the topically applied corticosteroid with the lowest potency that controls the lesions should be used.

Patients should be educated about sun avoidance and sun protection (e.g., wearing long sleeves and a hat and using broad-spectrum sunscreens, such as UVA guard, Johnson and Johnson Waterproof Sunscreen for Children SPF 30, or sunscreens with an SPF 30 and containing a physical sunblock, such as titanium dioxide). For patient support and information contact the Lupus Foundation of America.*

Chronic Cutaneous (Discoid) Lupus Erythematosus

For skin lesions, start with a low- to medium-potency topical corticosteroid (e.g., *triamcinolone* 0.1% cream) twice daily. Do not hesitate to use stronger topical steroids if no response is seen after 2 to 3 weeks. High-potency corticosteroids may even be necessary, including use on the face. Use cyclically (e.g., 2 weeks on, 2 weeks off) and monitor closely for skin atrophy. For isolated lesions unresponsive to potent topical corticosteroids, use intralesional corticosteroids (e.g., *triamcinolone* 2.5 to 5 mg/ml for

*Lupus Foundation of America, 1300 Piccard Dr. Ste. 200, Rockville, MD, 20850-303; 301-670-9292, 1-800-558-0121. Web site: http://www.lupus.org/lupus

TABLE 19–1.
Classification and Characteristics of Lupus Erythematosus*

	Chronic Cutaneous (Discoid) Lupus	Subacute Cutaneous Lupus	Systemic Lupus	Drug-induced Lupus
Incidence	Females; peaks in fourth decade	Young and middle-age white females	8:1 females/males; blacks	D-Penicillamine, hydralazine, procainamide
Distribution	Face, scalp, ears; rare below waist; asymmetric (see Fig.19-4)	Sun-exposed trunk and upper extremities, shoulders; less facial involvement; symmetric (see Fig. 19-5)	Sun-exposed areas butterfly rash: with nose and malar involvement, symmetric (see Fig. 19-6)	Sun-exposed, symmetric
Lesions	Violaceous-red papules, plaques with thick, adherent scales; plugged follicles with scales; telangiectasia; hyperpigmentation at margin; heal with central atrophy; scarring and hypopigmentation; if in scalp, scarring alopecia	Violaceous-red polycylic, annular plaques or papules with telangiectasia and scale; may resolve with hypopigmentation but *no* scarring	Violaceous-red, edematous plaques; may have fine scale; facial lesions have photodistribution with sparing of philtrum and nasolabial folds; generalized erythema	Rashes of DLE/SLE
Nonspecific skin manifestations	Oral ulcers, photosensitivity	Periungual telangiectasia marked photosensitivity, oral lesions, nonscarring alopecia, livedo reticularis	Oral ulcers, periungual telangiectasia, palpable purpura, livedo reticularis, urticaria, Raynaud's phenomenon, nonscarring alopecia, panniculitis, photosensitivity	Photosensitivity
Systemic involvement and special features	5%–10% will have evidence of SLE at some point during the disease course	Fever, arthralgias, malaise; renal, serositis, and CNS disease less common and less severe than in SLE	See Table 19–3, fever, arthralgias, malaise, hypocomplementemia; hypergammaglobulins, vasculitis; ≤ 25% develop chronic cutaneous lesions at some time	Fever, myalgias, arthralgias, serositis; rash, CNS, renal less often; related to liver metabolism of drug during course. Up to 10% will manifest chronic cutaneous lesions.

Differential diagnosis	*Polymorphous light eruption:* occurs in early spring without scaling and heals without scarring or atrophy *Lichen planus:* oral reticulate lesions; not photodistributed or photoexacerbated	*Psoriasis, eczema, and erythema multiforme:* not photodistributed or photoexacerbated; systemic signs may be helpful. *Photodrug eruption:* with drug exposure. *Dermatomyositis:* weakness; distribution includes knuckles and heliotrope rash	*Erysipelas:* acute onset, demarcated erythema, not photosensitive, responds to antibiotics. *Acne rosacea:* will have associated papules, pustules, and absence of systemic complaints. *Seborrheic dermatitis:* not photoexacerbated, absence of systemic complaints.	Same as DLE/SLE	Improves with drug withdrawal
Diagnosis	Punch biopsy of involved skin for routine light microscopy and DIF†	Punch biopsy of involved skin for routine light microscopy and DIF† in conjunction with systemic complaints and presence of autoantibodies	Punch biopsy of involved skin for routine light microscopy and DIF† (See Table 19–3.)		
Autoantibodies	5%–10% ANA+ <5% ds DNA+	>60% ANA+ 30% ds DNA+ 30%–60% SSA+	95% ANA+ 60% ds DNA+		Antihistone antibodies

* DLE = discoid lupus erythematosus; SLE = systemic lupus erythematosus; SCLE = subacute cutaneous lupus erythematosus; CNS = central nervous system; DIF = direct immunofluorescence; CCLE = chronic cutaneous lupus erythematosus; SCLE = subacute cutaneous lupus erythematosus.

†Skin biopsy requires special media for fixation and transport and reveals staining patterns for complement and immunoglobulins at the dermal-epidermal junction in LE. In CCLE (discoid/DLE), 85%–95% of sun-exposed skin lesions are abnormal. In SCLE, 60% of lesional skin and 25% of sun-exposed, nonlesional skin is abnormal. In SLE, 90%–95% of lesional skin and 70% of sun-exposed, nonlesional skin are abnormal.‡ The presence of immunoglobulins, particularly IgG, IgM, and IgA, or all three, strongly suggests SLE or certain bullous diseases. SLE is especially likely when IgG or C3 are present in a granular pattern with or without IgM. *False positive results may occur in ac-tinically damaged skin, dermatomyositis, rheumatoid arthritis and vasculitis.*

‡Sun-protected uninvolved skin tested by DIF (lupus band test) may serve to confirm the diagnosis of SLE and serve as a marker for increased renal disease.

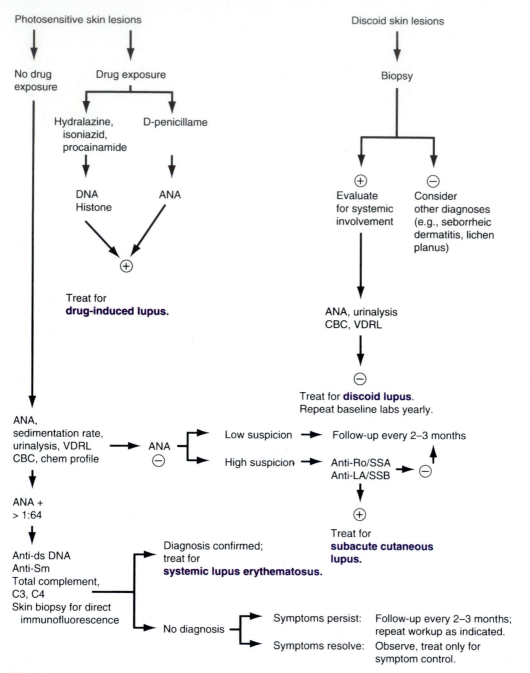

Fig. 19–3
Algorithm for workup and diagnosis of lupus erythematosus.

TABLE 19–2.

Positive Antinuclear Antibody Test Result*

Disease	Percent
Drug-induced lupus	100
Mixed connective tissue	100
Systemic lupus	95–100
Sjögren's syndrome	80
Scleroderma	60–95
Polymyositis/dermatomyositis	50–75
Rheumatoid arthritis	40–60
Normal population	0–4

*Modified from Harmon CE: *Med Clin North Am* 69: 547–563, 1985.

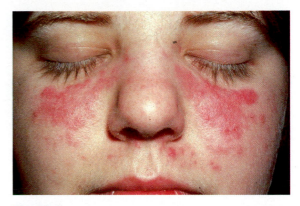

Fig. 19–6
Classic butterfly rash of systemic lupus erythematosus. (Courtesy Department of Dermatology, University of North Carolina at Chapel Hill.)

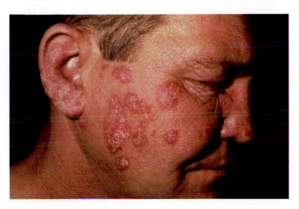

Fig. 19–4
Scaling plaques with thick scales on the ear and face of a patient who has discoid lupus. (Courtesy Department of Dermatology, University of North Carolina at Chapel Hill.)

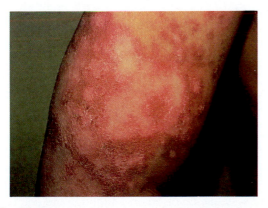

Fig. 19–5
Subacute cutaneous lupus with annular, scaling plaques and absence of scarring on sun-exposed arm. (Courtesy Department of Dermatology, University of North Carolina at Chapel Hill.)

the face or 5 to 10 mg/ml elsewhere, using approximately 0.5 ml for a 1-cm plaque).

For extensive or disfiguring disease unresponsive to other therapies, consider using antimalarial agents (e.g., *hydroxychloroquine sulfate* 200 mg PO twice daily for 3 to 4 weeks, then once daily). Before use, an ophthalmologic examination is necessary; repeat the examination at 4- to 6-month intervals to detect irreversible maculopathy. Atabrine has less retinal toxicity but gives an orange discoloration to the skin. Both can produce reversible corneal opacities. Low-dose oral corticosteroids occasionally may be necessary if patients do not respond to the previously mentioned treatments. If systemic complaints are present, a workup to rule out systemic lupus erythematosus is appropriate (see Fig. 19–3).

Explain that most disease can be controlled with therapy, that routine monitoring is important (baseline and yearly antinuclear antibodies, sedimentation rate, white blood cell count, creatinine clearance, urinalysis), and that most patients with discoid lupus do not develop systemic involvement. Educate patients on sun avoidance and sun protection and refer patients to one of the lupus support groups (see p. 261).

TABLE 19–3.

Antinuclear and Anticytoplasmic Antibodies*†

Antibody	Disease
ds DNA	Strongly suggests LE and is frequently found with SLE, hypocomplementemia, and renal disease.
	Seen with drug-induced LE caused by D-penicillamine. Low titers present in rheumatoid arthritis, Sjögren's syndrome, dermatomyositis, systemic sclerosis, and CCLE.
ss DNA	Common in LE but also seen in drug-induced LE, rheumatoid arthritis, and Sjögren's syndrome.
ENA	
Sm	Nearly specific for SLE but seen in only 20%–40% of patients. Presence, along with chronic cutaneous skin lesions, suggests systemic involvement.
RNP	Mixed connective tissue disease: overlap of scleroderma, SLE, and polymyositis. Seen in 30% of patients with SLE.
Ro (SSA)	Sjögren's syndrome. Seen in 35% of patients with SLE, especially ANA negative. Present in neonatal and SCLE.
La (SSB)	Seen in 15% of patients with SLE and 30% of patients with Sjögren's syndrome.
Jo-1	Polymyositis.
Scl-70	Scleroderma.
DNP (DNA-histone)	Drug-induced LE (except D-penicillamine). Seen in SLE and many other disorders.
Centromere	CREST syndrome.
ssRNA	Scleroderma.
PM-1(Mi)	Seen in poly-and dermatomyositis

* Modified from Dahl MV: *Clinical Immunodermatology,* ed 2, Chicago, 1988, Year Book Medical Publishers, p. 243.

†LE = lupus erythematosus; CCLE = chronic cutaneous lupus erythematosus; ENA = extractable nuclear antigen; SLE = systemic lupus erythematosus; ANA = antinuclear antibody; SCLE = subacute cutaneous lupus erythematosus; CREST = calcinosis cutis, Raynaud's phenomenon, esophageal dysmotility, sclerodactyly, and telangiectasia.

Drug-Induced Lupus Erythematosus

Serious, systemic signs should be treated in a manner similar to that of systemic lupus erythematosus. Cutaneous involvement is rare, and improvement should occur with discontinuation of the offending medication (see Table 19–1).

SCLERODERMA ICD-9 (LOCALIZED 701.0, DIFFUSE 710.1)

Scleroderma, derived from *skleros* meaning *hard* and *derma* meaning *skin,* refers to chronic, abnormal connective tissue fibrosis of unknown cause. It may occur as an isolated finding, known as *morphea,* in association with other connective tissue diseases (e.g., lupus erythematosus, rheumatoid arthritis, myositis, overlap syndrome) or, more classically, as *progressive systemic scle-* *rosis (PSS).* PSS is rare (2.7 cases per 1 million person-years) and more commonly affects women (3 to 4:1) in the fourth and fifth decades. Childhood forms tend to be more localized, without systemic involvement. Although the course is variable among patients, those with internal organ or generalized skin involvement and an older age at onset have increased mortality.

The most common initial clinical symptom is *Raynaud's phenomenon* (90%), an intermittent vasospasm of the terminal finger arterioles precipitated by stress and cold temperatures. Often patients may subsequently notice symmetric, painless edema of the fingers. A migratory polyarthritis or simple stiffness of the fingers or knees may be the first symptom, along with fatigue and myalgias.

Visceral fibrosis occurs in the lungs, heart, kidneys, or gastrointestinal tract. Gastrointestinal involvement with dysphagia, heartburn, and regurgitation is present in 80% to 90% of patients, sometimes preceding the onset of skin manifestations. Small bowel involvement is characterized by intestinal stasis, with cramping abdominal pain, diarrhea, and weight loss. Exertional dyspnea and respiratory failure occur in advanced disease secondary to pulmonary fibrosis. Cardiac abnormalities, such as pericarditis or myocardial fibrosis, occur late in the disease course and may lead to conduction defects or heart failure. Kidney involvement with proteinuria, severe hypertension, or azotemia is common and is the major cause of death in such patients.

Systemic sclerosis-like disease has been described in patients exposed to organic chemicals (e.g., benzene, xylene, toluene, epoxy resins, formaldehyde), medications (e.g., bleomycin, carbidopa, pentazocine, cocaine, appetite suppressants), adulterated rapeseed oil, silica dust, paraffin, processed petrolatum jelly, and L-tryptophan.

Classic Description

Skin thickening is characteristic, secondary to an imbalance in collagen metabolism, and initially presents as skin edema. Later the skin becomes indurated and bound down to the fascia, with subsequent atrophy, known as *sclerodactyly,* restricting the range of motion in the fingers and giving a clawlike deformity to the hands (Fig. 19–7). Concomitant pigment abnormalities include hyperpigmentation and depigmented areas, giving a "salt and pepper" appearance. Facial

skin involvement gives a pinched look to the face, with loss of facial skin lines, except perioral furrows, and narrowing of the lips and mouth opening (Fig. 19–8). Periungual telangiectasia and telangiectatic mats on the palms, lips, face, tongue, and mucous membranes are prominent (Fig. 19–9). Cutaneous and subcutaneous calcification may occur, especially on the fingertips, hands, and extensor surfaces of the extremities. Ulcerations may heal with scarring.

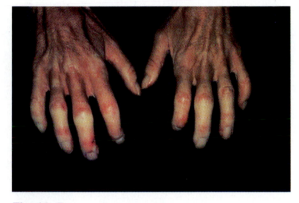

Fig. 19–7
Sclerodactyly of the hands in a patient with progressive systemic sclerosis. (Courtesy Medical College of Georgia, Division of Dermatology.)

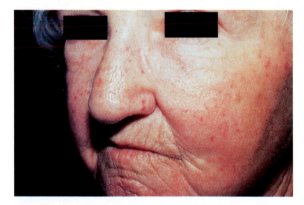

Fig. 19–8
Scleroderma. Note the pinched appearance of the face, matlike telangiectasia on the nose, and perioral furrows. (Courtesy Department of Dermatology, University of North Carolina at Chapel Hill.)

Localized scleroderma, or morphea, has one or more areas of indurated, hypopigmented plaques with a purplish-red edge (Fig. 19–10). Such lesions typically enlarge very little but may persist for years. Systemic signs are not seen.

Diagnosis

Diagnosis is made on clinical findings (Box 19–3). Nonspecific laboratory findings include anemia, elevated sedimentation rate, elevated immunoglobulin levels, and ANA (60% to 95%); Scl-70 autoantibodies are specific for PSS but not highly sensitive (55%) and are associated with an increased incidence of pulmonary fibrosis (see Tables 19–2 and 19–3). Decreased primary peristalsis and dilation of the lower two thirds of the esophagus are seen on barium swallow or manometry.

Differential Diagnosis

The differential diagnosis of finger and hand thickening includes the *cutaneous porphyrias,* but skin lesions in such patients will be sun sensitive and fragile and there will be a history of bulla formation. The two can be differentiated by skin biopsy. *Mixed connective tissue disease* is characterized by the presence of an extractable nuclear antigen, antiribonucleoprotein antibodies, and the clinical features of scleroderma, lupus erythematosus, and myositis. *Sclerodermatomyositis* produces features of scleroderma and polymyositis.

PM-Scl and Ku antibodies may be demonstrable in these patients. A subset of patients with scleroderma with *CREST syndrome* (*c*alcinosis cutis, *R*aynaud's phenomenon, *e*sophageal dysmotility, *s*clerodactyly, and *t*elangiectasia) tend to have milder systemic involvement compared with PSS; however, biliary cirrhosis, pulmonary hypertension, and Sjögren's syndrome may occur in this population.

Treatment

Obtaining symptom relief and maintaining optimal function are the most important current methods, inasmuch as no treatment is curative. Management of Raynaud's phenomenon includes protection from the cold, use of mittens or gloves, and *nifedipine* or topical *nitroglycerin* in refractory cases. Active physical therapy is vital to slow the rate of skin contractures. Manage other problems (e.g., intestinal overgrowth, arthralgias) as in any other illness. Systemic ther-

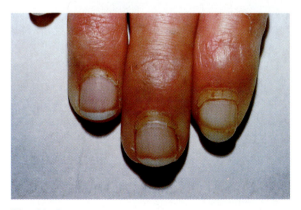

Fig. 19–9
Periungual telangiectasia in patient with scleroderma. (Courtesy Department of Dermatology, University of North Carolina at Chapel Hill.)

BOX 19–3.

Diagnostic Criteria for Scleroderma

MAJOR CRITERION*

Proximal diffuse truncal sclerosis (e.g., skin tightness, thickening, nonpitting induration)

MINOR CRITERION*

Sclerodactyly
Digital pitting scars
Loss of finger pad substance (pulp loss)
Bibasilar pulmonary fibrosis
Raynaud's phenomena

*The diagnosis is made in the presence of one major or two minor criteria.

A
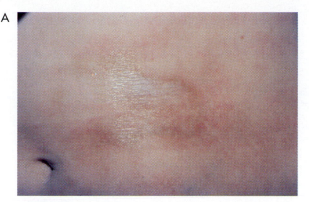
B
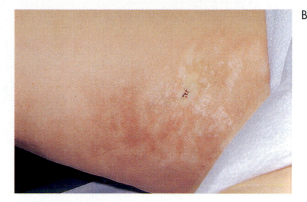

Fig. 19–10
Morphea. **A,** Atrophic, hypopigmented plaque with thin cigarette paper-like skin and a rim of inflammation.
B, Atropic plaque with mottled hypopigmentation and hyperpigmentation with biopsy site. (**A,** courtesy Department of Dermatology, University of North Carolina at Chapel Hill.)

apy with *D-penicillamine* or immunosuppressants is suboptimal but may slow the rate of visceral disease. Referral to a rheumatologist and to a pulmonologist is appropriate.

For information and support, contact the United Scleroderma Foundation.*

SUGGESTED READING

American Rheumatism Association: Preliminary criteria for the classification of systemic sclerosis (scleroderma): subcommittee for scleroderma criteria for the American Rheumatism Association diagnostic and therapeutic criteria committee, *Arthritis Rheum* 23:581–590, 1980.

Bernard P, Bonnetblanc J-M: Dermatomyositis and malignancy, *J Invest Dermatol* 100:1285–1325, 1993.

Boumpas DT et al: Systemic lupus erythematosus: emerging concepts. *Ann Int Med* 123:42–53, 1995.

Drake LA et al: Guidelines of care for dermatomyositis, *J Am Acad Dermatol* 34:824–829, 1996.

Drake LA et al: Guidelines of care for lupus erythematosus, *J Am Acad Dermatol* 34:830–836, 1996.

Mills JA: Systemic lupus erythematosus, *N Engl J Med* 330:1871–1879, 1994.

Perez MI, Kohn SR: Systemic sclerosis, *J Am Acad Dermatol* 28:525–547, 1993.

Provost TT, Watson R, Simmons-O'Brien E: Significance of anti-Ro (SSA Antibody in evaluation of patients with cutaneous manifestations of a connective tissue disease, *J Am Acad Dermatol* 35:147–169, 1996.

Rocco VK, Hurd ER: Scleroderma and scleroderma-like disorders, *Semin Arthritis Rheum* 16:22–69, 1986.

Smith CD, Marino C, Rothfield NF: The clinical utility of the lupus band test, *Arthritis Rheum* 27:382–387, 1984.

*United Scleroderma Foundation, Inc., P.O. Box 399, 734 East Lake Ave., Ste. 5 Watsonville CA, 95076; 1-800-722 HOPE, FAX 408-728-3328.

Web site: http://www.scleroderma.org

CHAPTER 20

Metabolic and Inherited Diseases

ACANTHOSIS NIGRICANS ICD-9 (701.2)

Acanthosis (*acantho* meaning *thorn*) nigricans (*black*) is a reactive, characteristic skin pattern seen in association with obesity and other systemic disorders (Box 20–1). The skin is thought to become thickened in response to a circulating growth factor. Lesions are gray-brown to black, rough, have thickened plaques and prominent skin lines, and occur most commonly in flexural areas (e.g., axillae, back and sides of neck, inguinal creases, inframammary) but may occur elsewhere (Fig. 20–1). The texture of lesions may be velvety because of small skin elevations. Internal malignancies are associated with extensive lesions, lesions that are rapidly progressive,

lesions with which there is mucous membrane involvement, and lesions with which there is prominent sole and palm involvement.

Treatment involves weight reduction for lesions in obese patients, particularly because insulin resistance plays a role in nonmalignancy-associated acanthosis nigricans. If a malignancy is discovered, it's successful treatment is correlated with improvement of the skin lesions. Extremely thick lesions may have a bad odor; treatment with antibacterial soaps (e.g., Phisoderm) and topical antibiotics (e.g., *erythromycin* 2% solution applied twice daily) may help in such cases.

BOX 20–1.

Disorders Associated With Acanthosis Nigricans Skin Lesions

Drug-induced: High-dose nicotinic acid, systemic corticosteroids, diethylstilbestrol, pituitary extract, fusidic acid, insulin
Endocrine disorders related to insulin resistance: Diabetes mellitus, thyroid disease, Cushing's syndrome
Hereditary: Benign without associations
Malignancy (rare): Adenocarcinoma
Obesity-associated

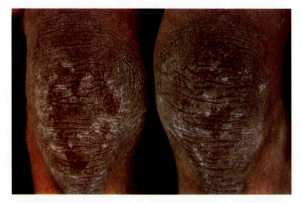

Fig. 20–1
Acanthosis nigricans with velvety-appearing plaques on the knees of a diabetic man. (Courtesy Medical College of Georgia, Division of Dermatology.)

EHLERS-DANLOS SYNDROME ICD-9 (756.83)

Ehlers-Danlos syndrome is a group of nine or ten heterogeneous, inherited disorders, all of which share similar abnormalities of connective tissue. Characterization often is made by the specific collagen synthesis abnormality, by the inheritance pattern, or on clinical findings. Subtypes range from those with very mild skin involvement (type 2) to those with life-threatening involvement of large blood vessels, such as aortic aneurysm (type 4). The common clinical feature is skin or joint hyperextensibility (Fig. 20–2). General features are shown in Box 20–2.

Ehlers-Danlos syndrome can be differentiated from *cutis laxa* by the latter's characteristic skin, which hangs in redundant folds, and the ab-

BOX 20–2.

Ehlers-Danlos Syndrome: Common Clinical Findings

Skin hyperextensibility and fragility
Poor wound healing
Broad, atrophic scars with a cigarette-paper appearance
Blood vessel fragility, ranging from easy bruisability to aortic aneurysm
Joint hypermobility (i.e., dislocated joints)
    Dorsiflexion of the fifth finger more than 90 degrees, with forearm flat
    Passive apposition of the thumb to the flexor forearm
    Hyperextension of the elbow or knee more than 10 degrees
    Forward trunk flexion, with palms resting easily on the floor

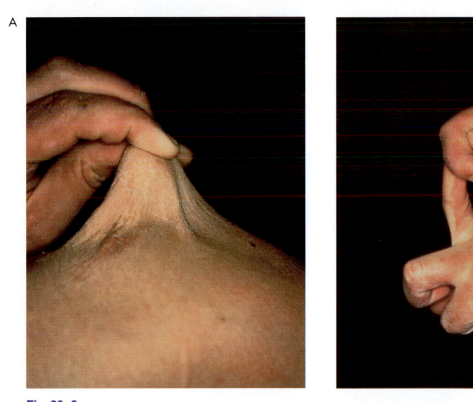

A   B

Fig. 20–2
Ehlers-Danlos syndrome with hyperextensibility of **A,** skin and **B,** joints. (Courtesy Medical College of Georgia, Division of Dermatology.)

sence of other findings, such as easy bruisability or joint hypermobility.

The best treatment is patient education and referral. Instruct patients to avoid unnecessary procedures, because of poor overall wound healing. When the diagnosis is suspected, refer patients for consultation and genetic counseling. The Ehlers-Danlos National Foundation provides patient support and information.

ICHTHYOSIS VULGARIS ICD-9 (757.1)

Ichthyosis vulgaris is a common (incidence 1:300), autosomal dominant, inherited disorder characterized by dry, scaling skin. So named because of its clinical appearance similar to fish scales (ichthyosis, fishlike), the onset is usually between ages 1 and 4, becoming more extensive with age, often at puberty. Ichthyosis is worse in dry weather, particularly winter. When it is associated with atopic dermatitis, increased palmar skin markings are seen, along with the keratin follicular plugging of keratosis pilaris.

Clinically, scales are generalized and are characteristically rectangular, often best appreciated with a magnifying hand lens. Lesions are usually most severe on the shin, back, or heels, sparing the flexural areas (Fig. 20–3).

Treatment consists of use of emollients and avoidance of dry environments. Instruct patients to use *urea* or *lactic acid* 10% to 20% creams or lotions chronically. Such creams (e.g., Carmol 10, Carmol 20, Ultramide, and Lachydrin 5) are available without a prescription. Lachydrin 12% is also available by prescription. Best results occur when such creams are applied to moist

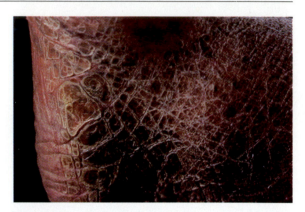

Fig. 20–3
Ichthyosis vulgaris. Note the characteristic fishlike scales on the heel. (Courtesy Medical College of Georgia, Division of Dermatology.)

skin directly after bathing. Humidifiers also may be helpful for patients who live in a dry environment.

For patient support or information regarding ichthyosis vulgaris or more rare ichthyotic diseases, contact the Foundation for Ichthyosis and Related Skin Types (FIRST).*

MYXEDEMA ICD-9 (HYPOTHYROIDISM 244.9; PRETIBIAL 242.9)

Myxedema is the broad term referring to a mucoidlike edema of the soft tissues associated with severe, generalized hypothyroidism. It is caused by excess dermal ground substance. Characteristic skin signs in generalized myxedema include cold, dry skin; puffy, nonpitting edema of the hands, face, and eyelids; broad nose; thick lips; macroglossia; coarse scalp hair; alopecia; loss of the lateral third of the eyebrows; and ivory-yellow skin. Often patients also have poor wound healing and frequent ecchymoses. The skin changes are usually reversible

*Foundation for Ichthyosis and Related Skin Types (FIRST), P.O. Box 669, Ardmore, PA 19003-0669; 1-610-789-4366, 1-800-545-3286.

with appropriate treatment of the underlying hypothyroidism.

Pretibial myxedema is a separate, distinct clinical entity that may be associated with hyperthyroidism, hypothyroidism, or euthyroidism. Lesions often occur after treatment of hyperthyroidism, or, rarely, they may be associated with the triad of Graves' disease (exophthalmos, hyperthyroidism, diffuse toxic goiter). Characteristic skin findings include bilateral, pretibial waxy nodules and plaques that are pink or salmon (Fig. 20–4). Such lesions have nonpitting edema and prominent hair follicles, giving a peau d'orange look to the skin. Clubbing of the fingers with osteoarthropathy, known as *thyroid acropachy,* occurs rarely. Treatment of pretibial myxedema skin changes involves the use of potent topical corticosteroids (e.g., *betamethasone diproprionate* 0.05% cream twice daily), monitoring for skin atrophy. Treatment of any underlying thyroid disease will not necessarily alter pretibial myxedema lesions.

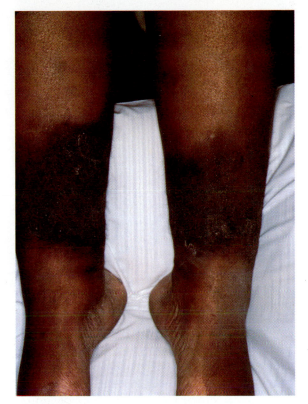

Fig. 20–4
Pretibial myxedema with hyperpigmented, indurated plaques. (Courtesy Medical College of Georgia, Department of Dermatology.)

NECROBIOSIS LIPOIDICA ICD-9 (709.3)

Necrobiosis lipoidica is an inflammatory skin disorder of unknown cause, occurring three times more often in females than in males. The name of this disease aptly describes its clinical findings: necrobiosis refers to the type of inflammation that occurs when lesions are examined histologically; lipoidica is the yellow appearance of lesions as a result of lipid deposits occurring secondary to inflammation.

The disease is frequently associated with diabetes. Although lesions occur in only 0.3% of all diabetics, more than three fourths of patients with the skin lesions either have or will develop diabetes mellitus, have a positive family history of diabetes, or have impaired glucose tolerance. There is no relationship to diabetic metabolic control.

Asymptomatic skin lesions usually occur on the lower extremities (15% of patients will have lesions elsewhere) in young or middle-age adults as oval or irregularly shaped, indurated plaques with central atrophy and yellow pigmentation (Fig. 20–5). Peripherally, along the margins, is either red-brown or violaceous pigmentation. Telangiectasia also may be seen. Ulceration may occur in one third of cases.

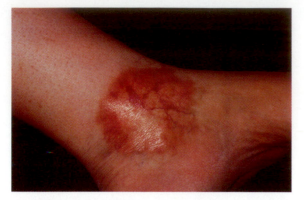

Fig. 20–5
Necrobiosis lipoidica. Note the thin, yellow, atrophic plaque with telangiectasia.

The differential diagnosis includes *granuloma annulare,* asymptomatic annular red plaques that occur more commonly on the dorsum of the extremities or posterior neck and that lack a yellow discoloration. Lesions of *sarcoidosis, rheumatoid nodules,* and *xanthomas* may appear quite similar and can be differentiated by biopsy.

Treatment is suboptimal at best, but initially try using a moderate-strength topical steroid (e.g., *triamcinolone acetonide* 0.1% cream 3 times daily). If there is no improvement after 2 weeks, consider using *betamethasone diproprionate* 0.05% twice daily, monitoring for skin atrophy. Intralesional *triamcinolone* 5 to 10 mg/ml can be attempted carefully. Avoid using topical corticosteroids if any ulcers are present. Referral or consultation often is indicated.

NEUROFIBROMATOSIS (VON RECKLINGHAUSEN'S DISEASE) ICD-9 (237.71)

Neurofibromatosis (von Recklinghausen's disease) is a neurocutaneous disease involving abnormalities of cells derived from the neural crest. It occurs with a frequency of 3 to 4:10,000, usually manifesting during late childhood. Multiple hamartomas occur in many organ systems, particularly the skin, brain, kidneys, and eyes. Patients must be montiored for conditions such as impaired vision, developmental disabilities, hearing problems, short stature, hypogonadism, and precocious puberty.

Fifty percent of cases are inherited in an autosomal dominant pattern; the rest are the result of spontaneous mutations. The defect has been localized to chromosome 17 for type 1 disease. Type 2 disease, localized to chromosome 22, refers to neurofibromatosis in which there are bilateral acoustic neuromas and much less skin involvement.

Typical skin findings include *café au lait spots,* which are hyperpigmented macules that often appear shortly after birth. Other skin findings include cutaneous and subcutaneous tumors. The cutaneous signs usually are the basis for an initial diagnosis (Boxes 20–3, 20–4, and Figs. 20–6 to 20–8).

Up to 5% of the skin tumors may eventually develop into malignancies (sarcomas), which, along with central nervous system involvement

BOX 20–3.
Skin Findings in Neurofibromatosis

Neurofibromas
  Discrete, soft papules to large nodules (Fig. 20–6)
    When pressed, the tumor may invaginate into the skin, causing a sign known as buttonholing (Fig. 20–7)
Café au lait
  Cutaneous hyperpigmented patches, light to dark brown spots appearing shortly after birth (Fig. 20–8). Frecklelike axillary pigmentation characteristic (Crowe's sign). Inguinal or inframammary freckling less common.
  Prepuberty: 6 lesions greater than 5 mm
  Postpuberty: 6 lesions greater than 15 mm
Plexiform neuromas
  Large, drooping tumors that have the consistency of soft neuromas.

BOX 20–4.

Diagnosis of Neurofibromatosis*†

Six or more café au lait macules
Two or more neurofibromas or one plexiform neuroma
Multiple freckles in the axillary or inguinal regions
Sphenoid wing dysplasia, congential bowing or thinning of long bone cortex, with or without pseudoarthrosis
Bilateral optic nerve gliomas
Two or more iris Lisch nodules (pigmented iris hamartomas) on slit examination
Neurofibromatosis in a first-degree relative

*Modified from Neurofibromatosis Res Newslett 2:2, 1986.
†Neurofibromatosis type 1 is present if ≥2 of the above are present in the absence of any other diseases causing the lesions.

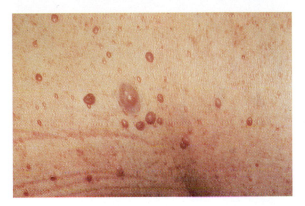

Fig. 20-6
Multiple papules and nodules in a patient with neurofibromatosis. (Courtesy Department of Dermatology, University of North Carolina at Chapel Hill.)

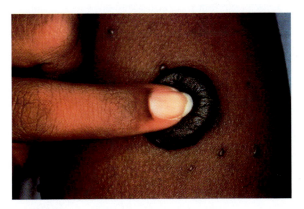

Fig. 20–7
Classic buttonholing of a neurofibroma. (Courtesy Medical College of Georgia, Division of Dermatology.)

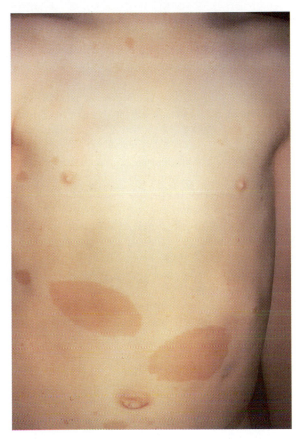

Fig. 20-8
Large, hyperpigmented macules (café au lait spots) in a child with neurofibromatosis. (Courtesy Department of Dermatology, University of North Carolina at Chapel Hill.)

(astrocytomas) or extramedullary spinal cord lesions, contribute to the shortened life span in patients with the disease. Although 10% to 20% of the normal population has café au lait spots, the presence of multiple lesions or a positive family history should warrant further investigation. There is no known cure, but affected individuals and parents of an affected child should be referred for genetic counseling and monitoring for potential sequelae.

For patient support and information contact the National Neurofibromatosis Foundation.*

*National Neurofibromatosis Foundation, 95 Pine St., 16th Floor, New York, NY 10005; 1-800-323-7938, 212-344-6633, FAX 212-747-0004; Website: http://nf.org/

PSEUDOXANTHOMA ELASTICUM ICD-9 (757.39)

Pseudoxanthoma elasticum is an inherited disorder of abnormal elastic tissue and calcification. The primary organ systems involved include the skin, eyes, and cardiovascular systems, with progressive skin lesions developing in 80% of individuals before age 20. The characteristic skin findings are 2- to 5-mm yellow to orange papules, which may coalesce into irregularly shaped plaques bounded by normal skin. Because such lesions have a pebbly appearance and are yellow, they are named *pseudoxanthomas*. The texture of the skin has been likened to plucked-chicken skin (Fig. 20–9). Lesions occur most commonly in flexural areas, such as the neck and axillary folds, periumbilically, and on the inner lower lip.

The primary ocular finding is that of angioid streaks, representing tears in Bruch's membrane, but this finding is seen in other disorders as well. Severe vision loss occurs in 3% to 8% of patients. Common cardiovascular manifestations include hypertension, peripheral vascular disease, and gastrointestinal bleeding.

Diagnosis is based on the clinical appearance and findings on histologic examination of lesional skin. Treatment consists of close ophthalmologic management, monitoring and treatment of any cardiovascular symptoms, and dietary consultation. Patients should be referred for genetic counseling.

For information and patient support contact the National Association for Pseudoxanthoma Elasticum.*

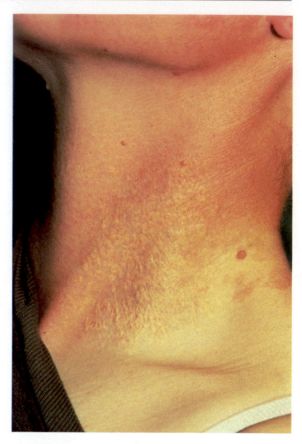

Fig. 20-9
Pseudoxanthoma elasticum with coalescing papules on the neck, giving a pebbly, plucked-chicken skin appearance. (Courtesy Marshall Guill, MD.)

TUBEROUS SCLEROSIS ICD-9 (759.5)

Tuberous sclerosis is an autosomal dominant, inherited disorder characterized by limited hyperplasia of both ectodermal and mesodermal cells. The incidence is 5 to 7:100,000, with one third of

patients having a positive family history and the remaining thought to represent spontaneous mutations. *The classic triad consists of adenoma sebaceum (which are actually angiofibromas), epilepsy, and mental retardation.* Central nervous system involvement includes calcified

*National Association for Pseudoxanthoma Elasticum, 1420 Augdon St., Denver, CO 80218; 303-321-6347.

gliomas, seizure disorders, retinal gliomas, and gray to yellow retinal plaques known as *phakomas*. Hamartomas of the kidney, heart, and liver may also be found. Variable expression occurs, and patients may manifest all or little of the syndrome (i.e., they may be of normal intelligence).

Skin findings are present in infancy as the earliest signs of the disease. *Hypopigmented macules,* accentuated with the use of Wood's light, are present in 85% of affected individuals. These macules, most commonly seen on the trunk or limbs, are in the shape of an ash leaf and may be single or multiple (Fig. 20–10). A *shagreen patch* is found in 80% of patients and actually is a connective tissue nevus clinically seen in the lumbosacral region as a yellow to flesh-colored plaque that has the texture of pig skin (Fig. 20–11). The *angiofibromas* occur as red to pink papules or nodules, predominantly in the nasolabial folds, cheeks, and forehead in 90% of patients over age 4. Periungual angiofibromas, known as *Koenen's tumors,* are also characteristic (Fig. 20–12).

The diagnosis is made on clinical findings and a skin biopsy specimen showing angiofibromas. A computed tomography scan is indicated to identify brain calcifications in an infant with ash leaf spots, shagreen patches, or other manifesta-tions. Angiofibromas may be removed for cosmetic purposes with excision, laser, cryosurgery, or dermabrasion. Patients and families should be referred for genetic counseling.

For patient information and support contact the Tuberous Sclerosis Association of America, Inc.*

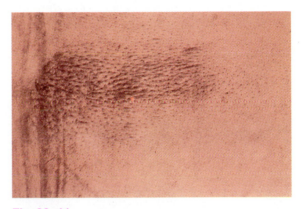

Fig. 20–11
Shagreen patch of tuberous sclerosis with pigskin appearance. (Courtesy Department of Dermatology, University of North Carolina at Chapel Hill.)

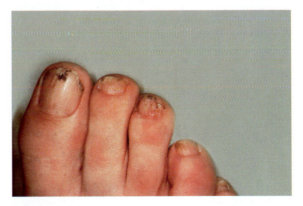

Fig. 20–12
Tuberous sclerosis. Periungual angiofibromas. (Courtesy Department of Dermatology, University of North Carolina at Chapel Hill.)

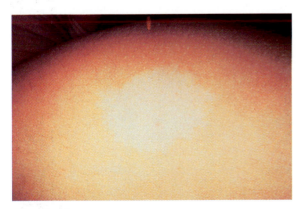

Fig. 20–10
Ash leaf spot in tuberous sclerosis. (Courtesy Beverly Sanders, MD.)

*Tuberous Sclerosis Association of America, Inc., 8181 Professional Pl., Ste. 110, Landover, MD 20785; 1-800-CAL-NTSA, 301-459-9888, FAX 301-459-0394.

XANTHOMAS ICD-9 (272.2)

Xanthomas represent skin, subcutaneous tissue, and tendon lipid deposits in response to abnormal lipid concentrations or other lipoprotein abnormalities. Primary dyslipidemias are associated with specific, genetically determined lipoprotein patterns, whereas secondary dyslipidemias result from other underlying diseases (Tables 20–1 and 20–2). Xanthomas are seen with primary and secondary dyslipidemias, and the diagnosis of a primary lipid disorder is made only after excluding secondary causes. Suspicion of a primary dyslipidemia should be heightened with any characteristic lesion in a patient younger than age 40 who has a family history of elevated lipid levels or associated cardiovascular disease.

Xanthomas are usually firm and yellow and involve characteristic sites (Table 20–3 and Figs. 20–13 and 20–14). Treatment involves a workup to exclude underlying diseases and treatment of the primary lipid disorder.

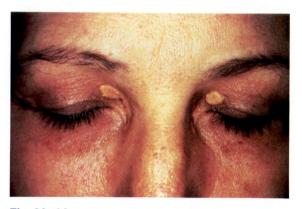

Fig. 20–14
Periorbital xanthelasmas in a woman with hypercholesterolemia. (Courtesy Medical College of Georgia, Division of Dermatology.)

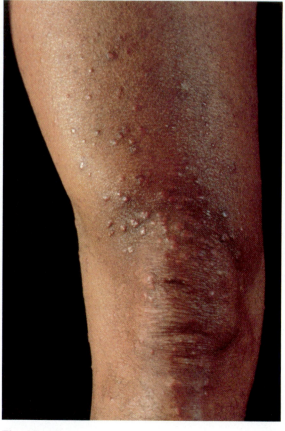

Fig. 20–13
Eruptive xanthoma with multiple yellow papules in a patient with new-onset diabetes and elevated triglyceride levels. (Courtesy of Medical College of Georgia, Division of Dermatology.)

TABLE 20–1.

Primary Hyperlipoproteinemias and Dermatologic Manifestations

Lipoprotein Phenotype	Lipoprotein Elevation*	Lipid Elevation	Skin Xanthoma(s)
I	Chylomicrons	Triglyceride	Eruptive
IIa	LDL	Cholesterol	Tendon, tuberous, xanthelasma
IIb	LDL, VLDL	Cholesterol, triglyceride	Tendon, tuberous, xanthelasma
III	IDL	Cholesterol, triglyceride	Palmar
IV	VLDL	Triglyceride	—
V	Chylomicrons VLDL	Triglyceride, cholesterol	Eruptive

*LDL = low density lipoprotein; VLDL = very low-density lipoprotein; IDL = intermediate-density lipoprotein.

TABLE 20–2.

Secondary Dyslipidemias

Lipid Disorder	Cause
Hypercholesterolemia	Diet, dysproteinemias, hypothyroidism, nephrosis, obstructive liver disease, porphyria
Hypertriglyceridemia	Diet, obesity, diabetes mellitus, alcohol abuse, renal failure, lupus erythematosus, glycogen storage disease, drugs-estrogens, isotretinoin

TABLE 20–3.

Types of Xanthomas

Xanthoma	Distribution	Description
Eruptive	Extensor surfaces: elbows, knees; pressure sites: buttocks, back; areas of trauma	Sudden appearance of discrete yellow papules with a red halo 1–6 mm (Fig. 20–13); usually asymptomatic but may be quite pruritic
Tuberous	Elbows, knees, digits, buttocks	Lesions are small, soft yellow-orange plaques and noninflammatory nodules
Tendinous	Achilles tendon, extensor tendons of digits	Firm, irregular, slow-growing nodules
Planar		
Palmar	Palmar creases	Yellow-orange macular discolorations
Planar	Hands, feet, or diffuse	Well-circumscribed macules or plaques
Xanthelasmas	Periorbital	Yellow macules of plaques (Fig. 20–14)

SUGGESTED READING

Heymann WR: Cutaneous manifestations of thyroid disease, *J Am Acad Dermatol* 26: 885–902, 1992.

Holt WS Jr, Harsha DM: Neurofibromatosis type 1: a case report and review of the literature, *J Fam Pract* 34:617–624, 1992.

Kuster W, Happle R: Neurocutaneous disorders in children, *Cur Opinion Ped* 5:436–440, 1993.

Lowitt MH: Dover JS: Necrobiosis lipoidica, *J Am Acad Dermatol* 25:735–748, 1991.

Neldner KH: Pseudoxanthoma elasticum, *Clin Dermatol* 6:1, 1988.

Patsch W, Patsch J: The hyperlipidemias, *Med Clin North Am* 73:859–883, 1989.

Prockop DJ, Kivirikko KI: Hereditable disease of collagen, *N Engl J Med* 311:376–386, 1984.

Riccardi VN, Von R: Neurofibromatosis, *N Engl J Med* 305:1617–1627, 1981.

Schaefer E, Levy R: Pathogenesis and management of lipoprotein disorders, *N Engl J Med* 312:1300–1310, 1985.

Schwartz RA: Acanthosis nigricans, *J Am Acad Dermatol* 31:1–19, 1994.

Sorensen SA, Mulvihill JJ, Nielsen A: Long-term follow-up of von Recklinghausen neurofibromatosis, *N Engl J Med* 314:1010–1015, 1986.

Williams ML, Elias PM: Genetically transmitted, generalized disorders of cornification: the ichthyoses, *Dermatol Clin* 5:155–178, 1987.

CHAPTER 21

Cutaneous Signs of Internal Malignancies

Virtually any internal malignancy may produce cutaneous skin manifestations. Most of these manifestations are nonspecific findings and can be related to a host of disorders; many are discussed elsewhere in this book. Paget's disease of the nipple and extramammary Paget's disease are associated with ductal breast carcinoma or adenocarcinoma (discussed fully in Chapter 13), as is metastatic melanoma, which usually has primary skin findings but may have secondary skin metastases. Generalized pruritus, often with few skin findings other than excoriations, is an important marker for internal malignancies, particularly leukemia and lymphoma (workup and discussion are presented in Chapter 23).

Many inherited diseases, such as Peutz-Jeghers syndrome (multiple small bowel polyps and pigmented macules), are associated with both primary skin findings and a propensity for an internal malignancy. Skin findings associated with many inherited diseases and paraneoplastic dermatoses are shown in Table 21–1. Skin findings in paraneoplastic dermatoses also may or may not be associated with various internal neoplasms (e.g., patients with acanthosis nigricans may or may not have underlying carcinoma, whereas those with necrolytic migratory erythema always have an underlying glucagonoma).

The internal malignancies discussed in this chapter exhibit clinical skin findings for which clinicians should maintain a high index of suspicion. Recognition of these disorders at their earliest stages may allow for improved patient survival or cure.

LANGERHANS' CELL HISTIOCYTOSIS ICD-9 (277.8, EXCEPT LETTERER-SIWE DISEASE 202.5)

Langerhans cell histiocytosis is a group of disorders characterized by granulomatous proliferation of histiocytic (Langerhans') cells. All of these disorders exhibit a proliferation of histiocytes in various organ tissues, such as the skin, liver, lymph nodes, and bones. Manifestations vary from chronic ulcerations to leukemic forms. Histiocytosis X occurs most commonly in children age 1 to 4. Although it is classified into three forms, overlap occurs between categories.

Eosinophilic granuloma is the chronic form, in which patients develop either solitary or multiple bone lesions involving only the axial skeleton. It usually occurs in children age 2 to 5, but may occur in adults. Skin lesions are rare and usually noduloulcerative.

Hand-Schüller-Christian syndrome involves lesions in bone plus lesser involvement of other tissues. It occurs most commonly in children age 2 to 6. Chronic otitis media may be the initial

TABLE 21–1.
Cutaneous Signs of Internal Neoplasms

Syndrome/Marker	Skin Findings	Internal Neoplasm
Genodermatoses:		
Primary immunodeficiency syndromes	Recurrent infections; some with severe eczema	Leukemia; lymphoma
Chromosomal instability syndromes	Photosensitivity, sclerodermoid changes, reticulate hyperpigmentation	Lymphoreticular malignancies, Squamous cell carcinoma
Gastrointestinal polyposis syndromes:		
Gardner's syndrome	Osteomas, epidermoid cysts, desmoid tumors, fibromas, lipomas	Gastrointestinal carcinoma
Peutz-Jeghers syndrome	Pigmented macules of lips; acral and periorificial	Gastrointestinal, genitourinary carcinomas
Cowden disease (multiple hamartomas)	Facial trichoepitheliomas, lipomas, oral papillomatosis, acral keratoses, angiomas	Breast, thyroid, uterine carcinomas
Muir-Torre syndrome	Multiple sebaceous neoplasms; with or without keratoacanthomas	Gastrointestinal and genitourinary carcinomas
Howel-Evans' syndrome	Palmoplantar keratoses	Esophageal carcinoma
Multiple endocrine neoplasia type III	Multiple neuromas, especially of lips, tongue, buccal mucosa, eyelids, and conjunctivae	Medullary thyroid carcinoma, pheochromocytoma
Nevoid basal cell syndrome	Multiple basal cell carcinomas, odontogenic cysts; palmar/plantar pits	CNS tumors (medulloblastoma)
Neurofibromatosis	Multiple café au lait macules, neurofibromas, iris hamartomas	Neural crest tumors
Hemochromatosis	Gray-brown pigmentation, skin atrophy	Hepatoma
Paraneoplastic dermatoses:		
Acanthosis nigricans	Pruritic, symmetric hyperpigmentation with thickening of skin in flexural areas, mucosal papillomas	Gastrointestinal, liver, lung, and breast carcinoma
Acanthosis palmaris	Epidermal thickening, hyperkeratosis of palms and volar fingers	Stomach and lung carcinoma
Amyloidosis	Eyelid and periorbital purpura; waxy, smooth papules and plaques of face, eyelids, oral mucosa; tongue enlargement	Multiple myeloma
Bazex's syndrome	Paronychia, nail dystrophy, erythematous to violaceous psoriasiform plaques on dorsal digits, nasal bridge, helices of ears	Squamous cell carcinoma (gastrointestinal and upper respiratory tract)
Carcinoid syndrome	Deep or purple flushing of head/neck; telangiectasia, pellagra-like rash	Carcinoid tumor

Condition	Description	Associated malignancy
Cronkhite-Canada syndrome	Hyperpigmented macules up to 10 cm dia.; extremities, palms, soles, face, buccal mucosa	Colon carcinoma
Cryoglobulinemia	Acral cyanosis, purpura, urticaria, Raynaud's, superficial or deep ulceration	Myeloma
Cushing's syndrome	Hyperpigmentation, edema, muscle wasting	Small cell lung carcinoma, carcinoid tumor
Dermatitis herpetiformis	Intensely pruritic vesicles of extensor surfaces; elbows, knees, buttocks	Intestinal lymphoma
Dermatomyositis	Heliotrope periobital eruption with edema; periungual telangiectasia; poikiloderma; scaling erythematous papules on extensor bony prominences	Variety; age-related
Digital clubbing	Soft tissue hypertrophy of distal phalanges	Intrathoracic neoplasms
Erythema gyratum repens	Irregular urticarial bands of erythema with fine scale in a polycyclic (grain of wood) pattern	Lung, breast carcinoma
Erythroderma	Generalized erythema with scaling, often pruritic	Lymphoproliferative
Extramammary Paget's disease	Erythematous scaling plaque with erosion of the perineum/genitalia	Adnexal, gastrointestinal, genitourinary carcinomas
Hypertrichosis lanuginosa	Fine hypertrichosis; face, then generalized; glossitis; acanthosis nigricans	Colon, lung carcinoma
Ichthyosis, acquired	> age 20; dry scaling eruption of trunk and legs; may generalize	Lymphoma, sarcoma
Leser-Trélat	Multiple seborrheic keratoses appearing over a few weeks to months	Stomach, leukemia, lymphoma, breast carcinoma
Multicentric reticulohistiocytosis	Yellow or red papules on hands and mucous membranes; ears, nose, scalp may be involved; arthritis (mutilans)	Multiple
Necrolytic migratory erythema	Erythematous erosive plaques with serpiginous borders in groin, thighs, acral; painful glossitis and angular stomatitis	Glucagonoma
Paraneoplastic pemphigus	Pruritic polymorphous papules, bullae with erosions, often mucocutaneous	Lymphoreticular, sarcoma, lung carcinoma
Pyoderma gangrenosum	Pustule or papule evolves into nodule that ulcerates, with an undermined irregular violaceous border. Usually on extremities	Leukemia
Sweet's syndrome (Acute neutrophilic dermatosis)	Erythematous to violaceous papules, nodular plaques on arms, head, or neck; may develop vesiculopustules	Leukemia
Trousseau's syndrome	Superficial migratory thrombophlebitis, tender nodules along the course of a superficial vein	Pancreas, lung, stomach, and colon carcinoma

sign. The classic triad of defects of cranial bone, exophthalmos, and diabetes insipidus is found only rarely. Skin lesions include chronic ulcerations, especially of the inguinal region, and lesions similar to those found in Letterer-Siwe disease. These patients have a 50% mortality rate.

Letterer-Siwe disease, the most serious form of histiocytosis X, occurs as the rapid onset of a petechial, seborrheic-like eruption in children age 3 months to 3 years, associated with extensive multiple organ involvement (i.e., hepatosplenomegaly, lymphadenopathy, pulmonary infiltration, fever, anemia, and thrombocytopenia). The skin eruption appears as small, scaly papules or vesicles with yellowish scale and petechiae and has a predilection for the scalp and intertriginous areas (Fig. 21–1). Other problems include chronic external otitis, peridontal disease, and loss of teeth.

If skin lesions are present, multiple biopsy specimens should be submitted from several lesions. The presence of *Birbeck granules,* an ultrastructural component in the histiocytes, is diagnostic for the disorder and is seen only on electron microscopy. Staining for CD1a antigen (T6) on the lesional cell will be positive.

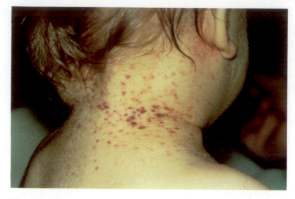

Fig. 21–1
Scaling papules with hemorrhagic areas in an infant with Letterer-Siwe disease. (Courtesy Medical College of Georgia, Division of Dermatology.)

Treatment ranges from radiation therapy for a single lesion to chemotherapy for more than one lesion. The natural history of the skin disease is for involution in 1 to 3 years. Bone marrow failure may ensue, with a dismal prognosis for many patients, particularly those who are younger at diagnosis.

For more information contact the Histiocytosis Association of America, Inc.*

LYMPHOMA/LEUKEMIA ICD-9 (BY TYPING OF LYMPHOMA OR LEUKEMIA)

Non–T-cell lymphomas or leukemias rarely are initially found in the skin. When they are found, the initial manifestation is usually nonspecific (Box 21–1), such as generalized pruritus, vasculitis, erythroderma, or purpura related to thrombocytopenia. In addition, certain skin infections, such as herpes zoster, fungal infections, and other opportunistic infections, are seen more often because of decreased cell-mediated immunity.

Skin involvement occurs in 17% of patients with B-cell lymphomas, either by direct extension from an involved node, hematogenous dissemination or, very rarely, initially in the skin. Four percent to 12% of Hodgkin's lymphomas eventually involve the skin, manifesting as purplish papules, plaques, or nodules. Leukemic

BOX 21–1.
Nonspecific Skin Conditions Associated With Lymphoma/Leukemia

Generalized pruritus
Vasculitis
Erythroderma
Purpura
Erythema multiforme
Pyoderma gangrenosum
Acanthosis nigricans
Urticaria
Dermatomyositis
Sweet's syndrome
Stomatitis
Erythema nodosum
Ichthyosis

*Histiocytosis Association of America, Inc., 302 N. Broadway, Pitman NJ 08071; 609-589-6606.

infiltration of the skin occurs in up to 20% of patients with chronic lymphocytic leukemia and less commonly in other forms. Such infiltration manifests as red to plum plaques or nodules that show atypical cells on skin biopsy (Fig. 21–2).

Biopsies of involved skin may require evaluation with special markers to diagnose lymphoma, which also may require special considerations for tissue handling (e.g., fresh tissue or frozen tissue for flow cytometry or immunologic marker studies at specialized facilities).

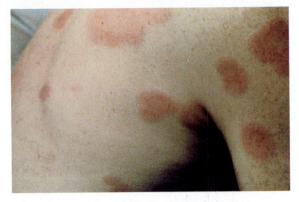

Fig. 21–2
Leukemic infiltration of the skin. Note the widespread indurated plaques on the trunk. (Courtesy John Cook, MD.)

METASTATIC CARCINOMA ICD-9 (199.1)

Three percent to 5% of all carcinomas metastasize to the skin, although rarely does a carcinoma initially manifest solely in the skin (with the exception of melanoma). Breast and colon cancer in women and lung and colon cancer in men are most frequently associated with skin metastasis. Ovary, stomach, and kidney cancers also metastasize to the skin, but at lower rates. Melanoma is the most common skin cancer to metastasize to other organs.

Cutaneous metastases appear as firm papules or nodules of recent onset. They may occur individually or in clusters. The color often is yellow, purple, blue, or brown, and lesions have a predilection for the scalp and trunk (Fig. 21–3). Direct extension to skin on the chest wall is not uncommon in breast carcinoma. Almost all lesions are associated with a poor prognosis because they herald dissemination.

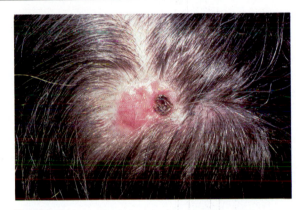

Fig. 21–3
Adenocarcinoma metastatic to the scalp, manifesting as a new nodule with ulceration and alopecia. (Courtesy Department of Dermatology, University of North Carolina at Chapel Hill.)

SUGGESTED READING

Egeler RM, D'Angio GJ: Langerhans' cell histiocytosis, *J Pediatr* 127:1–11, 1995.

Poole S, Fenske NA: Cutaneous markers of internal malignancy. I. Malignant involvement of the skin and the genodermatoses, *J Am Acad Dermatol* 28:1–13, 1993.

Poole S, Fenske NA: Cutaneous markers of internal malignancy. II. Paraneoplastic dermatoses and environmental carcinogens, *J Am Acad Dermatol* 28:147–164, 1993.

Schwartz RA: Cutaneous metastatic disease, *J Am Acad Dermatol* 33:161–182, 1995.

CHAPTER 22

Tropical Dermatology

Cutaneous diseases are common in the tropics, and multiple factors are important in the disease process, including specific geographic locations and habitats, natural environments that facilitate growth and survival of organisms, and, often, poor public health conditions; however, most parasitic diseases in the tropics are caused by disruption of host-agent-environment relationships and failure to control disease vectors. Overpopulation, poor nutritional status, inadequate water supplies, overcrowded living conditions, inadequate sanitation, lower education rates, social and political unrest, forceful evacuation, and mass exodus compound problems and lead to skin conditions that are unusual during peacetime. Finally, prolonged exposure to high temperature and humidity promote growth and survival of potentially pathogenic organisms.

Bacterial skin infections comprise one third of all cutaneous conditions in tropical areas. In most countries of Asia, Africa, and South and Central America, patients from rural areas have minimum health care facilities available. Patients are treated mainly on the basis of a clinical diagnosis. Microscopic examination of blood film preparations, cultures, and biopsies are usually done in referral hospitals. For practical purposes, patients are referred to hospitals in towns that may be many miles away. This chapter provides an overview on the recognition, diagnosis, and treatment of the most common bacterial, parasitic, and fungal tropical diseases.

For more information on a specific disease, contact the Centers for Disease Control, Division of Parasitic Diseases or the National Institutes of Health.*

PARASITIC DISEASES IN THE TROPICS

FILARIASIS ICD-9 (125.9)

Filariasis represents a group of diseases occurring in the tropics that are caused by infestation with parasitic round worms known as *filarial worms* that affect both humans and animals. The disease is endemic to tropical and subtropical countries in Asia, Africa, and Central and South America. Seventy-six countries with more than 90 million people are affected, and 905 million people are at direct risk. Various species of the filarial helminth, especially *Wuchereria ban-*

■Contributing authors: Hirak Behari Routh, MBBS, Former Research Associate, Department of Dermatology and Cutaneous Biology, Jefferson Center for International Dermatology, Jefferson Medical College, Thomas Jefferson University, Philadelphia, Pennsylvania
Lawrence Charles Parish, MD, Clinical Professor, Department of Dermatology and Cutaneous Biology, Director, Jefferson Center for International Dermatology, Jefferson Medical College, Thomas Jefferson University, Philadelphia, Pennsylvania

*Centers for Disease Control, Division of Parasitic Diseases, 1-404-488-7760; National Institutes of Health, Division of Parasitic Diseases, 1-301-496-2486.

crofti, Brugia malayi, and *Onchocerca volvulus,* all vector-borne (Table 22–1), cause clinical disease in humans.

Disease expression is related to host immune responses to the organism. A more vigorous immune response is often seen in individuals new to an infested area. Tolerance, manifested by little immune response and little clinically obvious disease, is more typically seen in individuals endemic to an area.

Lymphatic filariasis causes obstruction of the lymphatic system, leading to progressive enlargement, coarsening, corrugation, and fissuring of the skin and adjacent subcutaneous tissues. Warty, superficial excrescences proliferate, until the leg or other organ resembles that of an elephant; thus, *elephantiasis.* Recurrent and acute, rather than chronic, infections are thought to be the cause of elephantiasis. About 10% of patients suffering from lymphatic filariasis will develop elephantiasis, with resulting deformity and ultimate difficulty of even normal movement or function.

Classic Description

The distribution typically involves the leg, penis, scrotum, vulva, arm, or breast, although unilateral leg involvement is most common (Fig. 22–1). Filarial fever may be seen, more commonly, in Malayan and Timorian filariasis. Filariasis caused by *Wuchereria bancrofti* may be heralded by a

unique retrograde lymphangitis and lymphedema. Secondary lesions include excessive connective tissue proliferation, secondary infections, and regional lymphangitis or elephantiasis.

Diagnosis

Diagnosis is usually made by clinical examination and a history of travel to or living in an endemic area. Microfilariae may be detected in peripheral blood smears. Eosinophilia may be present in acute infections. Parts of worms in a skin biopsy may be seen in chronic infestation.

Differential Diagnosis

The differential diagnosis of filariasis includes *elephantiasis nostras,* which can be distinguished by a history of recurrent attacks of streptococcal lymphangitis, biopsy, and lymphangiogram.

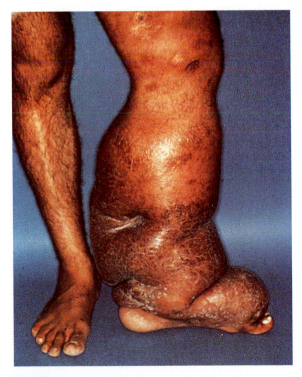

Fig. 22–1
Filariasis that eventually leads to elephantiasis. Note massive swelling of the extremity.

TABLE 22–1.

Filariasis: Vectors and Locations

Wuchereria bancrofti	Mosquito	Sub-Saharan Africa, Asia, South Pacific, western areas of the Pacific, Caribbean, Central and South America
Brugia malayi	Mosquito	Indonesia, Malaysia, Philippines
Onchocerca volvulus	Blackfly	Tropical Africa (99%), Yemen, Mexico, Central and South America

Chronic venous insufficiency is differentiated by dependent edema, stasis dermatitis, ulcers, and varicosities. *Deep fungal infections* are differentiated by culture and histologic findings. With *pretibial myxedema,* look for Graves' disease and the presence of mucin in the dermis.

Treatment and Patient Education

Medication and supportive measures are important in the management of elephantiasis. Give oral *diethylcarbamazine* 6 mg/kg for 12 days or use the following regimen: 50 mg PO on day 1, 50 mg 3 times a day on day 2; 100 mg 3 times a day on day 3, then 2 mg/kg 3 times a day on days 4 through 12. *Ivermectin* 150 g/kg in a single dose is used to suppress systemic microfilariae infections and reduce transmission, but the effect on the eradication of adult worms is unknown. Bed rest, elevation of the affected part, external compression stockings, and manual lymph drainage will help to relieve the massive swelling. Surgery is not always satisfactory. Patient education should emphasize regular cleaning of the affected part by washing and drying. Transmission may also be preventable by vector control and the use of ivermectin, as discussed above.

ONCHOCERCIASIS ICD-9 (125.3)

Onchocerciasis, or *river blindness,* is a devastating parasitic infestation of both the skin and eye that is caused by *Onchocerca volvulus* (Table 22-1). The vector, and hence the disease, usually affects people living near swiftly flowing rivers. An estimated 18 million people are affected, and 80 million more are at direct risk. The microfilariae tend to localize in the dermis, eyes, and regional lymph nodes. *Ocular damage is the most serious complication, but the skin lesions can prove disabling.*

Classic Description

Look for symmetric, pruritic papules or dermal nodules with secondary lichenification, involv-

ing the trunk, buttocks, thighs, legs, and axillae (Fig. 22–2). The manifestations of chronic disease vary by the geographic site of infestation. In Africa, chronic disease may be manifested as loss of skin elasticity, hypopigmentation, atrophy, scaling, development of furrows, and thickening of skin. In Yemen, patients may develop a condition known as *sowdah,* characterized by solitary extremity or anatomic quarter involvement, with edema, adenopathy, a pruritic papular eruption, and increased pigmentation. In Africa, encapsulated adult worms may develop in lower extremity or pelvic dermal or subcutaneous nodules. Scarring from microfilariae residing in lymph nodes may lead to the "hanging groin" phenomenon caused by atrophy and fibrosis. In Central America the head and upper body are more typically involved.

Ocular involvement in acute disease involves corneal opacities. Chronic disease results in keratitis, uveitis, and retinitis, with up to 15% of individuals in heavily infested areas being functionally blind.

Diagnosis

Microfilariae can be demonstrated with a skin-snip from a clinically involved site or bony prominence. The specimen should be placed in

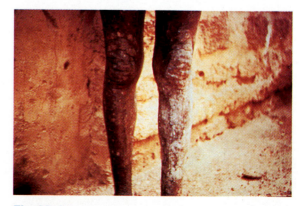

Fig. 22–2
Dermatitis often occurs in onchocerciasis. Note the pigmentary changes. (Courtesy Michel Larivière, MD, Paris, France.)

physiologic saline for several hours before microscopically examining it for microfilariae. Adult worms will be demonstrable by biopsy of an involved nodule. Slit lamp eye examination may also demonstrate microfilariae. Look for relative eosinophilia.

Differential Diagnosis

In early stages of *scabies* or *pyoderma,* look for the specific organisms. In chronic disease, consider *lichen simplex chronicus, vitiligo, pinta, yaws, leprosy, streptocerciasis (a rarer form of a different type of filariasis), cutis laxa, fibroma, or lipoma.* Snip biopsy or nodule biopsy will demonstrate evidence of infestation.

Treatment

Have patients take *ivermectin* 100 to 200 μg/kg in a single daily oral dose every 6 months for 10 to 15 years, to eradicate microfilariae. Ivermectin is contraindicated in patients with significant systemic disease, in lactating or pregnant women, and in children under age 5. *Prednisone* 1 mg/kg PO should be given for several days before treatment if ocular microfilariae are present. *Diethylcarbamazine* is an alternative drug for patients in whom ivermectin is contraindicated.

LEISHMANIASIS

The three cutaneous entities caused by the protozoa *Leishmania* are cutaneous leishmaniasis, post–kala-azar dermal leishmaniasis, and American mucocutaneous leishmaniasis. Leishmaniasis is most often transmitted by the sandfly *Phlebotomas* in various parts of the tropics.

CUTANEOUS LEISHMANIASIS ICD-9 (085.9)

Cutaneous leishmaniasis, also known as *Oriental sore, Delhi sore,* or *Baghdad boil,* is endemic in most of the tropics, extending from the Middle East to India and from the central Asian republics to China. It also occurs in the coastal areas of the Mediterranean. It is caused by the protozoa *Leishmania major* and *Leishmania tropica.*

The two forms of cutaneous leishmaniasis are the major, or wet, type that occurs mainly in rural areas and the minor, or dry, type that occurs in urban areas. Granulomatous changes are found in the disease, although the condition is usually self-healing.

Classic Description (Fig. 22–3)

After a typical incubation period of 1 to 12 weeks (but may extend to 1 year), pruritic, erythematous, and indurated papules form on exposed parts of the body, especially the face, nose, arms, and eyelids. Lesions are single or multiple and may slowly become crusted and develop into a shallow ulcer. Satellite nodules may develop at the ulcer edge. A *painless* nodule, up to 5 cm, forms within 3 to 4 months; healing occurs slowly, leaving a hypopigmented scar at the infestation site.

Diagnosis

The parasite can be seen in tissue fluid obtained by skin-slit (nonbloody) technique or by typical skin biopsy. Amastigotes (Leishman-Donovan bodies) may be detected both intracellularly and

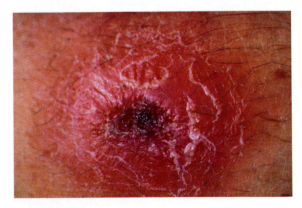

Fig. 22–3
Crusted lesions occurring in cutaneous leishmaniasis.

extracellularly with either Giemsa or Wright's stain. The leishmanin, or Montenegro, test (not available in the United States), an intradermal test for cell-mediated immunity, is positive in the early stages, but it is not clinically helpful in endemic areas. Culture media (NNN) overlaid with Schneider's *Drosophila* medium and fetal bovine serum) is not widely available but may be useful when organisms are not readily demonstrable with the staining techniques.

Differential Diagnosis

Cutaneous leishmaniasis is distinguished from *pyoderma, carbuncles, furuncles, deep fungal infections, mycobacterial infection, anthrax,* and *erysipelas* by bacteriologic cultures and the characteristic painless nodule. *Basal cell carcinoma, squamous cell carcinoma,* and *sarcoidosis* can be differentiated by biopsy.

Treatment

Isolated lesions of cutanous leishmaniasis may be self-limited and not require therapy. Systemic therapy is indicated for multiple lesions, for facial involvement, where cicatrix development may interfere with movement, or if visceral disease is evident. Pentavalent antimonials remain the drugs of choice. Use *sodium stibogluoconate* 20 mg/kg daily or *meglumine antimoniate* 20 mg/kg daily for up to 4 weeks or clinical or parasitologic cure. *Ketoconazole,* cryotherapy, surgical excision, or curettage may be used for smaller lesions.

POST–KALA-AZAR DERMAL LEISHMANIASIS ICD-9 (085.0)

Post–kala-azar dermal leishamaniasis usually follows an attack of visceral leishmaniasis, also known as *kala-azar* or *black fever.* It appears to be an extension of internal disease to the skin. The disease is confined mainly to Bangladesh, India, Nepal, Pakistan, and China, but foci are also found on the coasts of the Mediterranean, central Africa, the central Asian republics, and eastern Brazil. Cutaneous manifestations occur after several months or years of treatment for the internal signs of kala-azar.

Classic Description (Fig. 22–4)

Macules, papules, and nodules may be found on the face, nose, cheeks, trunk, or extremities. Secondary changes include hypopigmentation, erythema, and pigmentary changes from earth gray to typical black. Mucous membrane involvement may lead to blindness and dysphonia as a result of corneal and laryngeal lesions.

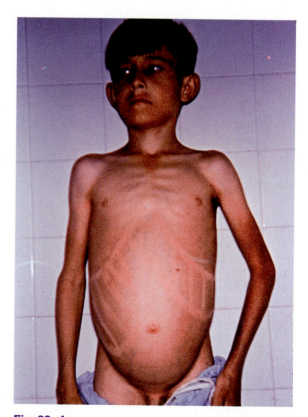

Fig. 22–4
Post–kala-azar dermal leishmaniasis. Note the skin pigmentation and hepatosplenomegaly.

Diagnosis

Rapid diagnosis and treatment are necessary to prevent the severe consequences of the disease, such as hypersplenism with anemia, thrombocytopenia, and heptomegaly. Slit-skin smears of nodular forms, stained with Giemsa stain, will reveal the causative organism. Macrophages, plasma cells, and lymphocytes are seen on biopsy.

Differential Diagnosis

Leprosy closely resembles post–kala-azar dermal leishmaniasis but is differentiated clinically and through skin biopsy findings of Lepra bacilli. *Diffuse cutaneous leishmaniasis* may be distinguished by massive dissemination of skin lesions and findings of many organisms. *Secondary syphilis* involves the skin and mucous membranes, contains many treponemes (seen on darkfield microscopy), and is confirmed by serologic tests. *Sarcoidosis, vitiligo,* and *rosacea* may be ruled out clinically and through biopsy. *Tinea versicolor* should be ruled out by KOH examination, showing fungal hyphae.

Treatment

The World Health Organization recommends *sodium stibogluconate* 20 mg/kg up to a maximum of 850 mg/day intramuscularly for 4 months. *Ketoconazole, allopurinol,* or *amphotericin* are alternative treatments in cases of serious adverse effects or resistance of pentavalent antimony preparations.

AMERICAN MUCOCUTANEOUS LEISHMANIASIS ICD-9 (085.5)

American mucocutaneous leishmaniasis is caused by the protozoa *Leishmania brasiliensis* and *L. mexicana,* transmitted by the bite of species of the sandfly *Lutzomyia* or *Psychodopygus.*

The disease is endemic in Central and South America, especially Brazil, Peru, and Venezuela.

After an incubation period that ranges between 2 and 10 weeks, a cutaneous lesion forms, most commonly at the bite site. In most infections of *L. mexicana* the lesion does not spread but rather resolves in a few months. However, a chronic ulcer, *chiclero ulcer,* may occur, whereby the lesion persists and is locally destructive for years. In one third of cases of *L. tropica* infections, lesions may involve the mucous membranes of the upper respiratory tract, with a chronic, mutilating, and even fatal disease known as *espundia*.

Classic Description (Fig. 22–5)

Papules or firm, indurated plaques are found on the nose, mouth, anus, or vulva. Destruction of the nasal septum, lip, back of nasopharynx, tongue, floor of the mouth and buccal mucosa may subsequently occur. These secondary changes may lead to infection, sepsis, difficulty in swallowing, lung infection, and respiratory failure.

Diagnosis

A definitive diagnosis can be made by finding parasites in a slit-skin smear. Cultures can be done on NNN medium. The leishmanin test may be positive for present or past infestation.

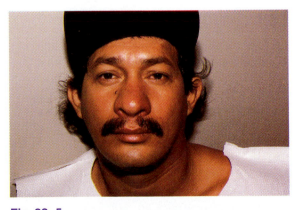

Fig. 22–5
Involvement of the mucocutaneous area with destruction in American mucocutaneous leishmaniasis.

Differential Diagnosis

Pyogenic infections may have an appearance similar to that of American mucocutaneous leishmaniasis but are ruled out by finding specific organisms. *Sporotrichosis, chromomycosis,* and *paracoccidiodomycosis* need to be distinguished by clinical findings and fungal cultures. *Squamous cell carcinoma* and *carcinoma of the oral cavity* are differentiated by biopsy. *Syphilis, yaws,* and *post–kala-azar dermal leishmaniasis* are also part of the differential diagnosis.

Treatment

Although not always satisfactory, *sodium stibogluconate* 20 mg/kg/day is given intramuscularly for 21 days; if there is mucosal involvment, it is given for 28 days. *Amphotericin B,* starting with 0.1 mg/kg in 500 ml of isotonic glucose up to 1 mg/kg/day, is recommended for pentavalent antimony-resistant patients. *Ketoconazole* 600 to 800 mg/day for 20 to 28 days may be used for less severe cases. Rifampicin, cycloguanil pamoate, allopurinol, emetine, and local heat may also be used. Patient education in all cases includes public awareness programs about disease transmission, vector control to reduce new cases, and preventive measures against bites, using nets, repellents, and antibite coils.

SCHISTOSOMIASIS ICD-9 (120.9)

The skin is involved only incidentally in this serious helminthic infestation. Human and other animals are definite hosts, although fresh water snails are the intermediate host. Schistosomiasis is caused by three distinct species of Schistosoma with different geographic distributions: (1) *Schistosoma haematobium,* commonly found in Africa and the Middle East, (2) *Schistosoma japonicum,* in the Far East, and (3) *Schistosoma mansoni,* in Africa and South America. About 200 million people in 75 countries are affected. The young parasites, cercariae, penetrate the skin or mucous membranes, then enter the lymphatic system, blood stream, and liver.

Individuals who live in endemic areas often have chronic, low-grade, asymptomatic infestations, with acute illness seen in those who acquire a large parasite burden. Acute schistosomiasis is more typically limited to travelers in an endemic area. Chronic schistosomiasis may result in varices, hepatosplenomegaly, and other systemic complications, primarily as a result of granulomatous responses to the deposition of eggs in tissues. *S. haematobium* frequently is found in the bladder; *S. japonicum* and *mansoni* are found usually in the liver, bowel, and venous plexuses.

Classic Description

Cutaneous involvement manifests in one of four ways:

1. *Schistosomal dermatitis:* Penetration of cercariae with a pruritic eruption called *swimmer's itch,* with discrete red papules
2. *Bilharzides* or *schistosomides:* An allergic reaction, 1 to 2 months after exposure, associated with fever, malaise, arthralgia, diarrhea, abdominal cramps, and hepatosplenomegaly (also known as *Katayama syndrome*)
3. *Bilharzia cutanea tarda:* Visceral schistosomiasis causes deposition of schistosome eggs, anogenital lesions, communicating sinuses and fistulas, and systemic involvement, including hematuria, papillomas, ulceration, splenomegaly, and hepatic cirrhosis
4. *Lesions related to complications of schistosomiasis.*

Dislodgement of ova or flukes, with deposition to the lung, central nervous system, skin, or conjunctiva, may lead to firm, ovoid, flesh-colored papules, nodules, or plaques, with scaling, ulceration, and hyperpigmentation. The infestation initally affects exposed parts of the body, trunk, anogenital region, and buttocks.

Diagnosis and Differential Diagnosis

Diagnosis is made by demonstration of ova in urine or stool. Skin biopsy is useful. Complement fixation and enzyme-linked immunosorbent assay (ELISA) tests help to confirm the diagnosis but are not readily available. The differential diagnosis includes *scabies, onchocercal dermatitis, toxic erythema, urticaria,* and *allergic vasculitis.*

Treatment and Patient Education

Treatment is *praziquantal* 40 mg/kg/day orally every 4 hours for two doses, except for *S. japonicum* and *S. mekongi,* which require 60 mg/kg/day every 4 hours for three doses. Patient education involves instructions on strict hygiene, with appropriate sterile disposal of urine and stool whenever possible. Water supplies in endemic areas should be considered contaminated and treated by heating to 122° Fahrenheit for 5 minutes or using chlorine or iodine treatments before use in bathing. Patients may also thoroughly dry their body with a towel after swimming and rub the body with alcohol for additional protection against infestation. Controlling snail hosts will help avoid cercariae-infested water.

BACTERIAL DISEASES IN THE TROPICS

MYCOBACTERIAL INFECTIONS

Mycobacteria are slow-growing, facultative, intracellular, aerobic organisms. They are called *acid-fast bacilli* because they retain carbolfuchsin despite decolorization with acid-alcohol. Classified according to the disease, they produce cutaneous tuberculosis, leprosy, and atypical mycobacterial infections. Alternatively, they can be classified on the basis of the types of organisms that cause diseases or tuberculosis caused by *Mycobacterium tuberculosis* and *Mycobacteroses* for other mycobacteria. The latter is also known as *MOTT,* Mycobacteria other than tuberculosis.

CUTANEOUS TUBERCULOSIS ICD-9 (017.0)

Cutaneous tuberculosis is primarily caused by *M. tuberculosis,* and *M. bovis. M. bovis* (attenuated) is also known as *Bacillus-Calmette-Guérin.* An increased incidence of cutaneous tuberculosis occurs in immunocompromised patients, with reactivation of "persisters" in immunocompromised hosts or in patients with impaired cellular immunity.

Immunologic anergy facilitates infection with normally low-virulence mycobacteria. Although mainly humans are affected, cats, dogs, cattle, and monkeys may also contract disease. Transmission is chiefly through inhalation, ingestion, and inoculation. Any age group may be affected, but a higher incidence is found in people younger than age 30.

Classic Description and Differential Diagnosis

Types and characteristics of cutaneous tuberculosis, along with their mode of spread, are classified through cutaneous involvement by inoculation from an external source, endogenous spread, and hematogenous spread.

Inoculation

Tuberculous chancre (Fig. 22–6) occurs with the first exposure to *M. tuberculosis* and requires an injury. Papules, nodules, and plaques, with secondary erythema, develop into an ulcer with a hemorrhagic base. Regional lymphadenopathy follows in 3 to 6 weeks. Lesions typically heal slowly without treatment, although, rarely, chronic infections may occur. Initially, the purified protein derivative (PPD) test is negative but later becomes positive. The differential diagnosis includes *syphilitic chancre, anthrax, sporotrichosis, tularemia,* and *atypical mycobacterial* or *fungal infections.*

Warty tuberculosis (tuberculous verrucosa cutis) (Fig. 22–7) occurs in immunocompetent

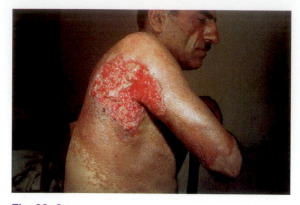

Fig. 22–6
Tuberculous chancre. Note the ulcer with a heaped-up border.

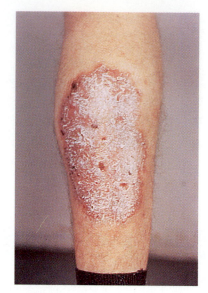

Fig. 22–7
Extensive involvement of the extremity in a patient with tuberculous verrucosa cutis.

people with previous exposure to *M. tuberculosis* and requires an injury. The disease is an occupational hazard to pathologists, butchers, and farmers. A papule or pustule evolves into a slowly growing (over years) plaque with secondary hyperkeratosis. Lymphadenopathy is rare, and spontaneous resolution may occur. Acid-fast bacilli are difficult to demonstrate. The differential diagnosis includes *deep fungal infections, hypertrophic lichen planus, verrucous squamous cell carcinoma, verruca,* and *syphilitic gumma.*

Lupus vulgaris (Fig. 22–8) occurs through direct inoculation or direct extension from an underlying involved lymph node (especially cervical), lymphatic spread, and hematogenous dissemination (pulmonary). Lesions are found commonly on the nose, cheek, or site of BCG vaccination (extremities and trunk less commonly). Plaques are slow-growing and have secondary brown pigmentation. When lesions are pressed with a glass slide, they have an apple-jelly appearance. Lesions may also ulcerate and develop nodules, tumors, or vegetating forms. Progression may lead to significant disfigurement. Squamous cell carcinomas may develop in chronic lesions. The differential diagnosis includes *discoid lupus erythematosus, sarcoidosis, syphilis, tuberculoid leprosy,* and *deep fungal* or *atypical mycobacterial infections.*

Endogenous Source

Scrofuloderma occurs with contiguous spread, usually from a lymph node, with breakdown of the overlying skin. Lesions are most common in children, typically appearing on the neck or supraclavicular area but may occur over joints or even over the scrotum. Nodules, with secondary blue-red appearance and doughy center, evolve into ulcers and sinus formation, with subsequent scarring of lymph nodes and bone. The differential diagnosis includes *actinomycosis* or *sporotrichosis infections, syphilitic gumma,* and *severe acne conglobata.*

Orificial tuberculosis is rare and affects the mouth and other mucous membranes and the skin surrounding such orifices. Painful nodules develop, with secondary erythema, evolving into ulcers with a punched-out appearance. Lesions tend to progress and herald severe infection.

The differential diagnosis includes *syphilis* and *squamous cell carcinoma.*

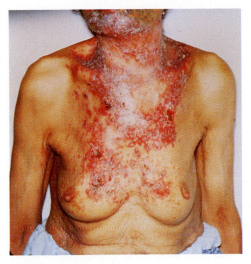

Fig. 22–8
Lupus vulgaris. Note the extensive involvement of the face, neck, and chest with plaques and atrophic scar formation.

Hematogenous Source

Acute miliary tuberculosis, with pulmonary and/or meningeal involvement, is rare and seen mostly in infants, young children, or immunocompromised patients. Papules, nodules, vesicles, or pustules are seen in these severely ill patients, and numerous mycobacteria are demonstrable on skin biopsy.

Metastatic tuberculous abscess or ulcer occurs through hematogenous dissemination from a primary focus, with subcutaneous abscess and subsequent ulceration. Mycobacteria are found on biopsy, and the differential diagnosis includes *sporotrichosis.*

Tuberculids are lesions that occur as a result of hematogenous spread where there is a high degree of immunity. Mycobacteria are not demonstrable in these lesions by conventional methods. **Lichen scrofulosorum** is rare, with yellow to pink, flat-topped papules that appear on the trunk in patients with either *M. tuberculosis* lymph node or bone infections. Lesions may resolve spontaneously but more typically respond to chemotherapy. The differential diagnosis includes *lichen planus* or *lichen nitidus* and *sar-*

coidosis. **Papulonecrotic tuberculids** appear on the lower extremities as multiple, symmetric, necrotic papules that may ulcerate. Extracutaneous sources may not be demonstrable, and lesions respond to chemotherapy. The differential diagnosis includes *lymphocytic vasculitis.* **Erythema induratum** is found on the lower extremities of middle-age women, with tender nodules and secondary dusky erythema. Exogenous sources may not be apparent, but a vigorous response to a skin test is typical. Lesions may persist, recur, or spontaneously heal and respond to chemotherapy. The differential diagnosis includes *nodular vasculitis.*

Diagnosis

A high index of suspicion is tantamount to making the diagnosis, particularly in the presence of clinical findings and factors such as prior exposure or living in areas with a high incidence of the disease. Histopathologically, these are granulomatous processes. Special stains will illustrate acid-fast bacilli. Tubercle bacilli may grow on special media culture in 3 to 4 weeks. In patients with a high degree of immunity, acid-fast bacilli may be very difficult to demonstrate.

Treatment

Multiple drug therapy (MDT), similar to that used for systemic tuberculosis, is indicated for cutaneous tuberculosis. Chemotherapy includes 9 months of a three-drug regimen:

1. *Rifampin* 10 to 20 mg/kg/day up to 600 mg/day
2. *Ethambutol* 15 to 25 mg/kg/day or *pyrazinamide* 1.5 g/day (less than 50 kg), 2 g/day (50 to 74 kg), 2.5 g/day (greater than 75 kg) or *streptomycin* 15 to 20 mg/kg/day up to 1 g/day
3. *Isoniazid* 5 mg/kg/day up to 300 mg/day with *pyridoxine* 10 mg/day to prevent peripheral neuropathy. Drainage, debridement, or surgical intervention may be necessary.

Patient Education

Emphasize immunoprophylaxis by BCG vaccination, when appropriate, and drug treatment of asymptomatic tuberculin "converters" with *isoniazid*. Early detection of cases and sources of infection by tuberculin testing, biopsy, and prompt initiation of treatment, along with isolation, when indicated, will decrease the burden of disease.

ATYPICAL MYCOBACTERIAL INFECTIONS ICD-9 (031.1)

The number of skin infections caused by atypical mycobacteria appears to be increasing. Factors such as drug use, invasive procedures, applications of topical steroids, and immunocompromised status play important roles in the disease process. Atypical mycobacteria are widely distributed in nature, being found in soil, water, vegetation, human skin and sputum, and human and animal excreta. Atypical mycobacteria are usually saprophytic, but under certain conditions they become pathogenic to man. They have been classified according to pigment changes with light and growth. The tropics are host to most of the atypical mycobacterial diseases.

Swimming pool granuloma (Fig. 22–9) is caused by *M. marinum,* following an injury or trauma to skin that has been in contact with contaminated fresh or salt water. It can be considered an occupational hazard of fishkeeping. Lesions are found on the hand and forearm. A localized papule or nontender nodule with secondary erythema develops 2 to 6 weeks following the injury. Ulceration subsequently occurs, and lesions spread along the lymphatics. Spontaneous healing usually occurs within a few weeks; however, a chronic lesion occasionally may result. Treatment includes *rifampin* with *ethambutol* or *minocycline* or *sulfamethoxazole/ trimethoprim*.

Buruli ulcer was first found in Australia, where it was referred to as *Bairnsdale ulcer,* although it also occurs in Africa. Caused by *M. ulcerans,* the greatest incidence occurs before age 25. Lesions are found on the elbow, leg, and hand (Fig. 22–10). Small, firm, pruritic nodules and necrotic ulcers form, ranging in size from a few millimeters to several centimeters. Although spontaneous healing may occur after 6 to 9 months, extensive ulceration may have already occurred. Surgery is the treatment of choice because drug therapy is typically not successsful. However, *rifampin* with *amikacin* or *ethambu-*

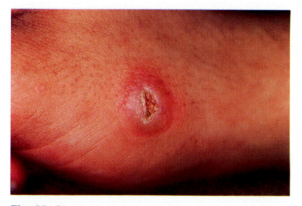

Fig. 22–9
Swimming pool granuloma. Involvement of the hand is common. Note nonhealing ulceration.

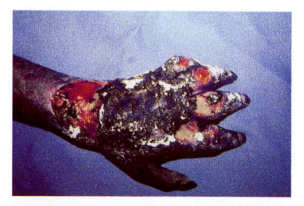

Fig. 22–10
Buruli ulcer. The wrist and hand are involved, with extensive ulceration.

tol with *sulfamethoxazole/trimethoprim* for 4 to 6 weeks may be helpful.

Sporotrichoid cutaneous infection is caused by *M. kansasii* or *M. fortuitum*. The disease is found as an extension of a primary lesion, as a postsurgical wound complication, or at the site of a penetrating wound injury. Primary lesions are variable, with verrucous nodules with papulopustules that evolve into ulcerations (Fig. 22–11). Infected cellulitis, pyoderma, or cervical lymphadenitis also occur. Clinicians should suspect sporotrichoid cutaneous infection in cases of chronic abscesses not responding to antimicrobial therapy. Treatment of *M. kansasii* infections includes *rifampin, isoniazid,* and *ethambutol* and surgical excision of involved lymph nodes. *M. kansasii* may be sensitive to *clarithromycin*. Treatment of *M. fortuitum* includes drainage (may cure 10% to 20%), *amikacin,* and *cefoxitin* with *probenecid* for 2 to 6 weeks, then oral *sulfamethoxazole/trimethoprim* or *doxycycline* for 2 to 6 months.

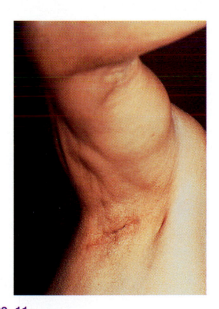

Fig. 22–11
An ulcer with adenopathy in a patient with *M. kansasii* infection.

Abscess formation is sometimes caused by *M. chelonei* or *M. fortuitum,* following trauma, injection, or surgery. Primary lesions exhibit inflammation and abscess formation after 4 to 6 weeks. Cellulitis and fistula formation may occur. Treatment may be guided by culture and sensitivity reports. Treatment of *M. chelonei* includes *clarithromycin* 500 mg bid for 6 months (see above for treatment of *M. kansasii* and *M. fortuitum*).

Mycobacterium avium-intracellulare complex infection is a common disease in both immunocompromised patients (e.g., patients with AIDS) and, increasingly, in non-AIDS patients. Primary lesions include papules, nodules, ulcers, and acnelike lesions. Secondary lesions include lymphadenitis and renal and bone involvement. For diagnosis, culture any drainage and examine a biopsy specimen. Smears of lesion may show acid-fast bacilli. Repeated bacteriologic tests may be necessary for confirmation of the particular atypical mycobacterial strain. Treatment regimens in HIV-positive patients should include two drugs, one of which should be *ethambutol*. Lifetime suppression is indicated with *rifabutin, clarithromycin,* and *ethambutol*. Avoid *rifampin*.

LEPROSY ICD-9 (030.9)

Leprosy is a chronic granulomatous disease that is also known as *Hansen's disease*. It is caused by *M. leprae* and is common in most tropical regions, particularly the Indian subcontinent, Southeast Asia, Africa, and Central and South America. About 2.5 million people are affected. Transmission is through inhalation or ingestion of infected nasal droplets, although the incubation period is apparently 5 to 20 years.

The three cardinal signs of leprosy are: (1) *sensory impairment* of the affected areas, (2) *tender, enlarged peripheral nerves, with signs of nerve damage,* (e.g., paralysis, sensory loss or sensory-motor dysfunction), and (3) *noncultivable acid-fast bacilli* from the affected areas.

There are four major types of leprosy: **tuberculoid, indeterminate, borderline,** and **lepromatous.** Cell-mediated immunity plays an active role in the presentation of the leprosy type.

Classic Description and Diagnosis (See Table 22–2 and Figs. 22–12 through 22–14)

Differential Diagnosis

Vitiligo is an idiopathic disease with depigmented areas of variable size and shape and no sensory impairment. Postinflammatory hypopigmentation may be the result of *discoid lupus erythematosus, dermatitis, psoriasis,* and *pyoderma,* with biopsy differentiating. *Pityriasis alba* is confined to the face, most commonly to the cheeks, with remission and relapses common. *Tinea versicolor* has hypopigmented, scaly macules and is confirmed by a positive KOH prep. *Tinea corporis* has scaly lesions with clear centers and positive KOH prep. *Post–kala-azar dermal leishmaniasis* is a clinical diagnosis made in a susceptible patient with hypopigmented macules of different sizes, primarily in the face. *Pityriasis rosea* is a self-limiting papulosquamous eruption, distributed over the trunk, with a herald patch that resolves in 6 weeks.

Treatment

Multiple drug therapy is indicated by the World Health Organization as a result of the emergence of secondary and subsequent primary dapsone-resistant mutants. Patients with negative slit-skin smear (i.e., paucibacillary) can be treated with *dapsone* 100 mg/day and 600 mg of *rifampicin* once a month for 6 months to a maximum of 9 months.

TABLE 22–2.

Features of Different Types of Leprosy

Conditions	Tuberculoid	Lepromatous	Indeterminate	Borderline
Skin lesion	Single, macules, plaques, dry hairless center, hypopigmented, erythematous edge	Numerous red macules, plaques, nodules, leonine facies, loss of eyelashes/brows, earlobe enlarged and pendulous	Usually single, hypopigmented, erythematous macule	Few to several macules, papules, nodules, plaques
Distribution	Trunk, face, extremities, lesions asymmetric	Earlobes, face, arms, buttocks, lesions, symmetric, bilateral	Lesions are asymmetric, ill-defined	Features of lepromatous and tuberculoid, multiple asymmetric lesions
Sensory	Marked impairment, anesthesia	No change in early stage	Normal or slightly impaired	None to total loss
Peripheral nerves	Enlarged, hard, palpable, tender	Symmetric, thin and fibrosed	Normal	Enlarged, hard, extensive neuropathy
Skin smear	Negative	Positive	Usually negative	Usually positive
Lepromin test	Strongly positive	Negative	Either positive or negative	Negative
Bacterial status	Few bacilli	Numerous bacilli	No bacilli	Bacilli only in smears
Consequences	Relatively stable, benign, prognosis good	Very infectious, poor prognosis if untreated	May regress or progress to definite type	Unstable, progress to lepromatous type

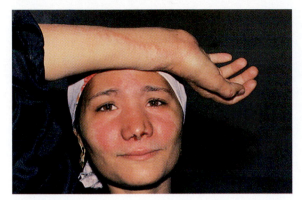

Fig. 22–12
Tuberculoid leprosy. Circumscribed lesion affecting the face.

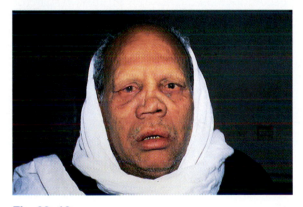

Fig. 22–13
Lepromatous leprosy. Involvement of the face, with destruction of the nasal bridge and loss of eyebrows.

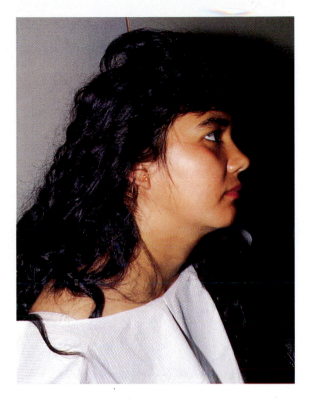

Fig. 22–14
Borderline leprosy involving the face.

For multibacillary patients (i.e., positive slit-skin smear) give *rifampin* 600 mg and *clofazimine* 300 mg once a month with *dapsone* 100 mg/day and *clofazimine* 50 mg/day. Duration of therapy should be for at least 2 years or until smears are negative. *Clarithromycin* 500 mg/day is a promising agent.

ANTHRAX ICD-9 (022.0)

Anthrax, or the disease of malignant pustule, is caused by *Bacillus anthracis,* a large, aerobic, spore-forming gram-positive rod. Anthrax is mostly found in the Middle East, especially in Iran, north and central Africa, central India, and some parts of South America. The virulent strains of anthrax are encapsulated and toxicogenic, and the toxin causes the characteristic signs and symptoms, including central nervous system dysfunction that leads to anoxia and respiratory failure. Anthrax is a zoonotic disease that primarily affects grazing animals; humans are accidental hosts. *Anthrax is an occupational hazard to workers who contact and handle animal products, such as wool, hide, hair, and bone or animal carcasses.*

The three types of anthrax that occur in humans are cutaneous, the most common; gastrointestinal; and pulmonary. Cutaneous anthrax is found in a dry form and an edematous form.

Classic Description and Diagnosis

Look for anthrax at sites of friction or trauma, such as hands, neck, lips, and exposed areas. Primary lesions include papules and vesicles that may form a necrotic ulcer or eschar. Local edema and lymphadenitis may be evident. Diagnosis is made clinically by observing a relatively painless, enlarging, nonhealing ulcer in a patient with a possible exposure and in conjunction with finding the causative organism in smears and culture. Biopsy shows a loss of epidermis, surrounding spongiosis, and intraepidermal vesicles.

Differential Diagnosis

Anthrax may resemble *carbuncles* and *furuncles* in their early stages. *Second-degree burns, bullous erysipelas, brown recluse spider bites, cutaneous leishmaniasis, bacterial abscesses,* and *cowpox* also need to be distinguished.

Treatment and Patient Education

Potassium penicillin V 30 mg/kg/day given orally 4 times a day for 5 to 7 days. Patients who are allergic or resistant to penicillin may take either *ciprofloxacin* 750 mg twice daily, *doxycycline* 100 mg orally twice daily, or *sulfadiazine* starting with 3 g and then 1 g every 4 hours. Systemic disease should be treated agressively with *penicillin G* 20 to 30 mg/kg/day intramuscularly in two equal doses for 1 week. Patients with pulmonary involvement should be treated intravenously. Emphasize that animal products should be decontaminated before handling and that animal carcasses should be burned or buried deeply. Protective clothing and gloves are needed for handling potentially infected materials.

Domestic animals in endemic areas should have active immunization with live attenuated vaccine, and people at high risk should be immunized with the cell-free vaccine.

CUTANEOUS DIPHTHERIA ICD-9 (032.85)

Cutaneous diphtheria is caused by *Corynebacterium diphtheriae,* a non–spore-forming gram-positive bacillus that is found with the normal flora of the skin and mucous membranes. The disease is found in the tropics and is a result of poor hygiene in combination with the hot, humid climate. Bacterial transmission occurs by respiratory spray or direct contact when bacteria invade skin traumatized by irritation, surgical wounds, insect bites, or scabies.

Classic Description

Single or multiple lesions are found on the legs, feet, and hands (Fig 22–15). Pustules or painful, nonhealing ulcers, with a gray-yellow or brown membrane that can be removed, appear, and the lesion then develops a thick, anesthetic eschar within 2 weeks, with associated surrounding bullous lesions and regional lymphadenopathy. The lesion persists for 6 to 12 weeks, then heals with a scar.

Diagnosis and Differential Diagnosis

Diagnosis is confirmed by the growth of the bacillus on culture and toxin production. The differential diagnosis includes other forms of nonspecific dermatitis.

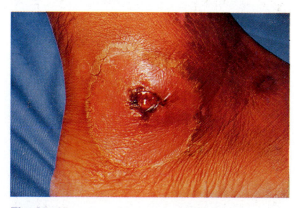

Fig. 22–15
Cutaneous diphtheria; eczematous lesion of the ankle.

Treatment and Patient Education

Antitoxin 2000 to 100,000 U intravenously, after skin testing, should be administered to neutralize unbound toxin. *Penicillin* 500 mg qid for 14 days, *erythromycin* 500 mg qid, or *rifampicin* 600 mg/day for 7 days are very effective. Use *erythromycin* 20 to 25 mg/kg intravenously every 12 hours for 7 to 14 days for systemic disease. Tell patients that close contacts should be cultured for the organism and should receive prophylactic antibiotics. Early childhood immunization with DPT vaccination and booster doses at 10-year intervals provide immunity.

GRANULOMA INGUINALE ICD-9 (099.2)

Granuloma inguinale, also known as *donovanosis,* is endemic in Southeast Asia, India, Australia, the Caribbean, Central America and Africa. Caused by *Calymmatobacterium granulomatis,* a gram-negative, facultative, intracellular, encapsulated bacillus, the disease is chronic and sexually transmitted.

Classic Description

The disease is found in the anogenital areas of both men and women, as well as extragenital sites (Fig. 22–16. There are four variants:

1. Ulcerative, or ulcerogranulomatous: Nontender and beefy red; bleeds easily; has a nonindurated ulcer, with increased formation of granulation tissue.
2. Hypertrophic or verrucous: Exuberant granulation tissue; irregular borders; bleeds easily with slight trauma.
3. Necrotic: Rapid and extensive tissue destruction; painful; gray, foul-smelling exudate.
4. Sclerotic, or cicatrical: Common in women; fibrous tissue formation results in a band-like scar. Sequelae include penile destruction, pseudoelephantiasis of external genitalia in women, and urethral, vaginal, or anal stenosis as a result of scarring.

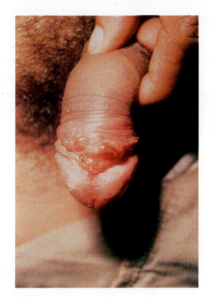

Fig. 22–16
Involvement of the penis, with a beefy red, granulomatous ulceration in a patient with granuloma inguinale.

Diagnosis and Differential Diagnosis

Donovan (intracellular organisms) bodies are seen in smears, with massive mononuclear infiltration of plasma cells in the dermis. Examine tissue either by routine histology or by crush prep, in which fresh biopsy tissue is crushed between two slides, allowed to air dry, and then stained.

The differential diagnosis includes *primary syphilis, genital herpes, chancroid, lymphogranuloma venereum, filariasis, cutaneous leishmaniasis, schistosomiasis, candidiasis,* and *traumatic ulcers.*

Treatment and Patient Education

Doxycyline 100 mg orally twice a day for 1 to 4 weeks or *sulfamethoxazole/trimethoprim* 80/400 mg bid, for 14 days are first-line therapies. Alternatives are *tetracycline* 500 mg qid for 3 to 4 weeks or *erythromycin* 500 mg for 3 to 4 weeks. Screen for other sexually transmitted diseases, including HIV disease, and discuss good wound (ulcer) care.

ERYTHRASMA ICD-9 (039.0)

Erythrasma is a superficial infection of any intertriginous area. The causative agent, *Corynebacterium minutissimum,* is gram-positive, aerobic in nature, and part of the normal skin flora. Hot and humid climates may contribute to the overgrowth of the organism.

Classic Description

The disease is found in the toewebs, groin, inframammary area, and axillae (Fig. 22–17). Primary lesions include brown patches with secondary scale. Patches are well defined, irregularly shaped, and often associated with itching. A generalized form may be found on the trunk and upper aspects of extremities.

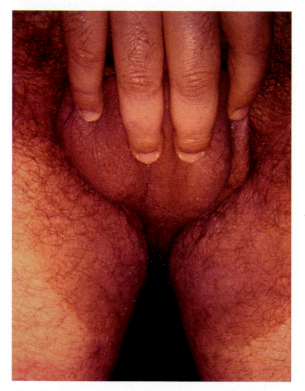

Fig. 22–17
Erythrasma and involvement of the groin. Note the bilateral, extensive brown plaques. (Courtesy Antar Padilha-Gonçalves, MD, Rio de Janerio, Brazil.)

Diagnosis and Differential Diagnosis

The diagnosis is confirmed by Wood's light examination, which reveals a coral-red fluorescence caused by the production of coporphyrin III by the bacteria. *Dermatophytosis,* especially *tinea cruris* and *candidiasis,* can be differentiated by KOH preparation or fungal culture.

Treatment

Use *erythromycin* 500 mg qid for 5 days. Topical application of *erythromycin, fusidic acid,* or broad-spectrum antifungal agents can be helpful as prophylactic measure for recurrences. Good hygienic care reduces the incidence of erythrasma.

PITTED KERATOLYSIS ICD-9 (040)

Pitted keratolysis is an uncommon, superficial, erosive disease of the stratum corneum of the sole. The causative organism is a *Corynebacterium,* but *Dermatophilus congolensis* and *Micrococcus sedantarium* may also be involved. Moisture caused by sweating in hot, humid weather plays an important role in the disease process.

Classic Description

Lesions, typically located on the sole or toe, are discrete, 1- to 3-mm rounded pits, with a brown or normal skin color. A fetid odor is common. Symptoms include burning, itching, and pain on walking or standing.

Diagnosis and Differential Diagnosis

Diagnosis is made by the clinical picture and the presence of gram-positive coccobacilli on a Gram's stain of a smear. Cultures are unreliable.

The differential diagnosis includes extensive *tinea pedis, basal cell nevus syndrome,* and *mosaic warts.* A negative KOH result and an absence of lesions elsewhere on the body help to distinguish this condition.

Treatment and Patient Education

Use Burow's compresses for 10 minutes, followed by topical *erythromycin* or *clindamycin* lotion, until the lesion resolves.

Explain the importance of properly fitting shoes, cotton socks, and sandals and educate patients about regular washing of the foot with soap.

TRICHOMYCOSIS AXILLARIS ICD-9 (039.0)

Trichomycosis axillaris is a discoloration, mainly of the axillary hairs. Other body hair is infrequently affected, and the skin is never involved. The causative agent, *C. tenuis,* is a gram-positive organism that proliferates in the presence of moisture on axillary hairs. In hot, humid areas of Australia, it is common among young adults.

Classic Description

Lesions involve a thickened hair shaft and discoloration, either yellow, red, or black, as a result of the production of porphyrin by the bacteria.

Associated characteristics include an offensive odor and discoloration of clothing. Lesions may coexist with those found in erythrasma and pitted keratolysis.

Diagnosis and Differential Diagnosis

Diagnosis is made with the clinical picture and Wood's light examination, showing fluorescence of the affected area. Bacterial culture will reveal the organism, if still in doubt. The differential diagnosis includes *chromihidrosis,* a rare functional sweat gland disorder. *Black piedra* should be differentiated by KOH preparation and culture.

Treatment and Patient Education

Regular shaving of the axillary hair and use of antibacterial soap will virtually eliminate the condition. Emphasis should be made on the necessity of good personal hygiene of the affected areas.

PASTEURELLOSIS ICD-9 (027.2)

Pasteurellosis is caused by *Pasteurella multocida,* as a result of animal bites, mainly from dogs or cats. *P. multocida* is part of the normal bacterial flora of the oropharynx of many domestic and wild animals. Humans are accidental hosts. *P. multocida* is a small nonmotile, gram-negative coccobacillus. Localized and systemic involvement may occur.

Classic Description

Lesions are typically found on the hand, arm, leg, or penis. Puncture wounds may be associated with erythema, edema, or exudate.

Regional lymphadenopathy may occur. Pain develops in lesions within a few hours of an animal bite, with subsequent wound infection characterized by cellulitis and systemic involvement, such as chills, malaise, and fever. The healing process is slow and the condition may persist for weeks.

Diagnosis and Differential Diagnosis

Diagnosis is usually made clinically in the context of a known exposure. Bacterial culture may reveal facultative anaerobes and aerobes. *Pyogenic cellulitis, cat scratch disease,* and skin manifestations of *tularemia* should be distinguished by clinical findings, as well as by finding the specific organism.

Treatment and Patient Education

Penicillin V 500 mg qid for 1 to 4 weeks, depending on response, is the choice of therapy. *Amoxicillin/clavulanic acid* 500 mg tid for 10 days or more is an alternative. *Tetracycline, erythromycin,* or one of the *quinolones* can also be used as alternatives in penicillin-resistant or allergic patients. Surgical drainage may be needed.

Proper wound care includes immediate, copious irrigation, early recognition of infection, prompt antimicrobial therapy initiation, and debridement of dead tissue.

YAWS ICD-9 (102.9)

Yaws is also known as *frambesia tropica, pian, parangi,* and *paru.* Yaws is a chronic, infectious, nonvenereal disease caused by a spirochete, *Treponema pertenue.* The disease is prevalent in South America, the Caribbean islands, Africa, India, Southeast Asia, and the Pacific islands. Transmission is through skin-to-skin nonvenereal contact and occurs as a result of damage of the skin by small abrasions, insect bites, or scratching. Children age 6 to 10 who live in rural areas and are scantily clothed are most commonly affected. Hot, humid climates, poor socioeconomic conditions, overcrowding, low standards of hygiene, and lack of sanitation also play important roles in the disease process and transmission.

Although *T. pertenue* is morphologically and serologically indistinguishable from *T. pallidum,* the causative organism of syphilis, yaws never affects the central nervous system, heart, or peripheral vascular system, nor does it ever cause congenital abnormalities. The incubation period ranges from 9 to 90 days.

Classic Description (Fig. 22–18)

Early yaws is found on exposed parts of the body (e.g., legs, face, trunk, natal cleft). Primary or "mother" lesions usually occur at the site of a preexisting skin lesion, such as traumatic injury. The lesion(s) is red and nontender. There may be an associated regional adenopathy. After several weeks, secondary yaws occurs as isolated or groups of papules in a generalized distribution. Crusted papillomas, constitutional symptoms, lymphadenopathy, and spontaneous healing with a depressed scar subsequently occur. Secondary lesions may also be accompanied by osteitis, periosteitis, and joint involvement, with healing and recurrences for 2 to 4 years. Late

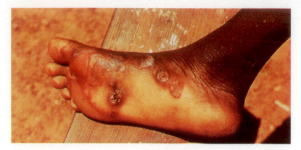

Fig. 22–18
Yaws and an early lesion on the sole. Note crusted papillomatous changes. (Courtesy Wolfram Höffler, MD, Tübingen, Germany.)

yaws develops in approximately 10% to 15% of patients with untreated disease. Lesions are found most commonly on the legs, initially as a painless nodule. Subsequent necrosis and deformity may be found, including gummatous osteitis, periosteitis, sabre tibia, ulcerative rhinopharyngitis mutilans (gangosa), and juxtaarticular contractures. Spontaneous healing may occur, with keloid formation.

Diagnosis and Differential Diagnosis

Diagnosis is made clinically by the history of recurrences and the characteristic morphology. *T. pertenue* can be seen on darkfield examination of an exudate. Skin biopsy and serologic tests will confirm the diagnosis, if still in doubt. The differential diagnosis includes bacterial and parasitic diseases, such as *impetigo, leprosy, anthrax, cutaneous leishmaniasis, scabies,* and *viral infections* (e.g., *molluscum contagiosum, warts*).

Treatment and Patient Education

Benzathine penicillin 2.4 million U in a single dose is sufficient. Children and contacts need half of the adult dose. *Erythromycin* and *tetracycline* can be used as alternatives if needed. All contacts, as well as active patients, must be treated. Improved personal hygiene and public health measures reduce the risk of recurrences. Continuous epidemiologic surveillance also helps to keep the disease in control.

FUNGAL DISEASES IN THE TROPICS

Several fungal diseases are predominantly found in tropical areas, where they cause significant suffering and morbidity. The diseases include sporotrichosis, coccidiodomycosis, mycetoma, and chromomycosis.

SPOROTRICHOSIS ICD-9 (117.1)

Sporotrichosis is endemic in, but not limited to, tropical countries. It is caused by a dimorphic fungus, *Sporothrix schenckii,* which is a saprophyte found on grass, shrubs, and plants. Sporotrichosis is an occupational hazard of farmers, gardeners, florists, and construction workers. Accidental trauma leads to infection at the site of the injury, with spread by the lymphatics. Systemic involvement can occur with skin, lung, central nervous system, and joint involvement, including cutaneous or subcutaneous abscesses on any part of the body. The outcome may be fatal if the disease is not properly managed.

Classic Description (Fig. 22–19)

Sporotrichosis is typically found on the hand or foot. Primary lesions involve papules at the infection site and nodules along lymphatics. Sec-ondary lesions include ulcers, regional lymphangitis, and cold abscesses.

Diagnosis and Differential Diagnosis

The diagnosis of sporotrichosis is made clinically and confirmed by fungal culture that grows rapidly, forming a firm chocolate-brown colony in culture media. *S. schenckii* can be difficult to identify by direct examination from an exudate. The differential diagnosis includes *cutaneous tuberculosis, syphilis, furunculosis, cat scratch disease, North American blastomycosis, anthrax,* and other *deep fungal infections.*

Treatment and Patient Education

Use *potassium iodide* starting with 5 drops tid and increase by 1 drop each day up to 30 to 40 drops daily for 4 to 6 weeks. Adverse effects include nausea, vomiting, parotid and eyelid swelling, coryza, and depression. *Itraconazole,* 200 mg/day for 3 months, until clinical and mycologic findings are negative, is an alternative treatment when allergy or intolerance to *potassium iodide* exists. Emphasize to patients that the disease is serious if it progresses.

COCCIDIOIDOMYCOSIS ICD-9 (CUTANEOUS; PRIMARY 114.1; DISSEMINATED 114.3)

Coccidioidomycosis is caused by a dimorphic fungi, *Coccidioides immitis,* and is endemic in Argentina, the Philippines, Mexico, Paraguay, Venezuela, and the southeastern United States. The disease is also known as *San Joaquin Valley fever* or *desert rheumatism. C. immitis* is found in the soil. Several clinical forms occur, including asymptomatic, self-limited pneumonia, chronic pulmonary involvement, and extrapulmonary diseases involving skin, bone, joint, and meninges. Filipinos, blacks, and pregnant women are particularly susceptible.

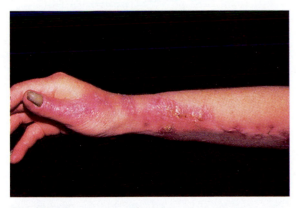

Fig. 22–19
Sporotrichosis and involvement of the arm. Note granuloma formation along the lymphatics. (Courtesy Roberto Arenas, MD, Mexico City, Mexico.)

Classic Description

Lesions are found on the face, nose, nasolabial fold, and extremities. Primary lesions include papules, pustules, nodules, and plaques, with secondary abscesses, draining sinuses, verrucous hyperkeratoses, and scars. Toxic erythema and erythema nodosum can occur within a few weeks of pulmonary coccidioidomycosis. The disease heals very slowly.

Diagnosis and Differential Diagnosis

A potassium hydroxide (KOH) preparation of sputum, pus, and CSF will be positive for *C. immitis,* with the presence of spherical or small endospores. *C. immitis* grows rapidly within 3 to 4 days on Sabouraud medium. Complement fixation, latex agglutination, and immunodiffusion tests are also helpful. Skin testing with coccidioidin spherulin is useful for documenting exposure but is not indicative of active disease. The differential diagnosis includes *folliculitis, furunculosis,* and *pyoderma,* all of which are ruled out by clinical grounds and bacteriologic culture. *North American blastomycosis* can be differentiated by fungal culture. In HIV-infected individuals, lesions may resemble *molluscum contagiosum.*

Treatment and Patient Education

Itraconazole 200 mg bid; *fluconazole* 200 to 400 mg/day for 12 to 18 months; or *amphotericin B* 0.5 to 0.6 mg/kg/day intravenously for 7 days, then 0.8 mg/kg/every other day until the lesion clears (average total dose 2.5 g) are the drugs of choice. Debridement is helpful in large lesions. Surgical intervention may be needed in chronic pulmonary, bone, joint, or meningeal involvement.

MYCETOMA ICD-9 (MADURA, MYCOTIC 117.4; ACTINOMYCOTIC 039.4)

Mycetoma, also known as *Madura foot* and *Madura mycosis,* represents a group of infections with similar clinical presentations. Two major groups of mycetoma are *eumycetoma,* caused by true fungi (e.g., *Madurella, Exophiala jeanselmei,* or *Pseudallescheria*), and *actinomycetomas,* caused by species of *Streptomyces, Nocardia,* or *Actinomyces.* The most common organisms are the fungi *P. boydii* and *M. mycetomatis. N. brasiliensis* and *Actinomadura madurae* also cause the disease. Acquired by accidental trauma, the disease is common in tropical areas of the Indian subcontinent, Africa, Mexico, and Brazil, but also may be found in the southern United States. Men are affected more than women, probably because of trauma to bare feet during work on farms. Three important clinical findings are tumefaction, sinus tracts, and visualization of grains of the causative organisms.

Classic Description (Fig. 22–20)

Lesions are found on the foot, hand, arm, chest, and buttock. Primary lesions include subcutaneous painless nodules. Secondary complications involve draining sinuses, grain production within a few months, new nodule formation, extension to deeper tissue and bone, swelling and deformity of affected parts, and loss of function. Secondary bacterial sepsis may lead to death.

Diagnosis and Differential Diagnosis

A potassium hydroxide (KOH) prep of exudate will reveal characteristic granules and hyphae. Gram's staining helps to detect the organism responsible for actinomycetoma. Eumycetomas grow on Sabouraud dextrose agar media. Bacterial or mycobacterial *osteomyelitis* needs to be differentiated from early stage mycetoma swelling. *Botryomycosis* may also mimic mycetoma.

Treatment and Patient Education

Use *sulfamethoxazole/trimethoprim* 80/400 mg for 6 months or *dapsone* 1.5 mg/kg bid for 6 to 24 months. *Itraconazole* 200 to 400 mg/day for 6 months can also be used. *Amikacin* 500 mg bid

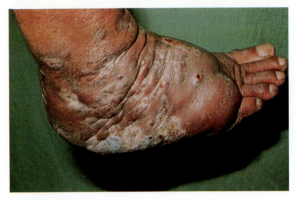

Fig. 22–20
Mycetoma. Subcutaneous nodules and sinus formation.

intramuscularly for 3 weeks or more may also help. Surgical excision helps cure smaller lesions, and amputation is necessary in progressive cases. Prompt diagnosis may prevent the severe consequences.

CHROMOMYCOSIS ICD-9 (117.2)

Chromomycosis is a chronic, warty, cutaneous and subcutaneous infection caused by several closely related dematiaceous fungi: *Fonsecaea pedrosoi, F. compactum, Phialophora verrucosa, Cladosporium carrionii,* and *Rhinocladiella aquaspera.* The disease is common in the tropical and subtropical areas of India; Southeast Asia; North, Central, and South America; and Africa. It is also found in Australia, Russia, and Cuba. Barefooted men are affected more than women, and agricultural workers, farmers, and gardeners are frequently infected.

Classic Description

Papules, nodules, and plaques are typically found on the leg, foot, hands, arms and trunk. Secondary erythema may range in color from pink to violaceous, with warty or cauliflower-like hyperkeratosis and a mixture of scarring and hypertrophy of the skin. Secondary bacterial infection, mossy foot, or lymphomatosis verrucosa may also occur.

Diagnosis and Differential Diagnosis

The diagnosis is confirmed by finding septate, dark brown cells in clusters or pairs in exudates and tissue. The causative organism can be grown on Sabouraud agar media. The differential diagnosis includes *tuberculosis verrucosa cutis, verruca vulgaris, lupoid leishmaniasis, late stage syphilis,* and *yaws,* all of which are ruled out clinically and by identification of specific organisms.

Treatment

Early stage chromomycosis is treated by deep and wide excision, followed by grafting. Cryosurgery or local heat may be used in small lesions. A combination of intravenous *amphotericin B,* 50 mg every other day, and *5 fluorocytosine* 3 g daily for 12 weeks is currently the best therapeutic approach. *Ketoconazole* 200 mg/day improves the condition, with *itraconazole* showing better results. Barring all else, amputation may be indicated in more advanced cases.

SUGGESTED READING

Amer M: Cutaneous schistomiasis, *Dermatol Clin* 12:713–717, 1994.

Anonymous: Expert committee on leprosy, Sixth Technical Series, no 768, Geneva, WHO, 1988.

Crissey JT, Lang H, Parish LC: *Manual of medical mycology,* Cambridge, Mass, 1995, Blackwell Science, 116–122.

Dutz W, Kohot-Dutz E: Anthrax, *Int J Dermatol* 20:203–206, 1981.

Goihman-Yahr M: American mucocutaneous leishmaniasis, *Dermatol Clin* 12:703–712, 1994.

Gross MI, Millikan LE: Deep fungal infections in the tropics, *Dermatol Clin* 12:695–700, 1994.

Hepburn NC: Cutaneous leishmaniasis, *Proc R Coll Phys Edin* 22:448–459, 1992.

Hobbs ER: Coccidioidomycosis, *Dermatol Clin* 7:227–239, 1989.

Hoffler W: Cutaneous diphtheria, *Int J Dermatol* 30:845–846, 1991.

Koff AB, Rosen T: Treatment of cutaneous leishmaniasis, *J Am Acad Dermatol* 31:693–708, 1994.

Lotti T, Hautman G: Atypical mycobacterial infection: a difficult and emerging group of infectious dermatoses, *Int J Dermatol* 32:499–501, 1993.

Milan CP, Fenske NA: Chromoblastomycosis, *Dermatol Clin* 7:219–225, 1989.

Murdoch ME et al: A clinical classification and grading system of the cutaneous changes in onchocerciasis, *Br J Dermatol* 129:260–269, 1993.

Niemel PLA et al: Donovanosis (granuloma inguinale) still exists, *Int J Dermatol* 31:244–246, 1992.

Parish LC, Millikan LE et al: *Global dermatology,* New York, 1994, Springer Verlag.

Parish LC, Witkowski JA, Vassilera S: *Color atlas of cutaneous infections,* 1995, Cambridge, Mass, Blackwell Science.

Ramesh V, Mukherjee A: Post–kala-azar dermal leishmaniasis, *Int J Dermatol* 34:85–91, 1995.

Routh HB, Bhowmik KR: Filariasis, *Dermatol Clin* 12:719–727, 1994.

Sehgal VN, Wagh SA: Cutaneous tuberculosis: current concepts, *Int J Dermatol* 29:237–252, 1990.

Sehgal VN et al: Yaws control/eradication, *Int J Dermatol* 33:16–20, 1994.

Shelley WB, Shelley ED: Co-existent erythrasma, trichomycosis axillaris, and pitted keratolysis: an overlooked Corynebacterium triad? *J Am Acad Dermatol* 24:752–757, 1982.

Weber DJ et al: Pasteurella multocida infection: report of 34 cases and review of literature, *Medicine* 63:133–154, 1984.

World Health Organization: Recommendations. Workshop on DNA diagnostics and filariasis and symposium on filariasis and onchocerciasis. Jakarta, Indonesia, 1989.

Zaias N: Pitted keratolysis: a review and update, *J Am Acad Dermatol* 7:787–791, 1982.

CHAPTER 23

Miscellaneous Lesions

CHONDRODERMATITIS NODULARIS HELICIS ICD-9 (380.00)

Classic Description

Chondrodermatitis nodularis helicis is a painful inflammatory papule or nodule of the ear, frequently involving the helix (Fig. 23–1). It occurs most commonly in elderly men, probably in relationship to trauma. *Patients often have a history of inability to sleep on the affected side because of discomfort.*

Diagnosis

The diagnosis is based clinically on a history of acute onset of a very tender lesion on the helix or antehelix of the ear and the appearance of a discrete nodule. Biopsy may be helpful in determining the diagnosis, especially if carcinoma is a concern.

Differential Diagnosis

The differential diagnosis includes *basal cell* and *squamous cell carcinomas;* however, these are usually slower growing and often are not so acutely tender. A *keratoacanthoma* may have an acute onset, similar to that of chondrodermatitis but has a central keratotic plug and rapidly enlarges. Other diagnoses to consider include *verruca* and *tophi.*

Treatment

Initial therapy consists of an intralesional injection with *triamcinolone acetonide* 10 mg/ml, 0.2–0.3 ml into the involved area. If the lesion

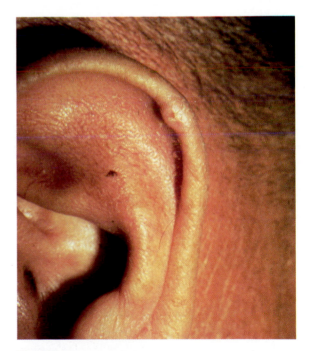

Fig. 23–1
Chondrodermatitis nodularis helicis with discrete, painful nodule on the helix of the ear. (Courtesy Department of Dermatology, University of North Carolina at Chapel Hill.)

persists, surgical removal of the affected area, including the cartilage, is indicated. The specimen should be sent for pathologic evaluation. Excisions on the ear often are quite disfiguring, and referral to a dermatologist or plastic surgeon is recommended.

CUTANEOUS LARVA MIGRANS ICD-9 (126.9)

Classic Description

Cutaneous larva migrans, or creeping eruption, as it is commonly known, is a self-limited pruritic skin infestation secondary to the presence of the dog, cat, or cattle hookworm, the most common of which is *Ancylostoma braziliense.* The ova are deposited into the soil by animal feces, and the larva subsequently penetrate human skin, usually through the feet or backs of children, gardeners, farmers, or people who bathe in the sea. Humans are not the primary host and are inadvertently infested. *Worms wander in the epidermis several millimeters each day in a bizarre configuration,* for up to 4 to 6 weeks before dying (Fig. 23–2).

Diagnosis

Diagnosis is based on the clinical appearance of pruritic, bizarre, tunnel-like lesions a few millimeters in diameter. Peripheral blood eosinophilia frequently is found.

Treatment

Treatment for cutaneous larva migrans is directed toward relieving the itching and treating

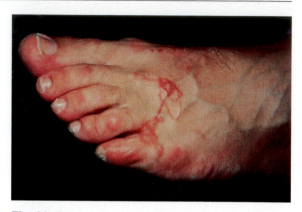

Fig. 23–2
Cutaneous larva migrans. Note the bizarre tunnel-like lesions on the dorsum of the foot. (Courtesy Department of Dermatology, University of North Carolina at Chapel Hill.)

the underlying infestation. Apply topical *thiabendazole* suspension 500 mg/5 ml 4 times daily for 1 week to the affected area. Extend coverage to include 2 cm of normal surrounding skin, because the actual location of the nematode can be anywhere in the area of the lesion. For pruritus control use *hydroxyzine hydrochloride* 10 to 50 mg every 6 hours or at bedtime. Mild topical corticosteroids, such as *hydrocortisone* 1% lotion (2 oz) with menthol 0.5%, also may be helpful.

ERYTHEMA NODOSUM ICD-9 (695.2)

Erythema nodosum is a well-circumscribed, acute, inflammatory disorder of the subcutaneous fat that is thought to represent an immune reaction occurring in response to a variety of underlying systemic disorders (Box 23–1). Seen most commonly in women age 20 to 30, the typical disease course has an acute onset, followed by resolution in 3 to 6 weeks, without sequelae.

Classic Description

The skin lesions are painful, erythematous nodules usually found on the extensor aspects of the legs (Fig. 23–3) but may also be seen on the thighs, forearms, and elsewhere. Lesions are usually bilateral but not necessarily symmetric in distribution. Single or multiple lesions that are

Conditions Associated With Erythema Nodosum

Drugs
  Oral contraceptives, sulphonamides, bromides
Infections
  Chlamydia infections (psittacosis, cat-scratch disease, lymphogranuloma venereum), fungal infections (histoplasmosis, coccidiodomycosis, blastomycosis), streptococcal infections, tuberculosis, viral infections (infectious mononucleosis), yersiniosis
Inflammatory bowel disease
Lymphoma
Pregnancy
Radiation therapy
Sarcoidosis
Idiopathic

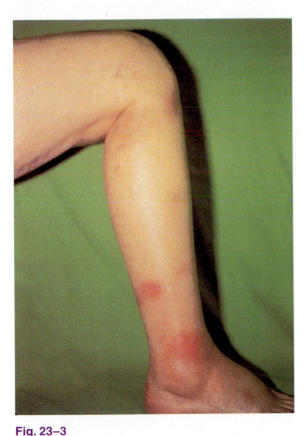

Fig. 23–3
Erythema nodosum, with erythematous tender nodules on the lower extremity. (Courtesy Beverly Sanders, MD.)

present often heal with overlying bruising. Arthralgias, fever, malaise, and pedal edema are associated in 50% of affected individuals.

Diagnosis

The initial evaluation of erythema nodosum includes a drug history; history of recent travel; exposure to animals; symptoms of underlying infections, particularly streptococcal infections; physical examination; and appropriate laboratory evaluation (Box 23–2). Diagnosis is based on the clinical appearance of erythematous tender nodules in the characteristic locations. *Biopsy occasionally is indicated and should be deep enough to include adequate subcutaneous fat for diagnostic purposes.* Use an ellipse excision with a no. 15 scalpel blade or a 6-mm punch biopsy.

Differential Diagnosis

The differential diagnosis includes *erysipelas* or other forms of *cellulitis,* but such lesions are unilateral and have increasing, expanding areas of erythema. *Phlebitis* will have a hard, irregular fibrotic area, as opposed to the discrete nodules of erythema nodosum. Lesions of *vasculitis* may be difficult to differentiate and require biopsy, although vasculitic lesions tend to be more chronic, and extensive systemic involvement

BOX 23–2.

Laboratory Evaluation in Patients With Erythema Nodosum

Chemistry profile and CBC count
Sedimentation rate
Throat culture
Antistreptolysin-O titer
Chest radiogragh*
Purified protein derivative
Stool culture for *Yersinia* (consider culture and/or serum titers if GI complaints predominate)

*Bilateral hilar adenopathy is present in sarcoidosis, coccidiodomycosis, histoplasmosis, and tuberculosis. Therefore, an abnormal chest radiograph alone is not a sufficient diagnostic confirmation for sarcoidosis in this population.

may or may not be present. Other types of panniculitis can only be ruled out by biopsy.

Treatment

Treatment consists of removal of any offending agent or the treatment of the underlying cause, frequent bed rest with elevation of the involved extremities, support hose or elastic bandage wraps during the day when walking, and aspirin and NSAIDs, such as *ibuprofen,* to control the discomfort. Resistant cases may respond to *potassium iodide* at 300 mg 3 times daily for 3 to 4 weeks, with monitoring of thyroid function. Refer difficult or chronic cases to a dermatologist.

GRANULOMA ANNULARE ICD-9 (695.89)

Granuloma annulare is a chronic, inflammatory, dermal disorder of unknown cause. The disease occurs most commonly in children and young adults, and there is a female predominance.

Classic Description

Lesions initially begin as small erythematous papules that evolve into annular plaques as they coalesce over a period of weeks into the characteristic pattern (Fig. 23–4). Lesions typically involve the dorsum of the hands or feet or the extensor aspects of the extremities, manifesting as solitary lesions 1 to 5 cm in diameter. The lesions may last for several months to several years before spontaneous resolution. Recurrences occur in approximately 40% of affected individuals. Rarely, a disseminated form occurs in adults, and there is a possible increased association of diabetes mellitus in such patients.

Diagnosis

Diagnosis is based on the clinical appearance of the characteristic lesions. A biopsy showing collagen degeneration will give a definitive diagnosis if there is any question.

Differential Diagnosis

The differential diagnosis includes *tinea corporis,* because of the annular configuration. However, granuloma annulare has no scales, and the results of the potassium hydroxide test are normal. *Lichen planus* is typically symmetric, often with associated buccal lesions. *Necrobiosis lipoidica diabeticorum, sarcoidosis,* and *rheumatoid nodules* can be differentiated by biopsy. *Late secondary* and *tertiary syphilis* can be ruled out with nontreponemal serologic tests (RPR/VDRL), if necessary.

Treatment

Treatment consists of reassurance that the majority of localized lesions will spontaneously involute within 2 years; however, recurrences and persistence are likely in the disseminated form. Intralesional *triamcinolone* 5 to 10 mg/ml injected into an elevated border may help resolve lesions that are cosmetically disfiguring. Referral to a dermatologist is indicated for symptomatic disseminated granuloma annulare.

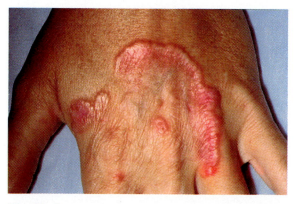

Fig. 23–4
Granuloma annulare. Note the nonscaling, annular plaque on the dorsum of the hands. (Courtesy Medical College of Georgia, Division of Dermatology.)

KAWASAKI SYNDROME ICD-9 (446.1)

Kawasaki syndrome, also known as *mucocutaneous lymph node syndrome,* is an inflammatory, reactional disorder that affects primarily children younger than age 5. Recently, some patients with a variant of toxic shock syndrome have presented with cases very similar to that found in Kawasaki syndrome. It is felt that the cause of Kawasaki syndrome may be an infectious agent that leads to an immune-mediated syndrome in genetically predisposed individuals. *Recognition of Kawasaki syndrome is essential because coronary artery aneurysms occur in as many as 30% of untreated children,* usually within 10 to 30 days. Fatal myocardial infarctions may occur in 0.6% of patients.

The disease is characterized by the presence of fever that is unresponsive to antipyretics and lasts at least 5 days, accompanied by several other characteristic signs (Box 23–3). Systemic features may include extreme irritability in infants, arthralgias, aseptic meningitis, hepatic dysfunction, hydrops of the gallbladder, otitis media, diarrhea, uveitis, pneumonitis, and peripheral gangrene. Laboratory findings include leukocytosis and elevated sedimentation rate. Thrombocytosis is present 2 weeks after disease onset.

Classic Description

The classic skin findings involve mucous membrane changes and a generalized rash. The mouth has red and fissured lips, often with strawberry tongue (Fig. 23–5). The exanthem may be discrete, morbilliform, scarlatiniform, or even urticarial, with generalized macules and papules that may coalesce into plaques. *Erythema and desquamation of the hands, feet, and perineal region are hallmarks of Kawasaki syndrome,* occurring 10 to 14 days after the onset of symptoms (Fig. 23–6).

Diagnosis

See Box 23–3 and Table 18–1.

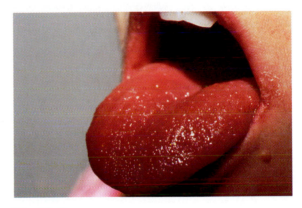

Fig. 23–5
Strawberry tongue in a patient with Kawasaki syndrome. (Courtesy Marshall Guill, MD.)

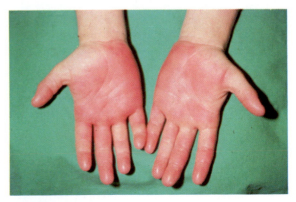

Fig. 23–6
Kawasaki syndrome. Note the erythema of the hands, to be followed by desquamation. (Courtesy Department of Dermatology, University of North Carolina at Chapel Hill.)

BOX 23–3.
Diagnosis of Kawasaki Syndrome

> Fever lasting >5 days, unresponsive to antipyretics
> Four of the following:
>   1. Bilateral nonexudative conjunctivitis
>   2. Generalized rash
>   3. Hand/foot erythema, edema, or desquamation
>   4. Mucous membrane changes: red or fissured lips, strawberry tongue
>   5. Cervical adenitis: >1.5 cm, nonpurulent

Differential Diagnosis

The differential diagnosis includes *measles, scarlet fever,* and *Stevens-Johnson syndrome.* Patients with *measles* will have an ocular and nasal discharge and a cough. Look for Koplik's spots early on in measles. Patients with *scarlet fever* will have an exudative pharyngitis, no conjunctivitis, and a culture positive for *Streptococcus.* Patients with *Stevens-Johnson syndrome* will have erythema multiforme skin lesions and prominent mucous membrane involvement with bullae, erosions, or both. *Staphylococcal scalded skin syndrome* has widespread lesions and superficial blisters, but mucous membrane involvement occurs less frequently.

Treatment

A suggested treatment regimen for Kawasaki syndrome is outlined in Box 23–4.

MASTOCYTOSIS ICD-9 (757.33; SYSTEMIC 202.6)

Mastocytosis is an uncommon spectrum of disorders linked by the presence of an increased number of mast cells. The skin is the most common organ system affected by the disease. Patients seek medical care for symptoms related to the release of mediators from mast cell granules, particularly histamine and heparin. In children younger than age 2, the disease occurs most commonly as a localized collection of mast cells in a *mastocytoma,* which typically resolves spontaneously.

Widespread cutaneous lesions are known as *urticaria pigmentosa* (Fig. 23–7). Such lesions are likely to spontaneously resolve in children, but are more chronic and associated with systemic disease in adults. When there is systemic involvement, with or without cutaneous involvement, the disorder is called *systemic mastocytosis,* and the bone, the liver, the central nervous system, and the gastrointestinal tract may be involved. The systemic form occurs in 10% of patients with mastocytosis and more commonly in adults. There is an increased incidence of peptic ulcer disease in systemic mastocytosis. Systemic adult mastocytosis carries a worse prognosis, with rare spontaneous resolution and a 10% to 30% incidence of malignant transformation. *Telangiectasia macularis eruptiva perstans* (generalized cutaneous mastocytosis) is a rare condition seen in adults and characterized by widespread telangiectatic macules occurring on an erythematous background.

Classic Description

Mastocytomas are usually characterized by solitary (but may be multiple) nodules 3 to 4 cm in

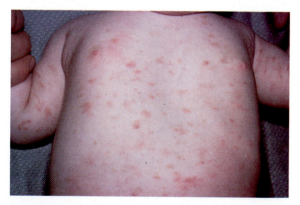

Fig. 23–7
Widespread erythematous macules, papules, and plaques of urticaria pigmentosa on the trunk of an infant. (Courtesy Department of Dermatology, University of North Carolina at Chapel Hill.)

diameter, associated with hyperpigmentation. The cutaneous rash presents with 0.5- to 1.0-cm reddish brown macules that urticate, or form wheals, on rubbing or scratching, a process known as *Darier's sign* (Fig. 23–8). Lesions may form vesicles or bullae. If many mast granules are released, systemic effects may include headache, flushing, bronchospasm, diarrhea, abdominal pain, and increased heart rate. Common events that may cause granule release are listed in Box 23–5.

Diagnosis

Diagnosis is based on the presence of urtication on rubbing or scratching of lesions. Biopsy is diagnostic, when there is any doubt. If skeletal symptoms coexist or there is widespread cutaneous involvement, a radiologic and/or bone survey should be done.

Differential Diagnosis

The differential diagnosis may include *ecchymoses,* as a result of child abuse, when there are multiple pigmented lesions on a child; however, Darier's sign will be absent. The flushing of *carcinoid syndrome* can be differentiated from the flushing of mastocytosis by the administration of epinephrine, which will precipitate flushing in carcinoid syndrome but not in mastocytosis.

Treatment

Treatment consists of avoiding precipitating factors (see Box 23–5). Patients unable to control symptoms with avoidance may benefit from potent topical corticosteroids (e.g., *clobetasol*

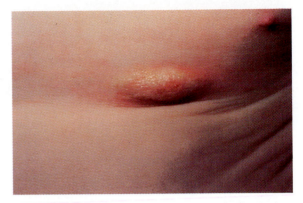

Fig. 23–8
Urticaria after scratching a macule in a patient with mastocytosis (Darier's sign). (Courtesy Department of Dermatology, University of North Carolina at Chapel Hill.)

BOX 23–5.
Agents Causing Granule Release in Mastocytosis

Rubbing or scratching of lesions
Exposure to extremes of temperature
Ingestion of certain foods (e.g., alcohol, cheese)
Drugs such as aspirin and codeine
Exercise
Stress

dipropionate or *betamethasone dipropionate* cream or ointment under occlusion twice daily). Antihistamines such as *hydroxyzine* or *chlorpheniramine* are useful to control pruritus and to prevent further aggravation of lesions. *Doxepin* may also be helpful. Anticholinergic agents (e.g., *propantheline bromide* [Pro-Banthine] 15 mg 4 times daily) have been used in combination with aspirin and antihistamines. *Cromolyn sodium* (100 mg 4 times daily) or *ketotifen* (2 mg every day) may prevent mast cell granule release. Refer difficult or systemic cases.

PRURITUS ICD-9 (698.9)

Pruritus (derived from *prurire,* meaning *to itch*) can be one of the most noxious sensations in the human experience, and patients with complaints of itching need extra emotional support and understanding from health care providers. Most patients will scratch an insect bite until it bleeds, because the sensation of pain is better tolerated than itching. *Also, generalized pruritus may be the first sign of an underlying malignancy; therefore never disregard a patient's complaint of itching.*

Pruritus is classified as local or generalized, and may be associated with an underlying skin disorder (e.g., scabies, dermatitis herpetiformis), may manifest with excoriations only, or may be a symptom with no objective skin findings.

Many systemic disorders can cause pruritus (Box 23–6). Emotional stress and, rarely, severe psychologic problems (e.g., monosymptomatic hypochondriasis in delusions of parasitosis) are associated with pruritus.

Skin lesions are variable, occurring as lichenified plaques from chronic rubbing, excoriations limited to where a person can scratch (e.g., the middle of the back will be spared), or with no identifiable lesions. An algorithm to assist in the workup of underlying systemic diseases in patients with generalized pruritus is shown in Fig. 23–9. Symptom control usually can be achieved by following simple treatment suggestions (Box 23–7).

Pruritus associated with uremia may respond to ultraviolet B light therapy, emollients, topical *capsaicin, cholestyramine,* and oral activated charcoal. Hepatobiliary-associated pruritus tends to improve with binding resins, such as *cholestyramine* or *colestipol.*

BOX 23–6.

Causes of Generalized Pruritus Without Specific Skin Lesions*

AIDS	
Drugs	Aspirin, cholestatic inducing agents (hormones, phenothiazines, erythromycin estolate), opiates (cocaine, morphine), quinidine, virtually any drug
External causes	Chemicals (fabric softeners, detergents), excessive bathing (hot tubs especially), fiberglass, low humidity, parasite exposures (birds, dogs, straw, old furniture)
Hematologic disorders	Iron deficiency, paraproteinemia, polycythemia vera
Infestations	Pediculosis corporis, scabies, trichinosis
Liver disease	Obstructive biliary disease, cholestasis
Malignancy	Lymphoma/leukemia, multiple myeloma, visceral carcinoma (adenocarcinoma and squamous cell carcinoma in particular)
Mastocytosis	
Metabolic	Carcinoid syndrome, diabetes mellitus, thyroid disease
Neurologic	Infarcts, abscess of brain, multiple sclerosis
Pregnancy	
Psychiatric	Delusions of parasitosis, stress
Kidney disease	Chronic renal insufficiency
Xerosis	

*Modified from Bernhard JD: Clinical aspects of pruritus, in Fitzpatrick TB et al, eds: *Dermatology in general medicine,* ed 3, New York, 1987, McGraw-Hill, pp 80–81.

BOX 23–7.

Pruritus Symptom Control

Mild cleanser for bathing (e.g., white Dove) or a soap substitute (e.g., Cetaphil, Aquanil, or CAM lotion)
Emollients after bathing or showering every day (e.g., Snow Drift shortening by Martha White, Lubriderm, Nutraderm, Complex 15, Moisturel, or Eucerin)
Lotions with menthol 0.5%, phenol (except in pregnancy) 0.5%, or camphor 0.5% (e.g., Sarna, Prax, Pramegel, or Itch X)
Oral antihisamines (e.g., hydroxyzine hydrochloride 10–50 mg q6h or qhs) if the patient is losing sleep
Mild topical corticosteroid (e.g., hydrocortisone 1% lotion 4 oz, with menthol 0.5%) or one with medium potency (e.g., triamcinolone 0.1%, cream or lotion, 4–8 oz, mixed 1:1 with Eucerin or Aquaphor with 0.5% menthol)
Avoid prolonged or multiple hot baths or showers

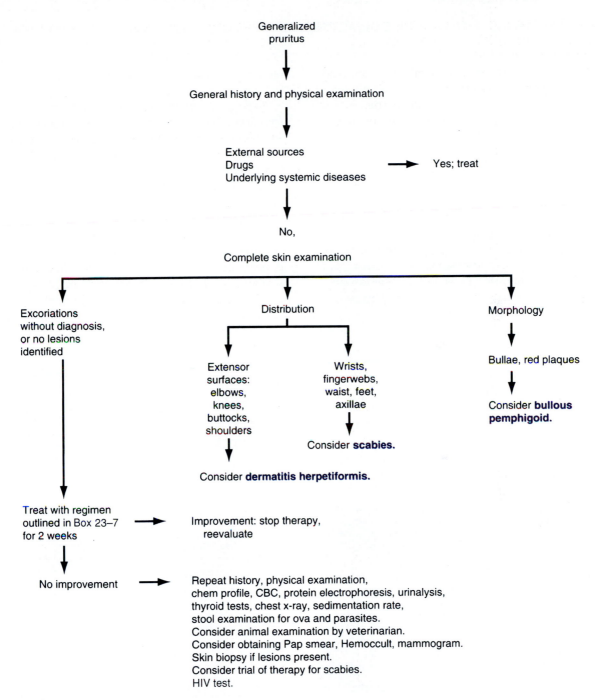

Generalized
pruritus

⬇

General history and physical examination

⬇

External sources
Drugs   ➡   Yes; treat
Underlying systemic diseases

⬇

No,

Complete skin examination

Excoriations without diagnosis, or no lesions identified	Distribution	Morphology

Distribution:

Extensor surfaces: elbows, knees, buttocks, shoulders

⬇

Consider **dermatitis herpetiformis.**

Wrists, fingerwebs, waist, feet, axillae

⬇

Consider **scabies.**

Morphology:

Bullae, red plaques

⬇

Consider **bullous pemphigoid.**

Treat with regimen outlined in Box 23–7 for 2 weeks   ➡   Improvement: stop therapy, reevaluate

⬇

No improvement   ➡   Repeat history, physical examination, chem profile, CBC, protein electrophoresis, urinalysis, thyroid tests, chest x-ray, sedimentation rate, stool examination for ova and parasites.
Consider animal examination by veterinarian.
Consider obtaining Pap smear, Hemoccult, mammogram.
Skin biopsy if lesions present.
Consider trial of therapy for scabies.
HIV test.

Fig. 23–9
Algorithm for workup and management of patients with generalized pruritis.

PURPURA ICD-9 (287.2 SENILE OR ACTINIC; 709.0 PROGRESSIVE PIGMENTED PURPURA; VASCULITIS BY ETIOLOGY)

Purpura (derived from the term *porpyra,* meaning *purple*) is caused by the hemorrhage of blood into the skin secondary to the loss of blood vessel integrity.

Classic Description

There are many different causes of purpura. Clinicians should initially classify purpura as either palpable or nonpalpable.

Nonpalpable purpura, with isolated and/or coalescing macules, has many causes, some benign and others life-threatening. *Actinic purpura,* or senile purpura, is a very common problem in older adults. It is characterized by areas of solar elastosis and accentuated by the use of agents such as aspirin, which decrease platelet aggregation properties (Fig. 23–10). Purpura may occur in response to minor trauma in any condition in which the clotting time is decreased, such as occurs with some *drugs,* such as aspirin, warfarin (Coumadin), and NSAIDs. In blood dyscrasias, such as *thrombocytopenia, disseminated intravascular coagulopathy,* and *leukemia,* petechiae, or minute areas of bleeding, are typically initially seen. Perifollicular petechiae, especially on the shins, are characteristic of *scurvy.*

Progressive pigmented purpura is a benign form of nonpalpable purpura most commonly seen on the lower extremities and thought to be caused by capillaritis. Petechiae are seen with hyperpigmentation as a result of breakdown of heme (Fig. 23–11). Also known as *Schamberg's purpura* and a multitude of other confusing terms, progressive pigmented purpura has no association with underlying systemic illnesses.

Palpable purpura is an inflammation-based purpura in which there is loss of the integrity of smaller blood vessels from many causes (Box 23–8). Palpable purpura may occur anywhere but is most common on the lower extremities.

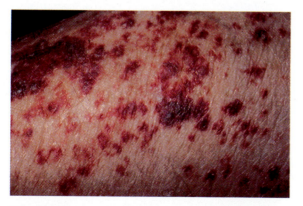

Fig. 23–10
Actinic purpura. Hemorrhagic areas on sun-exposed skin after minor trauma. (Courtesy Department of Dermatology, University of North Carolina at Chapel Hill.)

BOX 23–8.

Some Causes of Palpable Purpura

Connective tissue diseases	Rheumatoid arthritis, Sjögren's syndrome, systemic lupus erythematosus, etc.
Cryoglobulinemia	
Drugs	Aspirin, nonsteroidal antiinflammatory drugs, penicillins, phenothiazines, serum, sulfonamides, thiazides
Henoch-Schönlein purpura	History of upper respiratory tract infecton; joint, gastrointestinal, and renal involvement more common in children; IgA antibody seen with direct immunofluorescence of a skin lesion <24 hr old
Infection	Group A β-hemolytic *Streptococcus, Staphylococcus aureus,* Rickettsial infection, hepatitis B, urinary tract infection, literally any infection
Inflammatory bowel disease	
Malignancy	Lymphoma, leukemia, myeloma

A
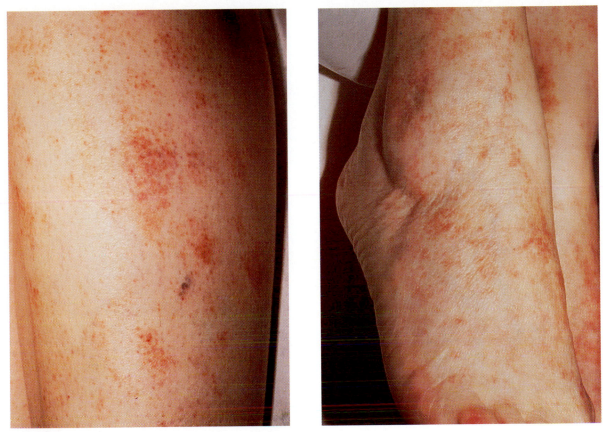
B

Fig. 23–11
Progressive pigmented purpura. Bronze hyperpigmentation of the skin with nonblanching erythema. (Courtesy Department of Dermatology, University of North Carolina at Chapel Hill.)

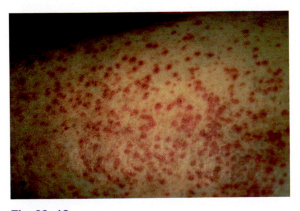

Fig. 23–12
Palpable purpura/vasculitis. (Courtesy Medical College of Georgia, Division of Dermatology.)

The skin lesions initially are nonblanching, erythematous papules, but if the necrosis is severe, lesions may be bullous and evolve into ulcers (Fig. 23–12). If deeper vessels are involved, look for nodules, pustules, urticaria, and edema, with prominent secondary ecchymoses. *Palpable purpura heralds vasculitis.* Systemic symptoms of fever, malaise, arthralgias, myalgias, and abdominal pain and systemic signs of microscopic hematuria, proteinuria, glomerulonephritis, peripheral neuropathy, pulmonary vasculitis, and myocardial involvement may complicate the disease course. General screening laboratory tests to consider in the workup for palpable purpura are given in Box 23–9.

BOX 23–9.

Evaluation of Palpable Purpura

Complete blood cell count with differential and platelets	Liver function tests
Serum creatinine	Hepatitis B surface antigen
Throat culture	Hepatitis C
Antistreptolysin O titer	ANCA (antineutrophil cytoplasmic auto-antibodies)
Erythrocyte sedimentation rate	Cryoglobulins
Urinalysis	Serum protein electrophoresis
Skin biopsy	Complement function
Stool examination for occult blood	Chest radiograph
Rheumatoid factor and antinuclear antibody	HIV test

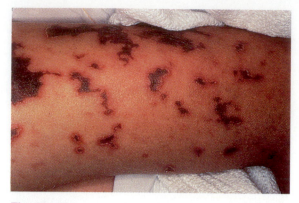

Fig. 23–13

Large hemorrhagic areas on the upper extremity in a patient with meningococcemia. (Courtesy Marshall Guill, MD.)

In certain diseases, such as *Rocky Mountain spotted fever,* petechiae classically begin on the wrists and ankles, then spread to involve the trunk and proximal extremities (Figs. 6–8 and 6–9). Cutaneous involvement, with fulminant *meningococcemia,* also occurs as palpable purpura (Fig. 23–13). There is a sudden onset of fever, headache, nausea, emesis, and petechiae, and bacteria are present in the skin and/or blood.

Diagnosis

The diagnosis of purpura often rests on the fact that purpuric erythematous macules or papules do not blanch with pressure because the blood has leaked out of the blood vessels and therefore cannot be pressed out with pressure. Palpable purpura always should signal vasculitis, and underlying causes should be sought, even if initially not evident. Skin biopsy usually is diagnostic; however, it may not be necessary, especially when palpable purpura is present in the absence of systemic findings. However, when a child is evaluated for possible *Henoch-Schönlein purpura* (Fig. 23–14), a 3- to 4-mm punch or deep shave biopsy of a new lesion less than 24 to 48 hours old for direct immunofluorescence to demonstrate IgA may be helpful.

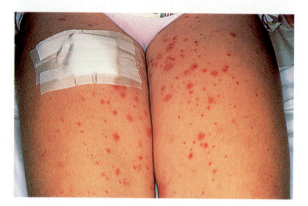

Fig. 23–14

Henoch-Schönlein purpura on the lower extremities of a child. (Courtesy Medical College of Georgia, Division of Dermatology.)

Differential Diagnosis

The differential diagnosis includes *cholesterol embolization,* although biopsy will usually differentiate. The nonblanchable nature of purpuric lesions in dark-skinned patients may be more difficult to discern clinically, and a biopsy may be necessary.

Treatment

Treatment consists of identifying and addressing any precipitating drug, infection, or other systemic illness. Short courses of *prednisone* (0.5 to 1.0 mg/kg/day, tapered over 2 to 3 weeks) usually are necessary only when lesions cause symptoms or when there is systemic involvement. *Colchicine* (0.6 mg daily, slowly increasing to 0.6 mg twice daily) also may be helpful in such cases. Refer chronic or recalcitrant cases for further management, including immunosuppressants.

PYODERMA GANGRENOSUM ICD-9 (686.0)

Pyoderma gangrenosum is a rare, painful, necrotizing, and ulcerative skin disease of unknown cause. Although it is often associated with an immune reaction and underlying systemic disorders (Box 23–10), 40% of cases have no associated systemic disease.

Classic Description

Single or multiple lesions begin as small, nonspecific, erythematous vesicles or papules that spread concentrically. Such lesions evolve into pustules, with significant induration, erythema, and subsequent ulceration. The borders usually are irregular, ragged, undermined, and violaceous (Fig. 23–15). Ulcers heal with cribriform, atrophic scars. The most common sites of involvement are the lower extremities, buttocks, and abdomen. Fever may accompany the lesions.

Diagnosis

Diagnosis is based on the clinical appearance of the lesions; a course lasting weeks to months, despite antibacterial or other therapies; and the exclusion of other ulcerative skin disorders, such as vasculitis and infections. Biopsy shows only

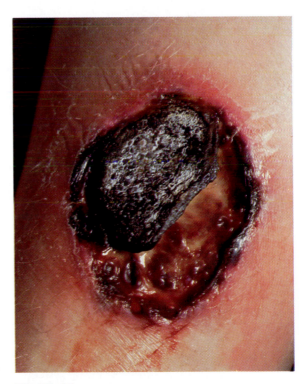

Fig. 23–15
Pyoderma gangrenosum. Large ulcer with indurated edges. (Courtesy Department of Dermatology, University of North Carolina at Chapel Hill.)

BOX 23–10.

Systemic Diseases Associated With Pyoderma Gangrenosum

Ankylosing spondylitis	Malignancies
Blood dyscrasias	Monoclonal
Chronic active hepatitis	gammopathies
Enteropathic	Myeloma
arthropathy	Rheumatoid arthritis
Granulocyte colony	Sarcoidosis
stimulating factor therapy	Psoriatic arthritis
Idiopathic (30%–40%)	
Inflammatory bowel	
disease (50%)	

nonspecific inflammation. Elevated sedimentation rate and leukocytosis usually are present. Cultures of bacteria from the lesions are thought to represent secondary invasion rather than primary infection.

Differential Diagnosis

The differential diagnosis includes *necrotizing vasculitis, brown recluse spider bites, echthyma gangrenosum, atypical mycobacterial and clostridial infections, deep fungal infections, amebiasis, tropical ulcers, and gangrene.* Demonstration of causative organisms and the clinical findings help to differentiate these diseases from pyoderma gangrenosum.

Treatment

General treatment involves control of any underlying systemic diseases and avoidance of trauma to the lesions. Needle punctures and other procedures, such as aggressive debridement, should be minimized because pathergy (a hypersensitivity reaction to minimal trauma) may occur in approximately 20% of patients. Specific treatments include intralesional injections of *triamcinolone diacetate,* ultrapotent corticosteroids under occlusion, or systemic *prednisone,* with initial doses of 0.5 to 1.0 mg/kg/day. Other treatments include sulfasalazine, dapsone, minocycline, and immunosuppressive agents. Gentle cleansing and debridement with whirlpool therapy, dilute hydrogen peroxide, and topical dressings also are helpful. Diagnosis and treatment should be coordinated in consultation with a dermatologist.

SARCOIDOSIS ICD-9 (135)

Sarcoidosis is a disease of unknown cause characterized by the presence of noncaseating granulomas in various organs, particularly the skin, lymph nodes, lungs, and eyes. It occurs more frequently in females, blacks, Scandinavians, and residents of the southeastern United States and has an incidence in the United States of 1 to 7:10,000.

Two clinical forms exist. The first occurs as an acute disorder, primarily in younger patients, with the sudden onset of skin lesions in association with eye involvement and hilar adenopathy. Serum angiotensin–converting enzyme and calcium levels may be elevated. Such disease typically remits spontaneously and has a good prognosis, although recurrences are possible.

The more chronic form occurs in patients over age 40, and although onset tends to be gradual, the disease tends to become progressive. Lung involvement is the predominant feature, and abnormalities of calcium or angiotensin–converting enzyme are less common. Lung involvement (87%) is followed in frequency by involvement of lymph nodes (27%), liver (25%), skin (25% to 30%), and eyes (20%). Other organs less frequently affected include the bones, spleen, heart, and salivary and lacrimal glands.

Classic Description

The skin lesions seen in sarcoidosis are erythema nodosum and noncaseating granulomas. Sarcoidosis can be likened to syphilis, because sarcoidosis' skin lesions mimic the skin findings of many other disorders. A violaceous nodule or plaque, *lupus pernio,* is seen on the nose, cheeks, or ears and may be associated with upper respiratory tract involvement and chronic fibrosis of the lungs (Fig. 23–16). More general-

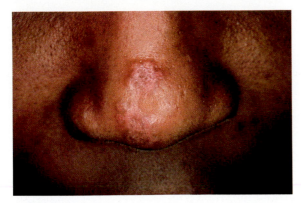

Fig. 23–16
Waxy plaque of lupus pernio on the nose of patient with sarcoidosis. (Courtesy Medical College of Georgia, Division of Dermatology.)

ized, symmetric, infiltrative papules and nodules that are annular or serpiginous have a predilection for the limbs, buttocks, shoulders, and face (Fig. 23–17). Scattered papules that coalesce into plaques occur on the face, characteristically along the eyelids and nasal ala, posterior side of the neck, shoulders, and extensor surfaces of extremities. Lesions also have a predilection for occurring in scars.

Diagnosis

The diagnosis of sarcoidosis is best made when widespread noncaseating graunulomas are present in more than one organ. The classic Kveim skin test is not standardized, nor readily available. *A strong suspicion for sarcoidosis should be maintained in any patient with symmetric infiltrative papules, nodules, or plaques; erythema nodosum; or systemic signs, such as bilateral hilar adenopathy, fever, uveitis, parotitis, or hypercalcemia. Biopsy of suspect lesions is essential.* Scars often are a common site of skin involvement and may provide the best specimen. Lymph nodes are often the next most accessible tissue source, although lung tissue will show noncaseating granulomas more than 90% of the time.

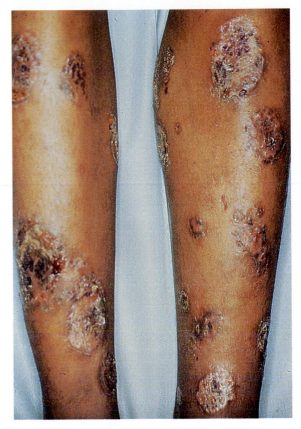

Fig. 23–17
Sarcoidosis. Note the symmetric, annular, infiltrative, scaling plaques on the lower extremities. (Courtesy Department of Dermatology, University of North Carolina at Chapel Hill.)

Differential Diagnosis

The differential diagnosis includes *syphilis,* but serology will distinguish the two. *Lupus vulgaris,* or tuberculosis of the skin, will reveal caseating granulomas and possible acid-fast bacilli on biopsy with special stains. *Lupus erythematosus* is easily differentiated by biopsy and a history of photosensitivity. *Berylliosis* and *foreign-body granulomas* are other considerations.

Treatment

Appropriate treatment should be coordinated with consultants. The workup includes baseline studies, such as routine chemistries, including calcium level and liver function tests, especially alkaline phosphatase levels, complete blood cell count, chest radiograph, pulmonary function tests, 24-hour urinalysis for calcium and hydroxyproline excretion, and a serum angiotensin-converting enzyme level.

Prednisone (0.5 to 1 mg/kg/day, tapering monthly to the lowest dosage that will control symptoms) is the mainstay of therapy. Prednisone is indicated for persistent systemic involvement, worsening chest radiograph findings, increasing shortness of breath, ocular disease, hypercalcemia or hypercalciuria, neurologic involvement, cardiac disease, dry eyes or mouth, severe arthritis, and disfiguring cutaneous lesions unresponsive to topical therapy. Other helpful agents may include antimalarials, methotrexate, or other immunosuppressant drugs.

For patient support and information contact the Sarcoidosis Family Aid and Medical Research Foundation.*

SUGGESTED READING

Dabski K, Winklemann RK: Generalized granuloma annulare: clinical and laboratory findings in 100 patients, *J Am Acad Dermatol* 20:39–47, 1989.

Edelglass JW et al: Cutaneous larva migrans in northern climates, *J Am Acad Dermatol* 7:353–358, 1982.

Jennette CJ, Milling DM, Falk RJ: Vasculitis affecting the skin, *Arch Dermatol* 130:899–906, 1994.

Jorizzo JL: Classification of vasculitis, *J Invest Dermatol* 100:106s–110s, 1993.

Longley J, Duffy TP, Kohn S: The mast cell and mast cell disease, *J Am Acad Dermatol* 32:545–561, 1995.

Lorette G, Vaillant L: Pruritus: current concepts in pathogenesis and treatment, *Drugs* 39:218–223, 1990.

Newburger JW: A single intravenous infusion of gamma globulin as compared with four infusions in the treatment of acute Kawasaki syndrome, *N Engl J Med* 324:1633–1639, 1991.

Pollack CV Jr, Jordan RC: Recognition and management of sarcoidosis in the emergency department, *J Emerg Med* 11:297–308, 1993.

Schwaegerle SM et al: Pyoderma gangrenosum: a review, *J Am Acad Dermatol* 18:559–568, 1988.

Shapiro JS: Sarcoidosis: current concepts and case reports, *J Am Board Fam Pract* 1:211–217, 1988.

Shulman ST, Inocencio JD, Hirsch R: *Kawasaki disease, Ped Clinic North America* 42:1205–1222, 1995.

*Sarcoidosis Family Aid and Medical Research Foundation, 460 Central Ave., East Orange, NJ 07018.

Patient Education Handouts

Use the following patient education handouts in whatever way is most appropriate or useful for your patients and practice setting. A practical suggestion is to give the handout to the patient and then go over the common questions, answering any new questions the patient may have. In addition, you may use the back of a handout to write down further appropriate detailed instructions on medication use, follow-up, and so on. Copies of each handout may be made without permission and adapted for clinical use.

Acne Vulgaris

What causes acne?

- Acne is caused by plugged pores on your skin. It affects many people just like yourself. Most acne can be made better.
- Pimples are not from having dirty skin, and they cannot be scrubbed off.
- Avoid picking and squeezing your bumps. This leads to scarring and also can cause more bumps to come out.

Will any foods that I eat make my acne worse?

- Foods that you eat, such as chocolate or fried foods, usually have little to do with your acne. However, eating the proper foods is good for your overall health.

How should I clean my skin?

- Use a mild soap, such as Dove, to gently wash your face. Avoid scrubbing your face.

How does the medicine help my acne?

- The medicines your provider is giving you will help keep most new bumps from forming. This will take about 6 to 8 weeks. The medicines will not "cure" your acne but will help keep it under control.
- Put a thin layer of the creams on all areas where you break out, not just on the bumps you see today.
- Once your face starts clearing up, it is important to keep using your medicines, or the acne may come back again.

What about using makeup?

- You may use makeup, but make sure it is water-based.

Atopic Dermatitis

What is atopic dermatitis?

- Atopic dermatitis, also known as atopic eczema, is common. Atopic dermatitis is often seen in children; its exact cause is not known. If someone in your family has asthma, hay fever, or eczema, other family members may have red, itchy skin. Your skin reacts too much to things you come in contact with every day.

What does atopic dermatitis look and feel like?

- Atopic dermatitis usually starts in the first year of life and almost always before age 5. In babies, you may see the rash on the face, elbows, and knees or all over the body.
- As you get older, the rash occurs where the elbows and knees bend and behind the neck or ears. On an adult, the rash often occurs on the hands.
- The rash is red, scaly, and very itchy.

What makes atopic dermatitis worse?

- Each person differs in what makes their atopic dermatitis worse. Some find they are worse in dry, cold weather, and others find sweating in the summer makes it worse. However, most find that stress, dry skin, harsh soaps or detergents, and infections make it worse.

What about allergies?

- Food allergies cause atopic dermatitis to get worse 10% to 15% of the time in children. Finding out which food is the cause is not easy. Talk with your provider about how to best tell if a certain formula or food is making your child's eczema worse. But do not hold out foods that are needed for good health.
- The most common foods that can cause allergies are eggs, cow's milk, peanuts, soy, wheat, and seafood. Some animals, dust, mites, molds, and pollens may also cause flare ups. Testing is only needed in the worst cases and is not always helpful.

How can I best take care of my skin?

- Use mild cleansers, such as plain White Dove, Cetaphil, or Aveeno.
- Use a good lotion or cream just after a luke-warm (not hot) bath (e.g., Eucerin, Eucerin Plus, Lubriderm, Moisturel)
- Avoid bubble baths, fragrances, or itchy clothes made out of wool. Use 100% cotton for babies.
- Use creams as instructed. Make sure you know exactly where to put the creams and at what times and for how long to use them. Rub a cream in until it is gone.

- If you see pus or scabs, there may be an infection that needs more treatment by your physician.
- Use medicines such as diphenhydramine syrup or capsules (Benadryl) to control itching, if you need it. Let your physician know if that medicine is not strong enough. Keep your fingernails short.

Do I need to use a special laundry detergent?

- Use a mild laundry detergent, such as Cheer Free or Ivory Snow Flakes. Avoid fabric softeners or static-free sheets.

Can atopic dermatitis be cured?

- Atopic dermatitis is a chronic problem that you should try to control rather than cure.

Most children will outgrow their eczema, but a few may have problems with their skin into adult years.

- Adults who had atopic dermatitis as a child may have problems in certain jobs in which there is a lot of wet work (hairdressers, hospital workers, food handlers, etc.).
- For the best control, both parents and patients must look to decrease stress in their lives. Ask your physician for ways to reduce stress.

Where can I can get more information and support?

- Contact the Eczema Association For Science and Education, 1221 S.W. Yamhill #303, Portland, OR 97205; 503-228-4430.

Callus

What is a callus?

- A callus is very thick skin on the feet or toes.

How do I keep from getting one?

- Shoes that do not fit right often cause a callus. Make sure your shoes are wide and long enough.

How do I treat the callus?

- You must have shoes that fit.
- You may also use a patch of 40% salicylic acid if you do not have diabetes. This patch can be bought at the drugstore. Cut the patch just to the size of the callus. Put the sticky side against the skin. It is best to just wear the patch at night so it does not slip.

- The medicine on the patch will cause the callus to thin, so put it only on the thicker area and not on the normal skin. Use tape to help keep it in place. The patch will turn the skin white.
- Each night before you put the patch back on, remove the white "dead" skin with either a metal nail file or a pumice stone. Stop using the patch when the skin is not thick anymore or if it starts hurting.

Contact Dermatitis (Poison Ivy/ Poison Oak)

What is contact dermatitis and how did I get it?

- Contact dermatitis is the way your skin reacts to something that has touched it and is now causing an allergic reaction. You get it by touching the substance or by touching clothing or an animal that recently touched it.

How long will it last?

- If you avoid new contact with the substance, the rash will be at its worst about 5 to 7 days after it first appeared, and, in 3 to 4 weeks, the rash should be gone.

Will medicine help?

- Some pills or creams can help control the rash until the 2 to 3 weeks are over. Even if you get several new lesions, the medicine may still be working.

What can I do to stop the itching?

- Avoid getting hot because this always makes itching worse. Do not take hot showers or baths and avoid the sun.
- Put cold, wet towels on any itchy area as often as you want.
- You can buy some lotions, such as Calamine, Sarna, PrameGel, Itch X, Aveeno Anti-Itch lotion, or Prax, without a prescription at most drugstores.

- If your itching is very bad, your physician may suggest a pill, such as Benadryl. If you still are not able to sleep because of the itching, let your physician know.

Does scratching make it spread and can other people get it from me by touching the rash?

- *Neither scratching the bumps nor others touching them will make it spread.* The rash is spread by having whatever you are allergic to touch the skin in different places. If it was on your hands and then you touched your face, then it will be on your face.
- It takes several days or even a week or so for all of the bumps or blisters to come out. You may still get a few new bumps or blisters each day.

How can I avoid getting it again?

- It is important that you know what you are allergic to so that you can avoid coming into contact with it again. Any clothes you wore that may have contacted the plant should be washed, avoiding contact with the skin. Know what poison ivy and poison oak look like.

Topical Corticosteroids: Proper Use and Possible Side Effects

What are topical corticosteroids?

- Topical corticosteroids are medicines that are used to help relieve the redness, swelling, itching, and pain of many skin problems. Most of these corticosteroids are available only with your physician's prescription.
- Hydrocortisone 0.5 and 1.0% (e.g., Cort-Aid) can be bought at the drugstore without a prescription.

How do I use the medicine?

- Use topical corticosteroids exactly as your physician tells you. Do not use the medicine more times, for a longer time, or on other places than your physician tells you to use them.
- Using the cream too much or for too long can increase the chance of problems, such as thinning out of the skin, stretch marks, blood vessels breaking, and acne. These problems may develop on areas with thinner skin (for example, face, armpits, groin). Creams can be as strong as pills, so it is very important for you to know how to use your cream safely.
- Be very careful not to get topical steroids in your eyes. Wash your hands after putting on the medicine. If you get this medicine in your eyes by mistake, wash them with water.

What other things should I do to make the medicine work better?

- Do not bandage or wrap the skin being treated unless told to do so by your physician.
- Avoid using tight-fitting diapers or plastic pants on a child if the medicine is being used on the child's diaper area. Plastic pants or tight-fitting diapers may make the medicine go deeper through the skin into the body and cause the skin to thin out.
- Do not use any leftover medicine for other skin problems without first checking with your physician. Topical corticosteroids should not be used on many kinds of skin infections because they can make them much worse.

Are there other side effects I should know about?

- All medicines can cause some side effects. Ask your physician about any of the following side effects: burning, dryness, irritation, itching, or redness of skin rash.
- When you use a gel, solution, lotion, or aerosol, a mild, short-term stinging may occur. If you notice any other effects, check with your physician as soon as possible.

Diaper Rash

What causes diaper rash?

- Diaper rash is the most common rash in babies. It is caused by contact with urine for a long time or contact with chemicals, soaps, or detergents in the diaper. Rubber or plastic diaper pants allow the chemicals to irritate the skin. Diarrhea also may make an infant more likely to get a diaper rash. Often, there is also an infection with a yeast.

How can I keep my baby from getting diaper rash?

- Keep the diaper area as dry as possible by changing the diapers often. Both cloth diapers and disposable diapers must be changed frequently.
- If your child is 6 to 12 months old, change the diaper 1 hour after the child goes to sleep at night. Avoid rubber or plastic diaper pants.
- Try to let your baby go without any diaper as often as possible.

How should I wash my child's diaper area?

- Wash the area gently with warm water after each diaper change.

- Do not use soap if the diaper area is raw or sore. Use a soap substitute, such as Cetaphil or Aquanil, in these cases.

How should I wash cloth diapers?

- Wash the cloth diapers in a washing machine half-filled with water. Add 1 cup of vinegar and let them sit for 30 minutes, then spin dry without rinsing. Dry as usual.

Are there any creams I can use?

- Use creams with zinc oxide, such as Desitin, with each diaper change.
- Your physician may give you a prescription cream or have you buy certain creams at the drugstore (Lotrimin A/F, Monistat Derm) to use carefully. Do not leave the cream on the surface; rub it in until it is gone.

How long should it take before it gets better?

- The rash should be better within a few days and gone in 2 weeks. Let your physician know if the rash is not getting better. You may need a different cream or medicine.

Eczema

What is eczema?

- Eczema is an itchy, often chronic rash that is seen commonly in young infants and children who have very dry and sensitive skin. Hand eczema is a chronic rash often seen in adults with dry, sensitive skin.

What causes eczema?

- The cause of eczema is not always known. Some rashes are caused by things that irritate the skin, such as soaps, chemicals, or frequent handwashing. Other rashes may be caused by the way the skin reacts to things that may be new, such as glue, dyes, some gloves, or inks.
- If one member of a family has eczema, others may be more likely to get it. Eczema is not spread from one person to another.

What makes eczema worse?

- Each person is different in what can make their rash worse. However, for most people with eczema, washing frequently with hot water or harsh soaps will make it worse.
- Some people find that stress makes their rash get worse. If you are allergic to something, getting even a little bit of that substance on your body or hands can make the rash stay itchy and inflamed.

How do I treat eczema?

- You should avoid frequent washing, especially with very hot water.
- Use a mild soap that will help to keep your skin moist. Several brands are White Dove, Tone, Basis, Neutrogena Unscented Soap, Purpose, and Caress. If you have very sensitive skin and cannot use soap, try using a soap substitute, such as Cetaphil, Aquanil, or Cam lotion. All of these products should be at your local pharmacy.

What can I use to keep my skin from getting dry?

- Use a moisturizer that does not have lanolin or much fragrance, such as Lubriderm, Nutraderm, Moisturel, or Purpose. Snow Drift shortening by Martha White is the least-expensive form of moisturizer and is found in the grocery store.
- Apply one of these lotions right after your bath or shower to help keep in your own moisture. If your skin is still dry, ask your physician for a prescription-strength moisturizer or steroid cream for your skin.

What else can I do when my skin gets very dry, especially in the winter?

- Use a humidifier if the air is very dry. Avoid wearing wool or using wool blankets.

My skin seems to itch sometimes. Are there any medicines I can get without a prescription to help relieve the itching?

- You can use a cool lotion to take the edge off of the itching, such as Sarna, Prax, PrameGel, Itch X, or Calamine. These will not cure your itching, but will make it feel better. If your skin still itches, despite using these lotions, contact your physician.

My hands are red and itchy. What can I do to protect them?

- It is very important to protect your hands as much as possible from chemicals and water. Use vinyl gloves for all wet work, such as housework or gardening, or at your job.

General Skin Care

What kind of soap is best for me to use?

- Use a mild soap that will help to keep your skin moist. Several brands are White Dove, Tone, Basis, Neutrogena unscented soap, Purpose, Oil of Olay unscented cleansing bar, and Caress. If you have very sensitive skin and cannot use soap, try using a soap substitute, such as Cetaphil bar or lotion cleanser, Aquanil lotion cleanser, Cam lotion, Lowila cake bar, or Aveeno cleansing bar. All of these should be at your local pharmacy.

What can I use to keep my skin from getting dry?

- Use a moisturizer (cream or lotion) that does not have lanolin or much fragrance, such as Eucerin Plus, Lubriderm, Nutraderm, Moisturel, or Purpose. Snow Drift shortening by Martha White is the cheapest form of moisturizer and is found in the grocery store. Apply one of these lotions right after your bath or shower to help keep in your own moisture. If your skin is still dry, ask your physician for a prescription-strength moisturizer for your skin.

Does it matter what kind of laundry detergent I use to wash clothes?

- Yes. Use a laundry detergent that does not have many extra chemicals. Two common store brands are Cheer Free laundry detergent and Ivory Snow Flakes.

What else can I do when my skin gets very dry, especially in the winter?

- Use a humidifier if the air is very dry. Avoid wearing wool or using wool blankets.

My skin seems to itch sometimes. Are there any medicines I can get without a prescription to help relieve the itching?

- You can use a cool lotion, such as Sarna, Prax lotion or cream, PrameGel, Itch X gel or spray, Aveeno Anti-Itch cream or lotion, or Calamine, to take the edge off of the itching. These will not cure your itching but will make it feel better. Hydrocortisone 1% cream is available without a prescription and may be used 1 to 3 times a day to stubborn areas of itching. You should not use hydrocortisone cream for more than a few weeks in the groin or on the face. If your skin still itches, despite using these lotions, contact your physician.

Impetigo

What is impetigo?

- Impetigo is a skin infection caused by germs known as *bacteria*. These bacteria are found all around us.

Who gets impetigo?

- Children often get impetigo, but adults also can get it. It usually comes from scratching the skin because of bug bites or rashes. The rash is contagious and can be spread from person to person.

How is impetigo treated?

- You must get a medicine from your physician to make the impetigo rash go away.
- Your physician will either give you an ointment or a medicine to take by mouth to treat the infection. It is important to use the medicine for the full time to keep the infection from coming back.
- Let your physicain know if the areas start to hurt, if you get a fever, if the rash is not get-

ting better after 4 or 5 days, or if it comes right back after your finish your medicine.

How do I take care of the sores?

- Wash the skin with a mild soap that helps to kill the bacteria, such as Lever 2000. Also, gently remove the crusts.
- Keep the draining sores covered, because they can cause the rash to spread to other areas or to another person.

Does my child need to stay out of school?

- Because impetigo can be spread from one child to another quite easily, children with impetigo should avoid children without the rash, until they have taken medicine for at least 1 day.
- If the scabs no longer have fluid coming out, the child probably will not infect others.

Lice–Pediculosis

What are lice?

- Lice are bugs that cause a disease known as *pediculosis*. These bugs cause a rash and itching in places on your skin where you may have a lot of hair, such as your scalp, eyelashes, or genital areas.

How did I get lice?

- Lice are spread from one infected person to another.
- In children, lice are usually found in the hair and come from another child or another family member. A comb, hat, or piece of clothing from an infected relative or friend can also carry the lice.
- In adults, lice on the genitals may also be given to another person through sex.

How can I get rid of the lice?

- Follow carefully the directions that your physician gives you for taking your medicine. After you have used the medicine, you will not infect others.

What are nits?

- Nits are the eggs from the lice. You must remove nits as best as you can to avoid getting the disease again.
- Nits are sometimes hard to remove from your hair, but your physician can suggest some ways to help you remove them, such as using white vinegar or Step 2 rinse (available at the pharmacy without a prescription).

How do I prevent the lice from coming back?

- All family members and close schoolmates of an infected child should be treated. The partner of an adult with lice in the pubic area should also be treated.
- Dirty clothes, linens, scarves, hats, combs, and brushes should be cleaned and washed in hot water and dried with a hot cycle or stored in a plastic bag for at least 30 days.

Moles and Melanoma

What is a mole?

- A mole, also known as a *nevus,* is a dark skin spot that you are either born with or may develop as you get older. Almost everybody has at least one mole. Most moles will never hurt you, but some moles can turn into cancers, known as *melanomas.*

What is melanoma?

- Melanoma is a type of skin cancer, which, if found very early, can be cured. If it is found late, however, it is deadly. Thousands of people die from melanoma each year.

Who gets melanoma?

- Anyone may get melanoma, but it occurs most often in light-skinned people, in people who were badly sunburned as children, in those that have a family member with melanoma, and in those who have many moles, especially large ones. The most common place for a melanoma to occur is on the back in a man and on the leg in a woman, but it can occur anywhere.

How can I tell if I have melanoma, and what do bad moles look like?

- Know the ABCDEFs of dangerous moles and look for any changes in any mole you have

now or any new moles you find. It may be hard to know if your mole is okay; if you have any mole that looks bad, you should show it to your physician.

UNUSUAL MOLES:

A = Asymmetry—If you draw a line down the middle of a mole, and one side does not look just like the other one, it may be abnormal.

B = Borders—Irregular. If the edge of your mole is not smooth but is irregular or blurred, point it out to your physician.

C = Color variation or change—Some people think that a mole must be very dark to be bad, but any change in the color of a mole is important, such as a brown mole turning red, white, or black.

D = Diameter—If your mole, *flat or raised,* is bigger than the size of a pencil eraser, it does not mean that the mole is a cancer. But if you have any mole that is growing bigger, you should ask your physician to look at it.

E = Elevation—If your mole was flat, but now it is raised, see your physician. But remember that flat moles can be bad, too.

F = Feeling—If your mole itches, tingles, or stings for 2 to 3 weeks, ask your physician to look at it.

How can I keep from getting melanoma?

- Do not stay out in the sun for very long between 10 AM and 3 PM when the sun is strong.
- *When you are in the sun, wear a hat, a shirt, and sunscreen that has a sun-protection factor (SPF) of 15 or higher.* Put on the sunscreen 30 minutes before going outside. After you swim or sweat, put sunscreen on again or use a sunscreen that will not come off in the water.
- Check all of your moles each month with a mirror under bright lights. Look for any change in the size, shape, or color of your mole. Be sure to look at your entire body.
- Have your physician look at any unusual moles as soon as possible.

Where can I get more information?

- For more information, write or call any of these groups:
- American Cancer Society, 1599 Clifton Road, N.E., Atlanta, GA 30329; 1-800-ACS-2345
- National Cancer Institute Hotline 1-800-4-CANCER
- Office of Cancer Communications, National Cancer Institute, Bldg. 31, Rm. 10A24, Bethesda, Maryland 20892
- The Skin Cancer Foundation, P.O. Box 561, New York, NY 10156

Scabies

What is scabies?

- Scabies is a skin disease caused by a very small bug known as a *mite*.
- People with scabies usually notice severe itching, usually on the hands, wrists, breasts, genitals, or waistline.
- The itching may be worse at night.

Is scabies contagious?

- Yes. Scabies is spread from one person to another through direct skin-to-skin contact.

How can I get rid of scabies?

- You can use medications from your physician that will get rid of scabies. *Medications for scabies must be used exactly as your physician tells you to use them.*
- It is very important to make sure you use the cream from your neck down.
- Make sure to use the cream between your fingers, toes, under your nails, and in the groin, not just where the rash is.

Who else needs to get treated?

- All family members or sexual partners need to be treated, even if they are not having a rash or itching. If you are pregnant, nursing, or have a small child, ask your physician about which medication to use.

What about my clothes and bed linens?

- Dirty clothes and all bed linens should be washed in hot water (or dry-cleaned) and dried on a hot dryer cycle. Hanging clothes dry will not kill the mites.

What about the itching?

- If you itch a lot, ask your physician about medications to help reduce your itching. Even after you get rid of all the mites, you may still have itching for a few more weeks. This will get better.

Seborrheic Dermatitis

What is seborrheic dermatitis?

- Seborrheic dermatitis, also known as *dandruff,* is very common. It usually causes your skin to flake and itch, often on your head, ears, and face. We do not know what causes dandruff.

How can I control the flaking in my scalp?

- For scalp problems, you need to use a special shampoo. You can get these without a physician's prescription. Look for shampoos containing either zinc pyrithione, salicylic acid, sulfur, selenium sulfide or coal tar (Sebulex, T/Sal, Denorex, etc).
- It is important to leave all shampoos on the scalp for at least 5 to 10 minutes before washing out, to give the medicine a chance to work. Use the shampoos at least 2 to 3 times a week.
- If these shampoos do not help your dandruff, let your physician know. There are also prescription lotions and shampoos that you can use to control your itching and flaking.

What about the red, flaking areas on my face and ears?

- There are several kinds of medications your physician may give you to use on your face. These medicines will not cure your problem but will help to keep it under control.
- Whenever your flaking or itching returns, feel free to use the medicines, but do not be surprised if the problem comes back after you stop using them.

Skin Cancers

What are skin cancers?

- Skin cancers are caused by abnormal growth of skin cells. The three main types of skin cancers are basal cell, squamous cell, and melanoma.
- *Basal cell cancers* are the most common, and they usually occur on sun-exposed areas, especially the face, arms, or back. They do not spread to other parts of your body but can cause a bad problem just where they are, especially if they are on your nose or near your eyes.
- *Squamous cell cancers* are the second most common and also occur on parts of your body that have been exposed to the sun for long periods of time. Rarely, they will spread to other parts of your body if they are not treated.
- *Melanoma* is the third type of skin cancer. Melanoma is less common, but it is the most serious type of skin cancer. It comes from an old mole that changes or from a new unusual mole. It is related to severe sunburns as a child, but anyone may get melanoma.

How do you get skin cancer?

- Most skin cancers occur as a result of too much sun exposure. Having a family member who has a skin cancer, especially melanoma, gives you a greater chance of also getting a skin cancer. Even people who do not burn but spend a lot of time out in the sun are at risk for getting skin cancer.

What do skin cancers look like?

- Skin cancers can look like many common bumps on the skin when they first show up. They may be red or itchy and look like a scar or like a scratch or pimple that will not heal.
- If you have any new skin bump or lesion that does not heal after 4 to 8 weeks and that you are worried about, call your physician. Skin cancers do not come and go, they stay and grow. Do not wait until a skin cancer hurts, bleeds, or bothers you before you have it checked.
- Melanoma skin cancers tend to be irregular in size, shape, or color. If you think you may have a melanoma, do not wait 4 to 8 weeks to have it looked at; contact your physician right away.

After I have had a basal cell or squamous cell skin cancer removed, will it ever come back?

- Almost one half of all patients with a basal cell or squamous cell skin cancer will get another one on their body at some time in the next 5 years. Therefore, you should see your physician every 6 to 12 months for a complete skin exam. You should also look over your entire body every month.

Do I need to protect myself from the sun?

- Yes. Use sunscreens with a sun-protection factor of 15 at all times when you go in the sun, along with a hat and shirt with long sleeves.

For more information, write or call any of these groups:

- American Cancer Society, 1599 Clifton Rd. N.E., Atlanta, GA 30329; 1-800-ACS-2345

- National Cancer Institute Hotline 1-800-4-CANCER
- Office of Cancer Communications, National Cancer Institute, Bldg. 31, Rm. 10A24, Bethesda, Md 20892
- The Skin Cancer Foundation, P.O. Box 561, New York, NY 10156

Sun Protection

Why do I need to protect myself from the sun?

- The number of cases of skin cancer increases each year. Almost all of these skin cancers are the result of too much outdoor time in the sun. A sunburn is the worst kind of sun damage because it increases the chance of you getting a very bad form of skin cancer called *melanoma*.

Who should wear sunscreens or use sun protection?

- Everyone should wear sunscreen. Children should always use it and so should anyone who has had a skin cancer, anyone that has a family member with a skin cancer, anyone whose skin is very light-colored, anyone who easily burns while in the sun, and anyone who works outdoors.
- Certain drugs can make you more likely to sunburn. Ask your physician if any medicine given to you can do this.

But I never burn in the sun...

- Anyone can get skin cancer, even people who do not usually sunburn.
- Most scientists worry that the ozone layer of our air (the part that helps block out the bad part of the sun) is getting smaller. This means that more harmful sun rays are getting to the ground, which increases everyone's chance of getting skin cancer. The sun rays may also cause your skin to get wrinkled and blotchy at a young age.

But it is cloudy outside...

- Do not let cloudy days fool you! Bad sun rays still reach your skin even on cloudy days, and you need to use sunscreen and sun protection just as you would on a sunny day.

What are sunscreens?

- Sunscreens are lotions that you put on your skin to protect you from the sun's harmful (ultraviolet) sun rays. Look for one that is a "broad spectrum" sunscreen with a *Sun-Protection Factor* (SPF) of at least 15.
- If you will be sweating or swimming, use a sunscreen that does not come off in the water.

How and when should I put on sunscreens?

- It is best to put on a sunscreen 30 minutes before going outdoors. Put it on again every 1 to 2 hours while in the sun, especially if swimming. Put lots of sunscreen on all areas of your body that are directly in the sun, even your ears and feet.

What else can I do to protect my skin from the sun?

- Wear a hat, sunglasses, and a T-shirt while in the sun.
- Wear a long-sleeved shirt and pants when you can.
- Sit in the shade or have your children play in the shade, but still wear sunscreen.

Tanning Salon Dangers

What are tanning salons?

- Tanning salons are sources of ultraviolet radiation (light). Usually, they give off a type of ultraviolet light called UVA. This type of radiation penetrates into the second layer of skin known as the *dermis*.

Are tanning salons safer than the sun?

- Absolutely not! The sun gives off ultraviolet rays, especially UVA and UVB. The UVA rays given off in high doses from tanning salons are not safer than the sun.
- Using a sunscreen with a sun-protection factor (SPF) of 8 or higher protects you just as much as a tan from a tanning salon. Therefore, it is much safer to use sunscreen with a sun-protection factor (SPF) of 15 or higher than to get a "base" tan from a tanning salon.

What are the dangers of using a tanning salon?

Short term dangers:

- Your eyes can be severely burned if not properly shielded during light therapy. Some medications, such as antibiotics and those for arthritis and diabetes, can make you much more sensitive to the tanning lights and cause a severe total body burn.
- The tanning light can trigger some light-sensitive illnesses that can be very serious (lupus erythematosus and porphyria).
- Some people get white splotches on their skin from using the tanning oils and beds.

Long term dangers:

- Dark freckling, or lentigines, wrinkling, and other signs of sun damage are seen especially from tanning salons, where the light penetrates into the deeper skin layers.
- Scientists have shown a direct link between skin cancers and tanning salon use.

What are my options to tanning?

- Using a tanning gel to get "color" does not increase your risk of skin cancer or wrinkling. Products made by Estee Lauder and Neutrogena, as well as many other companies, can give a "tanned" look without the risk. However, remember that those "tans" do not give any protection from the sun.

Tick Bites

Are tick bites dangerous?

- Tick bites cause a local reaction to the skin that is irritating. Disease can occur from some tick bites.

What is Lyme disease, and what are its symptoms?

- Lyme disease is an infection caused by a very small tick that is about the size of a pencil point. If you have been bitten by a tick and you think you may have Lyme disease, call your physician and, if possible, bring the tick to the physician's office.
- Patients with Lyme disease may notice, a few days after a tick bite, that they feel like they have the flu, with a high fever, runny nose, or cough.
- Some patients may also have a skin rash on their body that seems to be getting bigger. If you have these symptoms after a tick bite, call your physician for advice.

What is Rocky Mountain spotted fever and why is it serious?

- Rocky Mountain spotted fever is also caused by a tick bite, and patients may get a very

bad headache, high fever, sore muscles, and nausea. A rash on your hands and feet may appear a couple days later.
- If the disease is not treated, you may get very sick and die.

How can I prevent getting tick bites?

- The best way to avoid getting a tick bite is to use a good skin repellent, such as Deep Woods Off, Cutter, or Repel. Spray it on your exposed body parts and hair before going into the woods. Permanone is a good repellent for clothing.
- Be sure to wear light-colored clothing with long sleeves, pants (tucked into your shoes, if possible) and a hat.

If I find a tick on my body, how do I get it off?

- If you find a tick on your body, do not grab it with your hands. Use a thread or a pair of tweezers and very gently pull it off. Do not try to twist or burn it off.

Tinea Capitis

What is tinea capitis?

- Tinea capitis is also known as *"ringworm" of the scalp*. Tinea capitis is caused by a fungus, not a worm. The fungus is found on other people, animals, or even in the soil.

Is tinea capitis contagious?

- Yes. Sharing hats, combs, and brushes and close personal contact with playmates is the most common way it is spread. Check other children in your family and your pets as possible sources.
- Let school nurses or day care operators know if your child has tinea capitis, in order to keep it from spreading to your child again or to other children.

How is tinea capitis treated?

- You must take an oral medication to really get rid of the infection. Blue Star ointment and shampoos will *not* get rid of this infection.

- It is very important to take the medication for as long as it is prescribed. Keep your follow-up appointments with the physician to make sure the infection is all gone.
- Let your physician know if there are any new areas or if the rash is not better after 3 weeks of treatment.
- Medicated shampoos, such as Selsun Blue, should be used by everyone in the household to help keep tinea capitis from spreading. Disinfect all combs, brushes, and hats.

Will my hair grow back, and how long will it take?

- In most cases, your hair will grow back, but it will take at least 3 months to start seeing the fine "fuzz" of the new hairs coming in.
- If there is a lot of swelling and pus, there may be some permanent hair loss, but you cannot tell for sure for at least 3 to 4 months whether or not the hair will come back.

Tinea Corporis

What is tinea corporis?

- Tinea corporis is also known as *ringworm*. It is caused by a fungus, not a worm. The fungus is found on other people, animals (cats, especially), and in the soil.

Is tinea corporis contagious?

- Yes. It can be spread from one spot on your body to another, from one person to another, and from an animal to a person.

How is tinea corporis treated?

- If there are just a few spots, the rash is usually treated with creams. Lotrimin A/F is available without a prescription at the drugstore.

- All creams should be rubbed in until they disappear, once or twice a day for 1 to 4 weeks, depending on which cream you are given.
- You should use your cream for at least a full week after the scaling has gone. Sometimes another medicine must be taken by mouth if the rash is stubborn, in the hair, or widespread.

Tinea Cruris

What is tinea cruris?

- Tinea cruris is also known as *jock itch* or *ringworm of the groin area*. This is caused by a fungus, not a worm.

Is tinea cruris contagious?

- Yes. It usually comes from a fungal infection from the feet or toenails that spreads to the groin during hot weather or when you do a lot of exercising. It can spread to other areas of the body.

How is tinea cruris treated?

- If there are just a few spots, the rash is usually treated with creams. Lotrimin A/F, Mi-

catin, or similar creams are available without a prescription at the drugstore.
- All creams should be rubbed in until they disappear, once or twice a day for 1 to 4 weeks, depending on which cream you are given.
- You should use your cream for at least a full week after the scaling has gone. Sometimes another medicine must be taken by mouth if the rash is stubborn, in the hair, widespread, or keeps coming back.
- Use a nonprescription, drying powder (Zeasorb AF) over the cream and after the area has healed to prevent the area from becoming moist.

Tinea Pedis

What is tinea pedis?

- Tinea pedis, or athlete's foot, is a fungal infection. It is very common in teenagers and adults during warm weather.

Is tinea pedis contagious?

- Yes. It can spread to the toenails and to other parts of the body (jock itch).

How is tinea pedis treated?

- The rash is usually treated with creams. Lotrimin A/F, Micatin, or similar creams are available without a prescription at the drugstore. Your physician may give you a stronger prescription cream instead.

- All creams should be rubbed in until they disappear, once or twice a day for 1 to 4 weeks, depending on which cream you are given. You should use your cream for at least a full week after the scaling has gone.
- Sometimes another medicine must be taken by mouth if the rash is stubborn, in the nails, or keeps coming back.
- Use an antifungal powder (Zeasorb AF) daily to keep the feet dry. Spray your shoes once or twice a week, as well.
- Wear 100% cotton socks to help keep the feet dry.

Tinea Versicolor

What causes tinea versicolor?

- Tinea versicolor is a harmless skin infection caused by a yeast living on the normal skin. It is common in hot, humid climates.
- When you have a lot of the yeast growing in one area, it causes slightly scaly, pink patches that do not tan.
- It is most common on the back, chest, and arms, but may appear on the neck.
- In darker-skinned patients, the patches are much lighter than the normal skin.

Is tinea versicolor contagious?

- Tinea versicolor is not contagious to other people.

How can I treat tinea versicolor?

- If you just have a few small spots, you can use creams from the drug store, such as Lotrimin A/F twice a day for 2 to 3 weeks. If you have larger areas that need to be treated, you will need a prescription medicine from your physician. You may be given pills or a lotion.

Can I keep from getting tinea versicolor again?

- Avoid using oils, because the yeast thrives on oils and is more likely to come back.
- Use a soap containing sulfur and salicylic acid on a regular basis during warm weather.
- Your physician may prescribe a medicated lotion (selenium sulfide) for you to use on a monthly basis to keep tinea versicolor from coming back.

Urticaria (Hives)

What is urticaria or hives?

- Urticaria, or hives, is a very common skin rash that can be caused by many things. One out of every five people will get hives sometime in their lifetime.

What causes urticaria, or hives?

- Sometimes it is caused by a drug, such as aspirin or an antibiotic, but it can be caused by foods, especially eggs, seafood, chocolate, or nuts or by heat, exercise, stress, or, rarely, sunlight.
- A specific cause for hives is found in less than one half of all cases. In some people, stress may cause hives. If your hives last for more than 6 weeks, your physician may look for other causes of your hives.

Is there anything I can do to keep it from breaking out?

- You should avoid things that you think may be causing you to break out, such as a medicine or food. Ask your physician, if you are unsure.
- Even though you may not come in contact again with whatever caused your hives, the

hives may last for 2 to 4 weeks. You should follow your physician's advice carefully.

How can I tell what is causing the hives?

- Make a list of everything you eat and drink and any medicines you take or use, including creams, lotions, eyedrops, perfumes, sprays, soaps, etc., and try to see if there is any pattern to what you are being exposed to and when you get hives.

Is there any medicine I can get to help with the itching?

- Antihistamines (i.e., Benadryl) are used to treat urticaria or hives. You must know and follow exactly how your physician wants you to take the medicine. Let your physician know if your medicine is not working. Sometimes several medicines must be tried before the one you will respond to best is found.
- Some antihistamines may make you sleepy, so be very careful with driving or other such activities if you take one of these.

Warts

What causes warts?

- Warts are caused by a virus called the *human papilloma virus* that grows in the skin.

How did I get warts?

- The wart virus can be spread from person to person. It is more likely to infect your skin where there has been an open sore or even a scar.
- Some people can be around warts and never get one, while other people will get them very easily. We do not know why this happens.

Will they go away on their own?

- Some warts will go away without treatment. This is more common in young children. Other warts will appear but not change for years. Still others will spread quickly. Physicians cannot tell what your wart(s) will do.

What treatments are available?

- The available treatments do not directly kill the warts; they kill the surrounding skin. The goal is to kill the skin that has the wart virus in it and not damage much of the normal skin.
- Different ways of getting rid of warts include freezing, burning, cutting, or using certain medications. It is important to understand which treatment is best for you.

Can the wart come back?

- Because the wart virus is so small, it cannot be seen with the eye. It may be in other parts of nearby skin but has not yet made such skin grow a wart. Therefore, you may still get new warts while the ones already present are being treated.
- No treatment works 100% of the time; even though the wart looks like it is gone, it may still return several weeks or even months after it was "cured." It is very important to follow the physician's directions to try to prevent the warts from coming back.

Wound Care

Why is wound care important?

- Proper care of your wound is important to prevent it from becoming infected and to help it to heal.

What do I need to do to take care of my wound?

- Leave your dressing from the physician's office on for 24 hours. If it gets wet, replace it.
- Clean the wound _____ a day with dilute hydrogen peroxide. Mix a cup with ½ water from the sink with ½ hydrogen peroxide. Use a cotton-tipped swab (Q-tip) to remove any dried blood or crust.
- Dry the wound gently with a piece of gauze.
- Apply a very thin layer of antibiotic ointment, such as Polysporin or bacitracin.
- Apply a nonstick bandage, such as Telfa or a Band-Aid, if the wound is small. Tape it into place with nonallergenic tape.

- If bleeding occurs, put an ice pack on the wound for 20 minutes with firm pressure. (Do not dab, but keep constant pressure, and do not peek for 20 minutes.)

What about the bruises?

- A small amount of bruising is normal, but it should decrease each day.

What should I take for pain?

- Use acetaminophen (Tylenol), rather than aspirin, for pain.
- If the redness of your wound increases, if the pain gets very bad, or if pus comes out from the wound, please call the office at _____.

INDEX

I

Venereal warts; *see* Condyloma
    acuminata
Venous insufficiency, chronic,
    differentiation of, from
    filariasis, 288
Venous lake, 139
  in elderly, 215
Venous stasis ulcers, in homeless, 221,
    223
Verruca, 249-255
  classic description of, 249-250
  diagnosis of, 250
  differential diagnosis of, 250-251
    from chrondrodermatitis nodularis
      helicis, 309
    from molluscum contagiosum, 245
    from warty tuberculosis, 294
  patient education about, 254-255
  treatment of, 251-254
Verruca plana, 251
Verruca vulgaris, differentiation of, from
    chromomycosis, 307
Verrucous granuloma inguinale, 301
Verrucous squamous cell carcinoma,
    differentiation of, from warty
    tuberculosis, 294
Vesicle(s), 3
  differential diagnosis of, *endsheets*
  in newborns and neonates, 204
Vesicopustules, newborns with,
    differential diagnosis of,
    endsheets
Vicryl suture materials, 34
Viral diseases, 233-256
Viral exanthems, 255-256
  causes of, 256
  differential diagnosis of, 255
    from erythema multiforme, 85
    from measles, 244
    from pruritic urticarial papules and
      plaques of pregnancy, 226
    from secondary syphilis, 200
Viral infections
  differentiation of
    from Rocky Mountain spotted
      fever, 67
    from yaws, 304
  in HIV disease, 218-219
  rhinorrhea from, differentiation of,
    from congenital syphilis, 200
Viranol
  for molluscum contagiosum, 246
  for verruca removal, 253
Virus(es)
  Epstein-Barr, in HIV disease, 218

Virus(es)—cont'd
  herpes simplex; *see* Herpes simplex
  herpes zoster; *see* Herpes zoster
Vitamin A
  excessive, hair loss caused by, 116
  for measles, 244
Vitiligo, 213-215
  classic description of, 213
  diagnosis of, 213
  differential diagnosis of, 213-214
    from leprosy, 298
    from onchocerciasis, 289
    from post-kala-azar dermal
      leishmaniasis, 291
  patient education about, 214-215
  treatment of, 214
Vivagen for telogen effluvium, 116
von Recklinghausen's disease,
    274-275
Vytone for angular cheilitis in elderly,
    215

W

Warfarin, purpura caused by, 318
Wart-Off for verruca removal, 253
Warts, 249-255; *see also* Verruca
  cervical, treatment of, 192
  cryosurgery for, 29
  differentiation of, from yaws, 304
  genital or venereal; *see* Condyloma
    acuminata
  in homeless, 221
  mosaic, differentiation of, from pitted
    keratolysis, 302
  patient education handout for, 353
  plantar, differentiation of, from
    callus/clavus, 129
Warty tuberculosis, 293-294
Westcort; *see* Hydrocortisone valerate
Western immunoblot test to diagnose
    Lyme disease, 63-64
Wet dressings, 11
Wheal, 3
  of urticaria, 228
Whiteheads, 46
Whitlow, herpetic, 237, 238; *see also*
    Herpes simplex
  differentiation of, from paronychia, 121
Wickham's striae, 174
Wiskott-Aldrich syndrome,
    differentiation of, from atopic
    dermatitis, 159
Women, androgen excess syndrome in
  diagnosis of, 118

Women, androgen excess syndrome
  in—cont'd
  differentiation of, from androgenetic
    alopecia, 116-117
  treatment of, 120
Wood's lamp examination, 28
  to diagnose tinea capitis, 98
Worms, filarial, 286
Wound care, patient education handout
    for, 354
Wound lacerations in homeless, 221,
    223
Wuchereria bancrofti, 287

X

Xanthelasmas, 278, 279
Xanthomas, 278-279
  differentiation of, from necrobiosis
    lipoidica, 274
  eruptive, distribution of, 7
  types of, 279
Xeroderma pigmentosum, as precursor
    of squamous cell carcinoma,
    154
Xerosis, 171-172
Xerotic eczema, 171-172
  in elderly, 215
  in HIV disease, 220
Xylene, systemic sclerosis-like disease
    caused by, 267

Y

Yaws, 304
  differentiation of
    from American cutaneous
      leishmaniasis, 291
    from chromomycosis, 307
    from onchocerciasis, 289
Yeast infections, potassium hydroxide
    prep to diagnose, 23

Z

Zeasorb AF Powder for tinea cruris, 98
Zeasorb powder for intertriginous
    candidiasis, 108
Zinc deficiency, differentiation of, from
    seborrheic dermatitis, 185
Zinc oxide for diaper dermatitis, 206
Zinc pyrithione for seborrheic
    dermatitis, 185
Zincon for seborrheic dermatitis, 185
Zithromax; *see* Azithromycin
Zostrix; *see* Capsaicin
Zyrtec; *see* Cetrizine